Essentials of
NURSING RESEARCH
Methods, Appraisal, and Utilization

FIFTH EDITION

Essentials of
NURSING RESEARCH

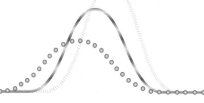

Methods, Appraisal, and Utilization

DENISE F. POLIT, PhD

President
Humanalysis, Inc.
Saratoga Springs, NY

CHERYL TATANO BECK, DNSc, CNM, FAAN

Professor
University of Connecticut School of Nursing
Storrs, Connecticut

BERNADETTE P. HUNGLER, RN, PhD

Visiting Lecturer
Regis College
Weston, Massachusetts

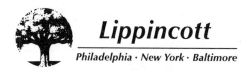

Lippincott

Philadelphia · New York · Baltimore

Acquisitions Editor: Margaret Zuccarini
Developmental Editor: Deedie McMahon
Editorial Assistant: Helen Kogut
Senior Project Editor: Erika Kors
Senior Production Manager: Helen Ewan
Production Coordinator: Nannette Winski
Design Coordinator: Brett MacNaughton
Manufacturing Manager: William Alberti
Interior Design: Melissa Olson
Cover Design: Melissa Walter

Edition 5

9 8 7 6 5 4 3 2 1

Library of Congress Cataloging-in-Publication Data
Polit, Denise F.
    Essentials of nursing research: methods, appraisals, and utilization/Denise F. Polit, Cheryl Tatano Beck, Bernadette P. Hungler.—5th ed.
      p. cm.
    Includes bibliographical references and index.
    ISBN 0-7817-2557-7 (alk. paper)
      1. Nursing–Research. 2. Nursing–Research–Evaluation. I. Beck, Cheryl Tatano. II. Hungler, Bernadette P. III. Title.

RT81.5 .P63 2001
610.73'07'2–dc21   00-044369

Care has been taken to confirm the accuracy of the information presented and to describe generally accepted practices. However, the authors, editors, and publisher are not responsible for errors or omissions or for any consequences from application of the information in this book and make no warranty, express or implied, with respect to the contents of the publication.

The authors, editors, and publisher have exerted every effort to ensure that drug selection and dosage set forth in this text are in accordance with current recommendations and practice at the time of publication. However, in view of ongoing research, changes in government regulations, and the constant flow of information relating to drug therapy and drug reactions, the reader is urged to check the package insert for each drug for any change in indications and dosage and for added warnings and precautions. This is particularly important when the recommended agent is a new or infrequently employed drug.

Some drugs and medical devices presented in this publication have Food and Drug Administration (FDA) clearance for limited use in restricted research settings. It is the responsibility of the health care provider to ascertain the FDA status of each drug or device planned for use in their clinical practice.

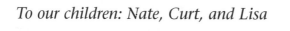

To our children: Nate, Curt, and Lisa

REVIEWERS

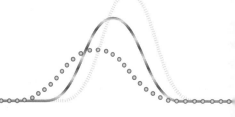

Valerie D. George, PhD, RN
Associate Professor
Cleveland State University
Cleveland, Ohio

Linda Goodfellow, RN, MNEd
Assistant Professor of Nursing
Duquesne University
Pittsburgh, Pennsylvania

Rhonda K. Hollis, RN, PhD
Assistant Dean, Nursing and Health
  Professions
Columbus State University
Columbus, Georgia

Joanne Profetto-McGrath, RN, BScN, BA, MEd, PhD
Assistant Professor
Faculty of Nursing, University of Alberta
Edmonton, Alberta
Canada

Mary Jo Regan-Kubinski, PhD, MSN, BSN
Chair, Department of Nursing
Saint Mary's College
Notre Dame, Indiana

Charlene Romer, MS, RNC, PhD candidate
Associate Professor
Blessing-Rieman College of Nursing
Quincy, Illinois

E. Ann Sheridan, EdD, RN
Associate Professor Emeritus
University of Massachusetts, Amherst
School of Nursing
Amherst, Massachusetts

Martha A. Spies, PhD (C), MSN, RN
Associate Professor
Deaconess College of Nursing
St. Louis, Missouri

Darlene Steven, RN, BScN, BA, MHSA, PhD
Associate Professor
Lakehead University, School of Nursing
Thunder Bay, Ontario
Canada

Catherine Turner, PhD, RN
Chair, Department of Nursing
Southwestern Adventist University
Keene, Texas

Patsy Yates, RN, BA MSocSc
Senior Lecturer, Nursing
Queensland University of Technology
Kelvin Grove, QLD
Australia

Donna L. Waddell, EdD, RN, CS
Associate Professor
North Georgia College and State University
Department of Nursing
Dahlonega, Georgia

PREFACE

This fifth edition of *Essentials of Nursing Research: Methods, Appraisal, and Utilization* presents a number of important changes to this award-winning textbook. This edition retains all of the features that have made the text popular in the past, while introducing revisions that we think will make it more useful to nurses and students who are learning to critically appraise research reports. There is a growing expectation that nurses—especially those in clinical practice—will utilize the results of scientific studies as a basis for their practice. A major purpose of this book is to assist consumers of nursing research in evaluating the adequacy of research findings in terms of their scientific merit and potential for utilization.

NEW TO THIS EDITION

Improved Readability

This textbook has been widely hailed for its clear, concise, and ``user-friendly'' presentation. It has been written in a style designed to be nonintimidating, without including any detailed information on the ``how-to's'' of conducting research. In this edition, however, we have gone to great lengths to write in an even simpler, more straightforward fashion, in recognition of the fact that research methods are an inherently complex topic. Additionally, the readability of the text is enhanced by several visual features, such as the use of two colors.

Greater Assistance to Consumers

This edition is more consumer-focused than ever before. It is designed to help consumers progress fairly slowly into the complexities of disciplined research. For example, we have added a separate chapter, early in the text, on how to read research reports. We have also reorganized the text to include such topics as the ethics of research earlier than in previous editions, in part because this enables readers to develop a fuller understanding of general research issues before delving into more technical material. Additionally, we have interspersed our consumer "tips" throughout the text, which not only high-lights the focus on consumer issues but also makes for a livelier presentation.

More Emphasis on Utilization

We have made two major changes to ensure that this textbook will better help to prepare students for utilizing research in their practice. First, we have made several important additions to the chapter on research utilization. Second, we repeatedly remind readers to think about the implications of research for uti-lization. In particular, we conclude each chapter with some actual research examples that highlight material discussed in the chapter (as before), and then we discuss the possible clinical implications of those research examples.

Better Coverage of Qualitative Research

Every new edition of this textbook has improved on the quality and quantity of information provided to students about qualitative research. This edition makes a major step forward in this tradition through the input of a new coau-thor, Cheryl Tatano Beck, who is well-known for her research and writing on qualitative methods.

ORGANIZATION OF THE TEXT

The content of this edition is organized into six main parts.

Part I—Overview of Nursing Research serves as the overall introduction to fundamental concepts in nursing research. Chapter 1 introduces and sum-marizes the history and future of nursing research, discusses the philosophi-cal underpinnings of qualitative research versus quantitative research, and describes the major purposes of nursing research. Chapter 2 presents an overview of the steps in the research process for both qualitative and quanti-tative studies and defines some key research terms. Chapter 3 provides an introduction to research reports—what they are and how to read them. Chap-ter 4 is devoted to a discussion of ethics in research studies.

Part II—Preliminary Steps in the Research Process includes three chapters and focuses on the steps that are taken in getting started on a research proj-ect. Chapter 5 focuses on the development of research questions and the for-mulation of research hypotheses. Chapter 6 discusses how to prepare and cri-tique literature reviews. Chapter 7 presents information about theoretical and conceptual frameworks.

Part III—Designs for Nursing Research presents material relating to the design of qualitative and quantitative nursing research studies. Chapter 8 describes some fundamental principles of research design and discusses many specific aspects of quantitative research design. Chapter 9 addresses the various research traditions that have contributed to the growth of naturalistic inquiry and qualitative research, and also describes integrated qualitative/ quantitative designs. Chapter 10 presents various designs for sampling of study participants.

Part IV—Collection of Research Data deals with the collection of research data. Chapter 11 discusses the full range of data collection options available to researchers, including both qualitative and quantitative approaches. The chapter focuses primarily on self-reports, observational techniques, and bio-physiologic measures, but other techniques are also mentioned. Chapter 12 explains methods of assessing data quality.

Part V—Analysis of Research Data is devoted to the organization and analysis of research data. Chapter 13 reviews methods of quantitative analysis. The chapter assumes no prior instruction in statistics and focuses primarily on helping readers to understand why statistics are needed, what tests might be appropriate in a given research situation, and what statistical information in a research report means. Chapter 14 presents a discussion of qualitative analysis, greatly expanded and improved in this edition.

Part VI—Critical Appraisal and Utilization of Nursing Research is intended to sharpen the critical awareness of consumers with respect to several key issues. Chapter 15 discusses the interpretation and appraisal of research reports. Chapter 16, the final chapter, is a guide to utilization for clinical practitioners.

KEY FEATURES

Many of the features successfully used in previous editions to assist consumers have been retained.

Research Examples: Each chapter concludes with one or two actual research examples designed to sharpen the readers' critical skills. In most chapters, there is an example of both a quantitative and a qualitative study. Students are asked to evaluate features of these studies according to the chapter's critiquing guidelines. Then, the clinical relevance of each example is explored. In addition, many real or fictitious research examples are used to illustrate key points in the text. The use of relevant examples is crucial to the development of both an understanding of and an interest in the research process. We also hope that the inclusion of many research ideas will stimulate an interest in further reading or pursuit of a utilization project of one's own.

Tips for Consumers of Nursing Research: Each chapter contains numerous tips on what to expect in research reports vis-a-vis the topics that have been discussed in the chapter. In these tips, we have paid special attention to helping students *read* research reports, which are often daunting to those without specialized research training. This feature will enable students to translate the material presented in the textbook into meaningful concepts as they approach the research literature. In this edition, these tips are located directly near related instructional material, rather than being placed at the end of the chapter.

Guidelines for Critiquing Research Reports: Each chapter has a section devoted to guidelines for conducting a critique. These sections provide a list of questions that walk the consumer through a study, drawing attention to aspects of the study that are amenable to appraisal by research consumers.

FEATURES FOR STUDENT LEARNING

To enhance and reinforce learning, several features are used to help focus the student's attention on specific areas of text content:

Chapter Objectives: Learning objectives are identified on the chapter opener to focus the reader's attention on critical content.

New Terms: Each chapter begins with a list of new terms that are defined in context when used for the first time.

Chapter Summary Points: A succinct list of summary points that focus on salient chapter content is included in each chapter. In this edition, the summary is presented as a bulleted list rather than, as in previous editions, in paragraph form.

Suggested Readings: Two lists of suggested readings, methodologic and substantive resources, are provided in each chapter to direct the student's further inquiry.

Actual Research Examples: This edition includes two recent full-length examples of research studies—one quantitative and the other qualitative—that students can read, analyze, and critique.

Critical Thinking Activities: Each chapter of the textbook now includes two or three questions or activities designed to reinforce student learning. The questions often relate specifically to the full research reports that are included in the appendix.

TEACHING-LEARNING PACKAGE

Essentials of Nursing Research: Methods, Appraisal, and Utilization, fifth edition has an ancillary package designed with both the student and the instructor in mind.

The Study Guide augments the text and provides the student with application exercises that correspond to each text chapter. This supports the learning of fundamental research terms that appear in research journals and provides the opportunity to practice the application of the concepts presented in the text and explore hundreds of research possibilities. This edition provides the answers to the selected exercises at the end of the study guide.

Free CD-ROM : The study guide also includes a CD-ROM providing 225 review questions to assist students in self-testing. This review program provides the rationale for both correct and incorrect answers, helping students to identify areas of strength and areas needing further study.

The Instructor's Manual and Testbank includes a chapter that corresponds to every chapter in the textbook. Each chapter of the instructor's manual contains the following: Statement of Intent, Comments on the Actual Research Examples in the Textbook, Answers to Selected Study Guide Exercises, and Test Questions and Answers.

It is our hope and expectation that the content, style, and organization of this fifth edition of *Essentials of Nursing Research* will be helpful to those students desiring to become intelligent and thoughtful readers of nursing research studies and to those wishing to improve their clinical performance based on research findings. We also hope that this textbook will help to develop an enthusiasm for the kinds of discoveries and knowledge that research can produce.

Denise F. Polit, PhD
Cheryl Tatano Beck, DNSc, CNM, FAAN
Bernadette P. Hungler, RN, PhD

ACKNOWLEDGMENTS

This fifth edition, like the previous four, depended on the contribution of many individuals. We are deeply appreciative of those who made all five editions possible. In addition to all those who assisted us with the earlier editions, the following individuals deserve special mention.

This edition of the book involved many revisions to more specifically address the needs of beginning students and to expand the discussion of qualitative research. We are indebted to the insightful comments of several anonymous reviewers, who contributed to the overall conceptualization of this edition.

We would also like to extend our warmest thanks to those who helped to turn the manuscript into a finished product, including Lisa Kachidurian and Chloë Kettlewell. The staff at Lippincott Williams & Wilkins has given us ongoing support and understanding. We would like to express our gratitude to many individuals, including Margaret Zuccarini, Deedie McMahon, Helen Kogut, Erika Kors, and all the others behind the scenes for their contributions.

Finally, we thank our friends and family, who were patient and supportive throughout this enterprise.

CONTENTS

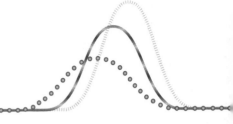

PART I

OVERVIEW OF NURSING RESEARCH

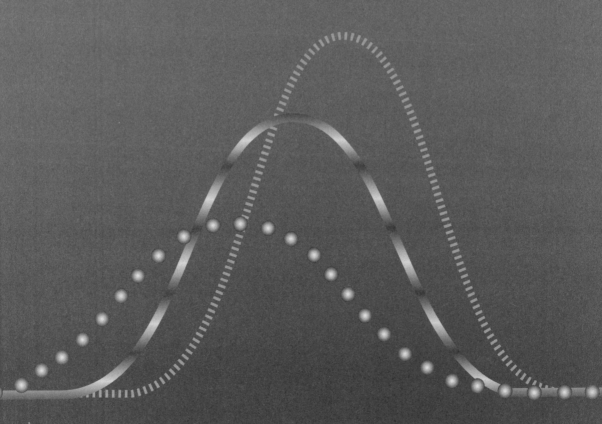

Exploring Nursing Research

Student Objectives

On completion of this chapter, the student will be able to:

- ○ describe why research is important in the nursing profession and discuss why evidence-based practice is needed
- ○ describe historical trends in the evolution of nursing research and identify several areas of current priority for nurse researchers
- ○ describe alternative means of acquiring knowledge
- ○ describe the major characteristics and assumptions of the two alternative paradigms used by nurse researchers
- ○ identify similarities and differences between the traditional scientific method (quantitative research) and naturalistic methods (qualitative research)
- ○ identify several purposes of qualitative and quantitative research
- ○ define new terms in the chapter

New Terms

Applied research
Assumption
Basic research
Control
Deductive reasoning
Determinism
Empirical evidence
Evidence-based practice
Generalizability
Inductive reasoning
Journal club
National Institute of Nursing Research (NINR)

Naturalistic paradigm
Nursing research
Outcomes research
Paradigm
Positivist paradigm
Qualitative research
Quantitative research
Replication
Research-based practice
Research methods
Research utilization
Scientific approach
Scientific research

AN INTRODUCTION TO NURSING RESEARCH

The purpose of this book is to provide you with the skills to read, understand, evaluate, and use nursing research. The goals of this introductory chapter are twofold: to highlight the important role of research in establishing a knowledge base for your nursing practice and to present an overview of nursing research approaches.

What Is Nursing Research?

Research is systematic inquiry that uses disciplined methods to answer questions or solve problems. The ultimate goal of research is to develop, refine, and expand a body of knowledge. Researchers have searched for knowledge and have made discoveries that aid us in our daily lives.

Nurses are increasingly engaged in disciplined studies that benefit the profession and its patients. **Nursing research** is systematic inquiry designed to develop knowledge about issues of importance to nurses, including nursing practice, nursing education, and nursing administration. In this book, we emphasize clinical nursing research, that is, research designed to generate knowledge to guide nursing practice and to improve the care and quality of life of clients.

Examples of nursing research questions

- What are the effects of physical and nonphysical abuse in an intimate relationship on women's physical and emotional health (Campbell & Soeken, 1999)?
- What are the reproductive and mothering experiences of HIV-positive women (Ingram & Hutchinson, 2000)?

The Importance of Research in Nursing

The development and utilization of nursing knowledge is essential for continued improvement in patient care. Nurses increasingly are expected to adopt a **research-based** (or **evidence-based**) **practice**, using research findings to inform their decisions, actions, and interactions with clients. Nurses are accepting the need to base specific nursing actions and decisions on evidence indicating that the actions are clinically appropriate, cost-effective, and result in positive outcomes for clients. Nurses who incorporate high-quality research evidence into their clinical decisions and clinical recommendations are being professionally accountable to their clients. They are also reinforcing the identity of nursing as a profession.

Another reason for nurses to engage in research involves the spiraling costs of health care and the cost-containment practices being instituted in health care facilities. Now, more than ever, nurses need to document the social relevance and the effectiveness of their practice not only to the profession but also to nursing care consumers, health care administrators, third-party payers (*e.g.,* insurance companies), and government agencies. Some research findings will help eliminate nursing actions that do not achieve desired outcomes. Other findings will help nurses identify the practices that alter health care outcomes and contain costs as well.

Nursing research is essential if nurses are to understand the varied dimensions of their profession. Research enables nurses to describe the characteristics of a particular nursing situation about which little is known, explain phenomena that must be considered in planning nursing care, predict the probable outcomes of certain nursing decisions, control the occurrence of undesired outcomes, and initiate activities to promote desired client behavior.

Roles of Nurses in Nursing Research

Undergraduate nursing students are sometimes puzzled by the requirement to take a course on nursing research. If you, too, are puzzled, you may be thinking that nursing research is not your responsibility. However, it is every nurses' responsibility to engage in one or more roles along a continuum of research participation. At one end of the continuum are those nurses whose involvement in research is indirect. Consumers of nursing research read research reports to keep up-to-date on relevant findings that may affect their practice. At a minimum, nurses are expected to maintain this level of involvement with research. **Research utilization**—the use of the findings from research in a practice setting—depends on intelligent nursing research consumers.

At the other end of the continuum are the producers of nursing research: nurses who actively participate in designing and implementing research studies. At one time, most nurse researchers were academics who taught in schools of nursing, but research is increasingly being conducted by practicing nurses who want to find what works best for their clients.

Between these two end points on the continuum lie a rich variety of research-related activities in which nurses engage as a way of improving their effectiveness and enhancing their professional lives. These activities include the following:

- Participating in a **journal club** in a practice setting, which involves regular meetings among nurses to discuss and critique research articles
- Attending research presentations at professional conferences
- Evaluating completed research for its possible use in practice
- Discussing the implications and relevance of research findings with clients
- Giving clients information and advice about participation in studies
- Assisting in the collection of research information (*e.g.,* distributing questionnaires to clients)
- Reviewing a proposed research plan with respect to its feasibility in a clinical setting and offering clinical expertise to improve the plan
- Assisting with the development of an idea for a clinical research project
- Participating on an institutional committee that reviews the ethical aspects of proposed research before it is undertaken
- Utilizing research by incorporating research results into nursing practice

In all these activities, nurses who have some research skills are in a better position to make a contribution to the nursing profession and to nursing knowledge; thus, most baccalaureate nursing programs include research methods as a requirement. A knowledge of nursing research can improve the depth and breadth of every nurse's professional practice. Learning about research methods allows you to evaluate and synthesize new information (*i.e.,* become an intelligent research consumer), develop knowledge that can be used in practice, and engage meaningfully in various research-related roles.

NURSING RESEARCH: PAST, PRESENT, AND FUTURE

Although nursing research has not always had the prominence and importance it enjoys today, its long and interesting history portends a distinguished future.

The Early Years: From Nightingale to the 1960s

Most people would agree that nursing research began with Florence Nightingale. Based on her skillful analyses of the factors affecting soldier mortality and morbidity during the Crimean War, she was successful in effecting some changes in nursing care—and, more generally, in public health. Her landmark publication, *Notes on Nursing* (1859), describes her early research interest in environmental factors that promote physical and emotional well-being—indeed, an interest of nurses that continues nearly 150 years later.

For many years after Nightingale's work, the nursing literature contained little nursing research. Some attribute this absence of research to the apprenticeship nature of nursing. The pattern of nursing research that eventually emerged at the turn of the century was closely aligned to the problems confronting nurses. For example, most studies conducted between 1900 and 1940 concerned nursing education. As more nurses received university-based education, studies concerning students—their problems, characteristics, and satisfactions—became more numerous. When the hospital staffing patterns changed, fewer students were available over a 24-hour period. As a consequence, researchers focused their investigations not only on the supply and demand of nurses but also on the amount of time required to perform certain nursing activities. During these years, nursing struggled with its professional identity, and nursing research took a twist toward studying nurses: who they were, what they did, how other groups perceived them, and what type of person entered the profession.

In the 1950s, a number of forces combined to put nursing research on the rapidly accelerating upswing it is on today. More nurses with baccalaureate and advanced academic preparation, the establishment of the *Nursing Research* journal, government funding to support nursing research, and upgraded faculty research skills are a few of the forces propelling nursing research. In the late 1950s, the need for studies addressing clinical nursing problems was recognized, and in the 1960s, practice-oriented research on various clinical topics emerged in the literature. Nursing research advanced worldwide: the *International Journal of Nursing Studies* began publication in 1963, and the *Canadian Journal of Nursing Research* appeared in 1968.

Nursing Research Since the 1970s

By the 1970s, the growing number of studies and the increased discussion of theoretical and contextual issues relating to nursing research created the need for additional communication outlets. Several additional journals that focus on nursing research were established in the 1970s, including *Advances in Nursing Science, Research in Nursing & Health*, the *Western Journal of Nursing Research*, and the *Journal of Advanced Nursing*. During that decade, there was a decided shift in emphasis from areas such as teaching, administration, and nurses themselves to the improvement of client care. Nurses also began to pay more attention to the utilization of research findings in nursing practice. A seminal article by Stetler and Marram (1976) offered guidance on assessing research for application in practice settings.

Several events in the 1980s provided impetus for nursing research. For example, the first volume of the *Annual Review of Nursing Research* was published in 1983. These annual reviews include summaries of current research knowledge on selected areas of nursing practice and encourage utilization of research findings. Of particular importance in the United States during the 1980s was the establishment in 1986 of the National Center for Nursing Research (NCNR) within the National Institutes of Health (NIH). The purpose of NCNR was to promote—and financially support—research training and clinical research focused on patient care. Additionally, the Center for Research for Nursing was created in 1983 by the American Nurses Association (ANA). The Center's mission is to develop and coordinate a research program to serve as the source of national information for the profession. Also in the 1980s, nurses began to conduct formal research utilization projects, and an important new journal was established: *Applied Nursing Research*. This journal includes research reports on studies of special relevance to practicing nurses.

After a long crusade by nursing organizations, nursing research was strengthened and given more visibility in 1993 when NCNR was promoted to full institute status within NIH. The birth of the **National Institute of Nursing Research** (NINR) helps put nursing research into the mainstream of research activities enjoyed by other health disciplines in the United States. Funding for nursing research is also growing. In 1986, the NCNR had a budget of $16.2 million, whereas in fiscal year 1999, the budget for NINR was about $70 million. In addition to the creation of NINR, several more research journals were inaugurated. They include *Qualitative Health Research* in 1990, *Clinical Nursing Research* in 1991, and *Clinical Effectiveness in Nursing* in 1996. These journals emerged in response to the growth in clinically oriented and in-depth research among nurses.

Some current nursing research is guided by priorities established by prominent nurse researchers, who were brought together by NCNR for two Conferences on Research Priorities (CORP). The priorities established by the first CORP for research through 1994 included low birth weight, human immunodeficiency virus (HIV) infection, long-term care, symptom management, nursing informatics, health promotion, and technology dependence.

In 1993, the second CORP established the following research emphases for a portion of NINR funding from 1995 through 1999: developing and testing community-based nursing models, assessing the effectiveness of nursing interventions in clients with HIV or acquired immunodeficiency syndrome (AIDS), developing and testing approaches to remediating cognitive impairment, testing interventions for coping with chronic illness, and identifying biobehavioral factors and testing interventions to promote immunocompetence.

Future Directions for Nursing Research

Nursing research continues to develop at a rapid pace and will apparently flourish in the 21st century. Broadly speaking, the priority for nursing research in the future will be the promotion of excellence in nursing science. Toward this end, nurse researchers and practicing nurses will be sharpening their research skills and using those skills to address emerging issues of importance to the profession and its clientele.

Certain trends for the beginning of the 21st century are evident from developments taking shape in the late 1990s:

- *Increased focus on outcomes research.* **Outcomes research** is research designed to assess and document the effectiveness of health care services. The increasing number of studies that can be characterized as outcomes research has been stimulated by the need for cost-effective care that achieves positive outcomes without compromising quality. Nurses are increasingly engaging in outcomes research that is focused both on patients and on the overall delivery system.
- *Promotion of research utilization.* Concerted efforts to translate research findings into practice will continue, and nurses at all levels will be encouraged to engage in evidence-based patient care. In turn, improvements will be needed both in the quality of nursing studies and in nurses' skills in understanding, critiquing, and utilizing study results.
- *Development of a stronger knowledge base through multiple confirmatory strategies.* Practicing nurses cannot be expected to change a procedure or adopt an innovation on the basis of a single, isolated study. Confirmation is usually needed through the deliberate **replication**, that is, the repeating of studies with different clients, in different clinical settings, and at different times to ensure that the findings are robust. Another strategy is the conduct of multiple-site investigations by a team of collaborating researchers in several locations.
- *Expanded dissemination of research findings.* The Internet and other modes of electronic communication have a great effect on the dissemination of research information, which in turn may help to promote research utilization. Through on-line publishing (*e.g.,* the *Online Journal of Clinical Innovation*), electronic document retrieval and delivery, e-mail, and electronic mailing lists, information about innovations can be communicated more widely and more quickly than ever before.

Priorities and goals for the future are also under discussion. In 1999, NINR established scientific goals and objectives for the 5-year period of 2000 to

2004. The four broad goals, and some examples of specific objectives and areas of research, are as follows:

1. Identify and support research opportunities that will achieve scientific distinction and produce significant contributions to health. For example, provide leadership in such areas of science as (a) end-of-life/palliative care research and (b) health-prevention and disease-prevention research.
2. Identify and support future areas of opportunity to advance research on high-quality, cost-effective care and to contribute to the scientific base for nursing practice. For example, identify promising avenues relating to (a) chronic illness and long-term care and (b) neurofunction and sensory conditions.
3. Communicate and disseminate research findings resulting from NINR-funded research.
4. Enhance the development of nurse researchers through training and career development opportunities.

SOURCES OF KNOWLEDGE

Think for a moment about a fact you have learned relating to the practice of nursing. Do you know the source of this information? Some facts are derived from research; some are not. Clinical knowledge used in nursing practice is a collage of sources that vary in their dependability and validity.

- *Tradition.* Within western culture and within the nursing profession, certain beliefs are accepted as truths—and certain practices are accepted as effective—simply based on custom. However, tradition may undermine effective problem solving. That is, traditions may be so entrenched that their validity or usefulness is not challenged or evaluated.
- *Authorities.* An authority is a person with specialized expertise and recognition for that expertise. Reliance on nursing authorities (such as nursing faculty) is, to some degree, inevitable; however, like tradition, authorities as a source of information have limitations. Authorities are not infallible (particularly if their expertise is based primarily on personal experience), yet their knowledge often goes unchallenged.
- *Personal experience.* We all solve problems based on observations and experiences. The ability to recognize regularities, to generalize, and to make predictions based on observations is a hallmark of the human mind. Nevertheless, personal experience has limitations as a knowledge source because each person's experience may be too restricted to be useful in general terms, and personal experiences are often colored by biases.
- *Trial and error.* Sometimes, we tackle problems by successively trying out alternative solutions. This approach may in some cases be practical, but

it is often fallible and inefficient. The method tends to be haphazard, and the solutions are, in many instances, idiosyncratic.

- *Intuition.* Intuition is a type of knowledge that cannot be explained on the basis of reasoning or prior instruction. Although intuition and hunches undoubtedly play a role in nursing practice—as they do in the conduct of research—it is difficult to develop policies and practices for nurses on the basis of intuition.
- *Logical reasoning.* Reasoning is the mental processing of ideas to solve problems. Two intellectual mechanisms are used in reasoning. **Inductive reasoning** is the process of developing conclusions and generalizations from specific observations. For example, a nurse may observe the anxious behavior of (specific) hospitalized children and conclude that (in general) children's separation from their parents is very stressful. **Deductive reasoning** is the process of developing specific predictions from general principles. For example, if we assume that separation anxiety does occur in hospitalized children (in general), we might predict that the (specific) children in Memorial Hospital whose parents do not room-in would manifest symptoms of stress. Both systems of reasoning are useful as a means of understanding phenomena, and both play a role in research. However, reasoning in and of itself is limited because the validity of reasoning depends on the accuracy of the information (or premises) with which one starts, and reasoning may be an insufficient basis for evaluating accuracy.
- *Disciplined research.* Research conducted within a disciplined format is the most sophisticated method of acquiring knowledge that humans have developed. Nursing research combines aspects of logical reasoning with other features to create systems of problem solving that, although fallible, tend to be more reliable than other sources of knowledge.

The current emphasis on evidence-based health care requires nurses to base their clinical practice to the extent possible on research-based findings rather than on tradition, intuition, or personal experience—although nursing will always remain a rich blend of art and science.

PARADIGMS AND METHODS FOR NURSING RESEARCH

A paradigm is a world view, a general perspective on the complexities of the real world. Disciplined inquiry in the field of nursing is being conducted mainly within two broad paradigms, both of which have legitimacy for nursing research.[1] This section describes the two paradigms and broadly outlines the research methods associated with them.

---

[1]Other inquiry paradigms exist, such as several that collectively have been labeled critical theory or critical inquiry (*e.g.,* feminism, neo-Marxism). It is beyond the scope of this book to discuss these other paradigms.

The Positivist Paradigm

The traditional scientific approach to conducting research has its underpinnings in the philosophical paradigm known as the **positivist paradigm.** Positivism is rooted in 19th-century thought, guided by such philosophers as Comte, Newton, and Locke. Although strict positivist thinking (sometimes referred to as *logical positivism*) has been challenged and undermined, a modified positivist position remains a dominant force in scientific research.

A fundamental assumption of positivists is that there is a reality out there that can be studied and known (an **assumption** is a basic principle that is believed to be true without proof or verification). Adherents of the scientific approach assume that nature is basically ordered and regular and that an objective reality exists independent of human observation. In other words, the world is assumed not to be merely a creation of the human mind. The related assumption of **determinism** refers to the positivists' belief that phenomena are not haphazard or random events, but rather have antecedent causes. If a person develops lung cancer, the scientist assumes that there must be one or more reasons that can be potentially identified and understood. Within the positivist paradigm, much of the scientific researcher's activity is directed at understanding the underlying causes of natural phenomena.

Because of their fundamental belief in an objective reality, positivists seek to be as objective as possible in their pursuit of knowledge. Positivists attempt to hold their personal beliefs and biases in check during their research. The positivists' scientific approach calls for orderly, disciplined procedures to test the researcher's ideas about the nature of the phenomena being studied and relationships among them.

The Naturalistic Paradigm

The **naturalistic paradigm** (which is sometimes referred to as the *phenomenologic paradigm*) began as a countermovement to positivism with writers such as Weber and Kant. The naturalistic paradigm represents a major alternative system for conducting disciplined inquiry in the field of nursing. Table 1-1 compares four major assumptions of the positivist and naturalistic paradigms.

For the naturalistic inquirer, reality is not a fixed entity. Instead, it is a construction of the individuals participating in the research; reality exists within a context, and many constructions are possible. Naturalists thus take the position of relativism: if there are always multiple interpretations of reality that exist in people's minds, then there is no process by which the ultimate truth or falsity of the constructions can be determined.

The naturalistic paradigm assumes that knowledge is maximized when the distance between the inquirer and the participants in the study is minimized. The voices and interpretations of those under study are key to understanding the phenomenon of interest, and subjective interactions are the pri-

TABLE 1-1. Major Assumptions of the Positivist and Naturalistic Paradigms		
PHILOSOPHICAL QUESTION	**POSITIVIST PARADIGM ASSUMPTIONS**	**NATURALISTIC PARADIGM ASSUMPTIONS**
Ontologic (What is the nature of reality?)	Reality exists; there is a real world driven by real natural causes.	Reality is multiple and subjective, mentally constructed by individuals.
Epistemologic (How is the inquirer related to those being researched?)	Inquirer is independent from those being researched; the findings are not influenced by the researcher.	The inquirer interacts with those being researched; findings are the creation of the interactive process.
Axiologic (What is the role of values in the inquiry?)	Values and biases are to be held in check; objectivity is sought.	Subjectivity and values are inevitable and desirable.
Methodologic (How is knowledge obtained?)	Deductive processes	Inductive processes
	Emphasis on discrete, specific concepts	Emphasis on entirety of some phenomenon, holistic
	Verification of researcher's hunches	Emerging interpretations grounded in participants' experiences
	Fixed design	Flexible design
	Tight controls over context	Context bound
	Emphasis on measured, quantitative information; statistical analysis	Emphasis on narrative information; qualitative analysis
	Seeks generalizations	Seeks patterns

mary way to access them. The findings from a naturalistic inquiry are the product of the interaction between the inquirer and the participants.

Paradigms and Methods: Quantitative and Qualitative Research

The two perspectives on the nature of reality have implications for the methods used to acquire knowledge. (Broadly speaking, **research methods** are the techniques used by researchers to structure a study and to gather and analyze information relevant to the research question.) The most common methodologic distinction focuses on differences between **quantitative research**, which is most closely allied with the positivist tradition, and **qualitative research**, which is most often associated with naturalistic inquiry—although positivists sometimes undertake qualitative studies, and naturalistic researchers sometimes collect quantitative information.

The Scientific Approach and Quantitative Research

The traditional **scientific approach** refers to a general set of orderly, disciplined procedures used to acquire information. The traditional scientist uses deductive reasoning to generate hunches that are tested in the real world. In **scientific research**—the application of the scientific approach to the study of a question of interest—the researcher moves in a systematic fashion from the definition of a problem and the selection of concepts on which to focus, to the solution of the problem. Systematic means that the scientific investigator progresses logically through a series of steps, according to a prespecified plan of action. The researcher uses, to the extent possible, mechanisms designed to control the study. **Control** involves imposing conditions on the research situation so that biases are minimized and precision and validity are maximized.

In addressing research questions, the scientist gathers **empirical evidence**—evidence that is rooted in objective reality and gathered directly or indirectly through the senses rather than through personal beliefs or hunches. In a scientific study, formal instruments are used to collect the needed information. Usually (but not always) the information gathered is quantitative (*i.e.,* numeric information that results from formal measurement and that is analyzed with statistical procedures). Scientists strive to go beyond the specifics of the research situation; the degree to which research findings can be generalized (referred to as the **generalizability** of the research) is a widely used criterion for assessing the quality and importance of a traditional research study.

The scientific approach has enjoyed considerable stature as a method of inquiry, and it has been used productively by nurse researchers studying a wide range of nursing problems. This is not to say, however, that scientific research can solve all nursing problems or that the scientific method has been without criticism. One important limitation of the scientific method is its inadequacy for addressing moral or ethical questions. Many of our most persistent and intriguing questions about the human experience fall into this area (*e.g.,* Should euthanasia be practiced? Should abortion be legal?). Given the many moral issues that are linked to medicine and health care, it is inevitable that the nursing process will never rely exclusively on scientific information.

The scientific approach also must contend with problems of measurement. In studying a phenomenon, the scientist attempts to measure it. For example, if the phenomenon of interest was patient morale, a researcher may want to know if a patient's morale is high or low, or higher under certain conditions than under others. Although physiologic phenomena such as blood pressure, temperature, and cardiac activity can be measured with high accuracy, the same cannot be said of psychological phenomena, such as patient morale, pain, or self-image.

A final issue is that nursing research tends to focus on human beings, who are inherently complex and diverse. The scientific method typically focuses on a relatively small portion of the human experience (*e.g.,* weight gain, depression, chemical dependency) in a single study. Complexities tend to be controlled and, insofar as possible, eliminated in scientific studies rather than studied directly. Sometimes this narrow focus obscures insights.

Naturalistic Methods and Qualitative Research
Naturalistic methods of inquiry deal with the issue of human complexity by exploring it directly. Researchers in the naturalistic tradition stress the inher-

ent complexity of humans, the ability of humans to shape and create their own experiences, and the idea that truth is a composite of realities. Consequently, naturalistic investigations emphasize understanding the human experience as it is lived by collecting and analyzing narrative, subjective (*i.e.,* qualitative) materials.

Some researchers reject the traditional scientific approach as reductionist (*i.e.,* it reduces human experience to the few concepts under investigation, with those concepts defined in advance by the researcher rather than emerging from the experience of those under study). Naturalistic researchers tend to focus on the dynamic, holistic, and individual aspects of phenomena and attempt to capture those aspects in their entirety, within the context of those who are experiencing them.

Flexible, evolving procedures are used to capitalize on findings that emerge in the course of the study. Naturalistic inquiry always takes place in the field (*i.e.,* in naturalistic settings), frequently over an extended period of time. The collection of information and its analysis typically progress concurrently. As the researcher sifts through the existing information and gains insight, new questions emerge, calling for additional evidence to amplify or confirm the insights. Through an inductive process, the researcher integrates the evidence to develop a theory or framework that helps explain the processes under observation.

Naturalistic studies result in rich, in-depth information that has the potential to clarify the multiple dimensions of a complicated phenomenon (*e.g.,* the process by which family caregivers adapt to their roles). The findings from in-depth qualitative research are typically grounded in the real-life experiences of people with first-hand knowledge of a phenomenon. However, the approach has several limitations. Human beings are the direct instruments through which qualitative information is gathered, and humans are intelligent and sensitive—but fallible—tools. The highly personal approach that enriches the analytic insights of a skillful researcher can sometimes result in petty and trivial "findings" among less competent ones.

Another potential limitation involves the subjective nature of the inquiry, which can raise questions about the idiosyncratic nature of the conclusions. Would two naturalistic researchers studying the same phenomenon in the same setting arrive at the same results? Moreover, most naturalistic studies involve a relatively small group of participants. Thus, the generalizability of findings from naturalistic inquiries can sometimes be challenged.

CONSUMER TIP:

When a study is qualitative or conducted within the naturalistic paradigm, you are likely to find an explicit statement to this effect early in a research report. This is less characteristic of quantitative studies. Researchers rarely discuss their paradigmatic orientation explicitly, but they may explain their methodologic approach in relation to the research problem. ■

Multiple Paradigms and Nursing Research

Paradigms are lenses that help us to sharpen our focus on a phenomenon of interest; they are not blinders that limit our intellectual curiosity. The emergence of alternative paradigms for studying nursing problems is, in our view, a healthy and desirable trend in the pursuit of new knowledge. The nursing knowledge base would be slim, indeed, without a rich array of approaches and methods available within the two paradigms—methods that are often complementary in their strengths and limitations and can be profitably used in tandem in a single investigation.

We have emphasized the differences between the positivist and naturalistic paradigms and their associated methods so that their distinctions would be easy to understand. Despite their differences, however, the alternative paradigms have many features in common. A few are mentioned below:

- *Ultimate goals.* The ultimate aim of disciplined inquiry, regardless of the paradigm, is knowledge. Both quantitative and qualitative researchers seek the truth about an aspect of the world in which they are interested, and both can make significant—and mutually beneficial—contributions.
- *External evidence.* Although the word *empiricism* is associated with the scientific approach, researchers in both traditions gather and analyze external evidence empirically, that is, through their senses. Neither qualitative nor quantitative researchers are "armchair" analysts, relying on their own beliefs and world views for their conclusions.
- *Reliance on human cooperation.* Because evidence for nursing research comes primarily from human study participants, the need for human cooperation is essential. To understand people's characteristics and experiences, researchers must persuade them to participate in the investigation and to act and speak candidly. In some areas of inquiry, the need for candor and cooperation is a challenging requirement—for researchers in either tradition.
- *Ethical constraints.* Research with human beings is guided by ethical principles that sometimes interfere with the researcher's ultimate goal. For example, if a researcher's aim is to test a potentially beneficial intervention, is it ethical to withhold the treatment from some people to see what happens? As discussed in Chapter 4, ethical dilemmas often confront researchers, regardless of paradigms or methods.
- *Fallibility of disciplined research.* Virtually all studies—in either paradigm—have limitations. Every research question can be addressed in many different ways, and inevitably there are tradeoffs. Financial constraints are universal, but limitations usually exist even when resources are abundant. This does not mean that small, simple studies have no value. It means that no single study can ever definitively answer a research question. Each completed study adds to a body of accumulated knowledge. If several researchers pose the same question and if each obtains the same or similar results, increased confidence can be placed in the

answer to the question. The fallibility of any single study makes it important for you as a consumer of research to understand the tradeoffs and decisions that researchers make and to evaluate the adequacy of those decisions.

Despite philosophical and methodologic differences, researchers using the traditional scientific approach or more naturalistic methods generally share overall goals and face many similar constraints and challenges. The selection of an appropriate method depends to some degree on the researcher's personal taste and philosophy but largely on the nature of the research question. If a researcher asks, "What are the effects of surgery on circadian rhythms (biologic cycles)?" the researcher needs to express the effects through the careful quantitative measurement of various bodily processes subject to rhythmic variation. On the other hand, if a researcher asks, "What is the process by which parents learn to cope with the death of a child?" the researcher may be hard pressed to quantify the process. Researchers' personal world views help to shape the types of question they ask.

In reading about the alternative paradigms for nursing research, you were probably more attracted to one of the two paradigms—the paradigm that corresponds most closely to your view of the world and of reality. Learning about and respecting both approaches to disciplined inquiry, however, and recognizing the strengths and limitations of each are important. In this textbook, we provide an overview of the methods associated with both qualitative and quantitative research and offer guidance on how to understand, critique, and use findings from both.

PURPOSES OF NURSING RESEARCH

The general purpose of nursing research is to answer questions or solve problems of relevance to the nursing profession, but there are more specific purposes of disciplined inquiry.

Specific Purposes of Quantitative and Qualitative Research

The specific purposes of nursing research include identification, description, exploration, explanation, prediction, and control. Within each purpose, various types of questions are addressed by nurse researchers, and certain questions are more amenable to qualitative than to quantitative inquiry, and *vice versa*.

Identification
Many qualitative studies focus on phenomena about which little is known. In some cases, so little is known that the phenomenon has yet to be clearly identified or named—or has been inadequately defined or conceptualized. The in-depth, probing nature of qualitative research is well suited to the task of answering such questions as, "What is this phenomenon?" and "What is its

name?" (Table 1-2). In quantitative research, by contrast, the researcher begins with a phenomenon that has been studied or defined previously, sometimes in a qualitative study. Thus, in quantitative research, identification typically precedes the inquiry.

Qualitative example of identification:

Roberts (1999) investigated illicit drug use in the lives of 32 drug-using inner-city women. Through in-depth interviews, Roberts identified the basic social process underlying the women's lives as *managing loss*, that is, dealing with painful feelings of loss resulting from separation of someone or something from their lives.

TABLE 1-2. Research Purposes and Research Questions

PURPOSE	TYPES OF QUESTIONS: QUANTITATIVE RESEARCH	TYPES OF QUESTIONS: QUALITATIVE RESEARCH
Identification		What is this phenomenon? What is its name?
Description	How prevalent is the phenomenon? How often does the phenomenon occur? What are the characteristics of the phenomenon?	What are the dimensions of the phenomenon? What variations exist? What is important about the phenomenon?
Exploration	What factors are related to the phenomenon? What are the antecedents of the phenomenon?	What is the full nature of the phenomenon? What is really going on here? What is the process by which the phenomenon evolves or is experienced?
Explanation	What are the measurable associations between phenomena? What factors caused the phenomenon? Does the theory explain the phenomenon?	How does the phenomenon work? Why does the phenomenon exist? What is the meaning of the phenomenon? How did the phenomenon occur?
Prediction and control	What will happen if we alter a phenomenon or introduce an intervention? If phenomenon X occurs, will phenomenon Y follow? How can we make the phenomenon happen, or alter its nature or prevalence? Can the occurrence of the phenomenon be controlled?	

Description

The main objective of many nursing research studies is the description and elucidation of phenomena relating to the nursing profession. The researcher who conducts a descriptive investigation observes, counts, describes, and classifies. Phenomena that nurse researchers have described vary. Examples include stress and coping, pain, health beliefs, rehabilitation success, and time patterns of temperature readings.

Description can be a major purpose for both qualitative and quantitative researchers. Quantitative description involves the prevalence, incidence, size, and measurable attributes of a phenomenon. Qualitative researchers, on the other hand, use in-depth methods to describe the dimensions, variations, importance, and meaning of phenomena. Table 1-2 compares some of the descriptive questions posed by quantitative and qualitative researchers.

Quantitative example of description:

Maguire (1999) performed a study to describe the problem of skin breakdown in extremely low-birth-weight infants. In the research report, Maguire described such factors as the percentage of infants with severe skin breakdown and the percentage of nurses using various products for skin breakdown prevention.

Qualitative example of description:

Robinson (2000) undertook an in-depth study to describe the psychosocial and behavioral aspects of living with urinary incontinence in a nursing home.

Exploration

Like descriptive research, exploratory research begins with some phenomenon of interest; however, rather than simply observing and describing the phenomenon, exploratory research investigates the full nature of the phenomenon and the other factors with which it is related. For example, a descriptive quantitative study of patients' preoperative stress might seek to document the degree of stress patients experience before surgery and the percentage of patients who actually experience it. An exploratory study might ask the following: What factors are related to a patient's stress level? Is a patient's stress related to behaviors of the nursing staff? Does a patient's behavior change in relation to the level of stress experienced?

Exploratory studies are undertaken when a new area or topic is being investigated, and qualitative methods are especially useful for exploring a little-understood phenomenon. Exploratory qualitative research is designed to shed light on the various ways in which a phenomenon is manifested and on underlying processes.

Quantitative example of exploration:

Parshall (1999) conducted a study to explore the role that dyspnea plays in the disposition and treatment of patients being treated for chronic cardiorespiratory diseases, using records from more than 25,000 adult patient visits to hospital emergency departments.

Qualitative example of exploration:

Banister (1999) explored women's midlife experience and perceptions of their changing bodies within the Western cultural context through interviews with 11 women aged 40 to 53 years.

Explanation

The goals of explanatory research include understanding the underpinnings of specific natural phenomena and explaining systematic relationships among phenomena. Explanatory research is often linked to a theory, which represents a method of deriving, organizing, and integrating ideas about the manner in which phenomena are interrelated. Whereas descriptive research provides new information, and exploratory research provides promising insights, explanatory research focuses on understanding the causes or full nature of a phenomenon.

In quantitative research, theories are used deductively as the basis for generating explanations that are then tested empirically. That is, based on previous theory or a body of evidence, the researcher makes specific explanatory predictions that, if upheld by the data, add further credibility to the theory. In qualitative studies, the researcher may search for explanations about how or why a phenomenon exists as a basis for developing a theory that is grounded in rich, in-depth, experiential evidence.

Quantitative example of explanation:

Lauver, Settersten, Marten, and Halls (1999) conducted a theoretically based study to explain women's use of hormones during menopause, based on quantitative indicators of the women's habits, beliefs, norms, and demographic characteristics.

Qualitative example of explanation:

Cohen (1999) undertook a study aimed at developing a comprehensive explanation of the process of transitioning technology-dependent children from hospital to home and community-based care.

Prediction and Control

Many research problems defy absolute comprehension and explanation. Yet it is possible to predict and control phenomena based on research findings, even without complete understanding. For example, research has shown that the incidence of Down syndrome in infants increases with the age of the mother. Therefore, we can predict that a woman aged 40 years is at higher risk of bearing a child with Down syndrome than a woman aged 25 years. The incidence of Down syndrome may be partially controlled by educating women about the risks and offering amniocentesis to women older than 35 years of age. Note, however, that the ability to predict and control in this example does not depend on an explanation of why older women are at a higher risk for having an abnormal child. There are many examples of nursing and health-related studies—typically, quantitative ones—in which prediction and control are key objectives.

Quantitative example of prediction:

The main purpose of a study by Brooks-Brunn (2000) was to identify risk factors that could predict postoperative pulmonary complications after total abdominal hysterectomy.

CONSUMER TIP:

Most nursing studies have multiple aims. Almost all studies have some descriptive intent. Some exploratory studies also have an expectation that the results will serve a predictive or control function. Truly explanatory studies are the least common in the nursing literature. ■

Basic and Applied Research

A study's purpose can also be characterized by the direct utility of the findings. **Basic research** is undertaken to accumulate information, extending the base of knowledge in a discipline to improve understanding, or to formulate or refine a theory. For example, a researcher may perform an in-depth study to understand better the normal process of grieving, without having an explicit nursing application in mind.

Applied research focuses on finding an immediate solution to an existing problem. The ultimate goal of applied research is the systematic planning of change in a problematic situation. For example, a study of the effectiveness of a specific nursing intervention to ease grieving would be applied research. Basic research is appropriate for discovering general principles of human behavior and biophysiologic processes, but applied research is designed to indicate how these principles can be used to solve problems in nursing practice.

In nursing, as in medicine, the feedback process between basic and applied research operates more freely than in other disciplines. The findings from applied research almost immediately pose questions for basic research, whereas the results of basic research often suggest clinical applications.

CONSUMER TIP:

Researchers rarely specify whether their intent is to address a pragmatic problem or to generate basic knowledge. The study's intent generally has to be inferred and, in some cases, may be ambiguous. ■

ASSISTANCE TO CONSUMERS OF NURSING RESEARCH

This book is designed to help you develop skills that will allow you to read, evaluate, and use nursing studies (*i.e.,* to become intelligent consumers and users of nursing research). In each chapter of this book, we present information relating to the methods used by nurse researchers and provide specific guidance to consumers in two ways. First, interspersed throughout the chapters, we offer tips on what you can expect to find, with regard to the material discussed in the chapter, in actual research reports. These tips are identified with this icon: ☑. Second, we include guidelines for critiquing those aspects of a study covered in each chapter. The questions in Box 1-1 are designed to assist you in using the information in this chapter in an overall preliminary assessment of a research report.

BOX 1-1 ☐ **QUESTIONS FOR A PRELIMINARY OVERVIEW OF A RESEARCH REPORT**

1. How relevant is the research to the actual practice of nursing? Can the study be described as *clinical* nursing research?

2. Does the study focus on a topic that is considered a priority area for nursing research?

3. Is the research qualitative or quantitative? What is the underlying paradigm?

4. What is the underlying purpose (or purposes) of the study—identification, description, exploration, explanation, or prediction and control?

5. Is the study fundamentally basic or applied in nature?

6. What might be the clinical applications of this research? To what type of people and settings is the research most relevant? How, if at all, can the results of this study be used by *me?*

RESEARCH EXAMPLES

Each chapter of this book presents brief descriptions of actual studies conducted by nurse researchers, followed by some comments on the study's clinical relevance. The descriptions focus on aspects of the study emphasized in the chapter. In most cases, a review of the full research report in the nursing journal will enhance your assessment and will be a useful supplementary assignment. In this chapter, you can use the guidelines in Box 1-1 to do a brief preliminary assessment of some of the features of the two studies we describe next.

RESEARCH EXAMPLE OF A QUANTITATIVE STUDY

Stevens and colleagues (1999) conducted a study to determine the effectiveness of developmentally sensitive nursing interventions for relieving procedural pain in very-low-birth-weight infants. Their report appeared in the journal *Nursing Research.*

Research Summary
Stevens and her colleagues, who had conducted earlier research on the topic of infant pain, exposed 122 low-birth-weight infants to four different pain-relieving interventions, in random order, during a heel lance procedure. The interventions included (a) prone positioning; (b) receipt of a pacifier with sterile water; (c) receipt of a pacifier with sucrose; and (d) the standard treatment, which was side-lying or supine positioning without pacifier. The researchers compared the infants' pain responses to the four treatments. The infants' pain was measured through a composite pain scale that involved both observed behavioral indicators (*e.g.,* the infants' eye squeeze) and physiologic ones (*e.g.,* their heart rate). The researchers found that the most effective intervention for reducing pain was the pacifier with sucrose. Positioning was unrelated to the neonates' pain responses.

Clinical Relevance
In the discussion of their study, the researchers note that further research is needed to determine the efficacy and safety of a sucrose intervention for infants undergoing repeated painful procedures. Nevertheless, this study offers strong evidence that the pain response of infants receiving a sucrose pacifier during a single painful procedure is lower than when they do not.

The strength of this evidence lies in several factors—several of which you will appreciate more as you become familiar with research methods. First and foremost, this study was scientifically rigorous. The researchers took extreme care to ensure that the infants in the study were treated in a comparable fashion, so that any differences in the pain responses reflected the interventions themselves and not some spurious factor. Second, by exposing the infants to all of the interventions and then comparing the pain responses, the researchers ruled out the possibility that the pain responses differed simply because different infants have different pain thresholds or pain manifestations. A third feature strengthened this study's clinical significance: the study was conducted in four separate hospitals—and the results were the same in all four settings. Finally, the findings are more persuasive because the team of researchers who conducted the study have developed a solid program of research on neonatal pain, and their research has contributed incrementally to our understanding of infants' pain responses and appropriate nursing interventions.

The findings from their study have implications for clinicians who strive to provide developmentally sensitive care to very-low-birth-weight infants. These fragile infants in newborn intensive care units experience large numbers of painful procedures daily and are vulnerable to the consequences of pain. Providing a pacifier dipped in sucrose is a noninvasive, low-cost treatment for reducing procedural pain in these infants. Clinicians, however, need to use caution in the widespread use of this nonpharmacologic intervention because the possibly adverse long-term effects of sucrose have yet to be assessed.

RESEARCH EXAMPLE OF A QUALITATIVE STUDY

Nehls (1999) conducted an in-depth study of the experience of living with the diagnosis of borderline personality disorder. Her study was published in *Research in Nursing & Health*.

Research Summary

Nehls' study was undertaken to understand the meaning of being diagnosed with borderline personality to the people who actually experience it. The researcher wanted to gain insight into what is unique about living with the diagnosis, to improve future caring practices for this illness. Thirty women diagnosed with this psychiatric illness were interviewed in depth, using two guide questions: "What does the diagnosis of borderline personality mean to you?" and "What is it like for you to live with the diagnosis of borderline personality?" The women's responses were analyzed to identify the common meanings and shared practices of women living with this disorder. The researcher identified three recurring themes in the participants' narratives. The first theme, living with a label, concerned the women's perception that mental health care providers held preconceived and negative opinions of people with borderline personality disorder. The ramifications of this negative labeling, even more than the diagnosis itself, were problematic for these women. The second theme was living with self-destructive behavior. Attempted suicide and self-mutilation were common experiences for these women. Finally, the third theme was living with limited access to care, including limited opportunity to engage in dialogue with mental health clinicians.

Clinical Relevance

Nehls' thorough and careful study provides a unique, first-hand perspective on the shared meaning of borderline personality disorder to those who have this diagnosis. The clinical implications of the study are strengthened by the fact that the researcher took steps to ensure its rigor. For example, Nehls audiotaped her interviews and transcribed them verbatim, used multiple stages of data analysis with her research team, and included people outside the team to provide feedback on the analysis. The powerful themes that were revealed in the study suggest ways to improve clinical practice.

The women in the study perceived that negative views of borderline personality adversely affected the delivery of not only mental health care services but also other health care services. They believed, for example, that health care providers viewed the self-harm behavior of these women as manipulative because of their prejudice of the diagnosis of borderline personality disorder and that this prejudice resulted in the clinicians' failure to identify the reasons underlying self-destructive behavior. The women also perceived that their access to health care was intentionally circumscribed as a result of this prejudice.

Thus, the themes that emerged from Nehls' study suggest that mental health care for individuals with borderline personality disorder can be improved by confronting prejudice toward this illness, by striving to better understand self-harm behaviors, and by increasing opportunities for dialogue and caring. The findings indicate that clinicians could enhance the quality of care they provide by offering their full attention, by listening more intently, and by caring about the day-to-day experiences of those with the disorder.

• • • • • SUMMARY POINTS

- **Nursing research** is systematic inquiry to develop knowledge about issues of importance to nurses and serves to establish a scientific base of knowledge for nursing practice.
- Nurses in various settings are adopting **a research-based** (or **evidence-based) practice** that incorporates research findings into their decisions and their interactions with clients.
- Knowledge of nursing research enhances the professional practice of all nurses, including both consumers of research (who read and evaluate studies) and producers of research (who design and undertake research studies).
- Nursing research began with Florence Nightingale but developed slowly until its rapid acceleration in the 1950s. Since the 1970s, nursing research has focused on problems relating to clinical practice.

- **The National Institute of Nursing Research (NINR)**, established at the U.S. National Institutes of Health in 1993, affirms the stature of nursing research.
- Future emphases of nursing research are likely to include **outcomes research**, research utilization projects, **replications** of research, multiple-site studies, and expanded dissemination efforts.
- Disciplined research stands in contrast to other sources of knowledge for nursing practice, such as tradition, voices of authority, personal experience, trial and error, intuition, and logical reasoning.
- Disciplined inquiry in nursing is conducted within two broad **paradigms**, or world views with underlying **assumptions** about the complexities of reality: the **positivist paradigm** and the naturalistic paradigm.
- In the positivist paradigm, it is assumed that there is an objective reality and that natural phenomena are regular and orderly. The related assumption of **determinism** refers to the belief that events are not haphazard but rather the result of prior causes.
- In the **naturalistic paradigm**, it is assumed that reality is not a fixed entity but is rather a construction of human minds, and thus "truth" is a composite of multiple constructions of reality.
- The positivist paradigm is associated with the traditional **scientific approach**, which is a systematic and controlled process. Scientists base their findings on **empirical evidence** (evidence collected by way of the human senses) and strive for **generalizability** of their findings beyond a single setting or situation. The scientific approach is associated with **quantitative research**—the collection and analysis of numeric information.
- Researchers within the naturalistic paradigm emphasize understanding the human experience as it is lived through the collection and analysis of subjective, narrative materials using flexible procedures that evolve in the field; this paradigm is associated with **qualitative research**.
- Research purposes include identification, description, exploration, explanation, prediction, and control.
- **Basic research** is designed to extend the base of information for the sake of knowledge. **Applied research** focuses on discovering solutions to immediate problems.

➤➤➤➤ CRITICAL THINKING ACTIVITIES

Chapter 1 of the accompanying *Study Guide to Accompany Essentials of Nursing Research,* 5th edition offers various exercises and study suggestions for reinforcing the concepts presented in this chapter. In addition, you can consider the following:

1. Read the abstracts from one or both of the actual research studies in the Appendix of this book, and then answer questions 1, 2, 4, 5, and 6 in Box 1-1. Do the results of the study, as summarized in the abstract, seem to be consistent with any "facts" you have learned in your nursing studies, or do they have the potential to challenge what you have learned?

2. Is your world view closer to the positivist or the naturalistic paradigm? Explore the aspects of the two paradigms that are especially consistent with your world view.

For additional review, see questions 1–15 on the study CD provided with Polit: Study Guide to Accompany Essentials of Nursing Research.

⊞ WORLD WIDE WEB SITES

National Institute of Nursing Research:
http://www.nih.gov/ninr

Nurse researcher mailing lists:
http://www.springnet.com/np/nplstsrv/htm

SUGGESTED READINGS

Methodologic and Theoretical References

American Nurses' Association Cabinet on Nursing Research. (1985). *Directions for nursing research: Toward the twenty-first century.* Kansas City, MO: American Nurses' Association.

Guba, E. G. (Ed.). (1990). *The paradigm dialog.* Newbury Park, CA: Sage Publications.

Lincoln, Y. S., & Guba, E. G. (1985). *Naturalistic inquiry.* Beverly Hills: Sage Publications.

Nightingale, F. (1859). *Notes on nursing: What it is and what it is not.* Philadelphia: J.B. Lippincott.

Schlotfeldt, R. M. (1992). Why promote clinical nursing scholarship? *Clinical Nursing Research, 1,* 5–8.

Stetler, C. B., & Marram, G. (1976). Evaluating research findings for applicability in practice. *Nursing Outlook, 24,* 559–563.

Substantive References

Banister, E. M. (1999). Women's midlife experience of their changing bodies. *Qualitative Health Research, 9,* 520–537.

Brooks-Brunn, J. A. (2000). Risk factors associated with postoperative pulmonary complications following total abdominal hysterectomy. *Clinical Nursing Research, 9,* 27–46.

Campbell, J. C., & Soeken, K. L. (1999). Women's responses to battering: A test of the model. *Research in Nursing & Health, 22,* 49–58.

Cohen, M. H. (1999). The technology-dependent child and the socially marginalized family: A provisional framework. *Qualitative Health Research, 9,* 654–668.

Ingram, D., & Hutchinson, S. A. (2000). Double binds and the reproductive and mothering experiences of HIV-positive women. *Qualitative Health Research, 10,* 117–132.

Lauver, D. R., Settersten, L., Marten, S., & Halls, J. (1999). Explaining women's intentions and use of hormones with menopause. *Research in Nursing & Health, 22,* 309–320.

Maguire, D. P. (1999). Skin protection and breakdown in the ELBW infant. *Clinical Nursing Research, 8,* 222–234.

Nehls, N. (1999). Borderline personality disorder: The voice of patients. *Research in Nursing & Health, 22,* 285–293.

Parshall, M. B. (1999). Adult emergency visits for chronic cardiorespiratory disease: Does dyspnea matter? *Nursing Research, 48,* 62–70.

Roberts, C. A. (1999). Drug use among inner-city African-American women: The process of managing loss. *Qualitative Health Research, 9,* 620–638.

Robinson, J. P. (2000). Managing urinary incontinence in the nursing home: Residents' perspectives. *Journal of Advanced Nursing, 31,* 68–77.

Stevens, B., Johnston, C., Franck, L., Petryshen, P., Jack, A., & Foster, G. (1999). The efficacy of developmentally sensitive interventions and sucrose for relieving procedural pain in very low birth weight neonates. *Nursing Research, 48,* 35–43.

Comprehending the Research Process

● ●

Student Objectives

On completion of this chapter, the student will be able to:

○ define new terms presented in the chapter
○ distinguish terms associated with quantitative and qualitative research
○ distinguish independent and dependent variables
○ describe the flow and sequence of activities in quantitative and qualitative research

● ●

New Terms

Associative relationship	Pilot study
Categorical variable	Population
Cause-and-effect (causal) relationship	Qualitative data
Coding	Quantitative data
Concept	Raw data
Conceptual model	Relationship
Constant	Representativeness
Construct	Research design
Continuous variable	Research proposal
Data	Research report
Dependent variable	Researcher
Functional relationship	Respondent
Gaining entrée	Sample
Hypothesis	Sampling plan
Independent variable	Saturation
Informant	Site
Interpretation	Statistical analysis
Investigator	Study participants
Literature review	Subjects
Operational definition	Theory
Outcome variable	Variable

BASIC RESEARCH TERMINOLOGY

Research, like nursing or any other discipline, has its own language and terminology—its own *jargon*. Some terms are used by both qualitative and quantitative researchers, whereas others are used predominantly in connection with one or the other approach.

The Study

When researchers address a problem or answer a question through disciplined research—regardless of the underlying paradigm—they are doing a **study** (or an **investigation** or **research project**). Research studies with humans involve two sets of people: those who conduct the study and those who provide information. In a quantitative study, the people being studied are referred to as the **subjects** or the **study participants**, as shown in Table 2-1. (When the subjects provide information to the researchers by answering questions, as in an interview, they may be called **respondents**). In a qualitative study, the individuals cooperating in the study play an active rather than a passive role and are therefore referred to as **informants** or study participants. The person who undertakes the research is called the **researcher** or **investigator** (or sometimes—more often in quantitative studies—the **scientist**).

Phenomena, Concepts, and Constructs

Research focuses on abstract rather than tangible phenomena. For example, the terms *pain, patient care, coping,* and *grief* are all abstractions of particular aspects of human behavior and characteristics. These abstractions are often referred to as **concepts** (or, in qualitative research, **phenomena** or topics).

Researchers also use the term construct. Kerlinger (1986) distinguishes concepts from constructs by noting that **constructs** are abstractions that are deliberately and systematically invented (or constructed) by researchers for a specific purpose. For example, *self-care* in Orem's model of health maintenance may be considered a construct. The terms *construct* and *concept* may be

TABLE 2-1. Key Terms Used in Quantitative and Qualitative Research

CONCEPT	QUANTITATIVE TERM	QUALITATIVE TERM
Person contributing information	Subject	—
	Study participant	Study participant
	Respondent	Informant
Person undertaking the study	Researcher	Researcher
	Investigator	Investigator
	Scientist	—
That which is being investigated	—	Phenomena, topics
	Concepts	Concepts
	Constructs	—
	Variables (independent, dependent)	—
System of organizing concepts	Theory, theoretical framework	Theory
	Conceptual framework, conceptual model	—
Information gathered	Data (numeric values)	Data (narrative descriptions)
Connections between concepts	Relationships (cause-and-effect, functional)	Patterns of association

used interchangeably, although by convention, a construct often refers to a slightly more complex abstraction than a concept.

Theory

A **theory** is a systematic, abstract explanation of some aspect of reality. In a theory, concepts are knitted together into a coherent system to explain some aspect of the world. Theories play a role in both qualitative and quantitative research.

In a quantitative study, the researcher starts with a theory or a **conceptual model** (the distinction is discussed in Chap. 7), and, using deductive reasoning, makes predictions about how phenomena will behave *if the theory were true.* The researcher's specific predictions are then tested through research, and the results are used to reject, modify, or lend credence to the theory.

In qualitative research, information from the participants is the starting point from which the researcher begins to conceptualize, seeking to explain patterns emerging from the researcher–participant interactions. The goal is to arrive at a theory that explains phenomena as they occur, not as they are preconceived. Inductively generated theories from a qualitative study are sometimes subjected to more controlled confirmation through quantitative research.

Variables

In a quantitative study, concepts are usually referred to as **variables.** A variable, as the name implies, is something that varies. Weight, blood pressure readings, preoperative anxiety levels, and body temperature are all variables (*i.e.,* each of these properties varies or differs from one person to another). In fact, nearly all aspects of human beings and their environment are variables. For example, if everyone weighed 150 pounds, weight would not be a variable; it would be a **constant.** But it is precisely because people and conditions *do* vary that most research is conducted. Most quantitative researchers seek to understand how or why things vary and to learn how differences in one variable are related to differences in another. For example, lung cancer research is concerned with the variable of lung cancer. It is a variable because not everybody has the disease. Researchers have studied what variables might be linked to lung cancer and have discovered that cigarette smoking is related to the disease. Again, smoking is a variable because not everyone smokes.

A variable, then, is any quality of a person, group, or situation that varies or takes on different values—typically, numeric values. Sometimes a variable can take on a range of different values (*e.g.,* height or weight); such variables are **continuous variables** because their values can be represented on a continuum. Other variables take on only a few discrete values (*e.g.,* pregnant/not pregnant, single/married/divorced/widowed). Variables of this type, which essentially place individuals into categories, are **categorical variables.**

Variables are often inherent characteristics, such as age, blood type, health beliefs, or grip strength. In some research situations, however, the investigator *creates* a variable. For example, if a researcher is interested in testing the effectiveness of patient-controlled analgesia as opposed to intramuscular analgesia in relieving pain after surgery, some patients would be given patient-controlled analgesia and others would receive intramuscular analgesia. In the context of this study, method of pain management has become a variable because different patients are given different analgesic methods.

CONSUMER TIP:

Every study focuses on one or more phenomena, concepts, or variables, but these terms *per se* are not necessarily used in research reports. For example, a report might say: "The purpose of this study is to examine the effect of primary nursing on patient satisfaction." Although the researcher has not explicitly labeled anything a concept, the concepts (variables) under study are *type of nursing* and *patient satisfaction.* ■

Dependent Variables and Independent Variables

Many quantitative studies are aimed at determining the causes of phenomena. Does a nursing intervention cause improved patient outcomes? Does a certain procedure cause stress? The presumed cause is referred to as the **independent variable**, and the presumed effect is referred to as the **dependent variable.**

Variation in the dependent variable is presumed to *depend on* variation in the independent variable. For example, the researcher investigates the extent to which lung cancer (the dependent variable) depends on smoking (the independent variable). In another study, a researcher might examine the effect of a special diet (the independent variable) on weight gain in premature infants (the dependent variable). The dependent variable (sometimes referred to as the **outcome variable**) is the variable the researcher is interested in understanding, explaining, or predicting. For example, in lung cancer and smoking research, it is the carcinoma that the researcher is trying to explain and predict, not smoking.

Frequently, the terms *independent variable* and *dependent variable* are used to designate the direction of influence between variables rather than cause and effect. For example, suppose a researcher studied urinary incontinence among community-dwelling older women and found that incontinence severity was greater among women with a slower gait. The researcher might be unwilling to take the position that the incontinence was caused by slower mobility. Yet the direction of influence clearly runs from gait to incontinence: it makes little sense to suggest that incontinence influenced the women's gait. Although in this example the researcher does not infer a cause-and-effect connection, it is appropriate to conceptualize incontinence as the dependent variable and gait as the independent variable.

Many of the dependent variables studied by researchers have multiple causes or antecedents. If we were interested in studying the factors that influence people's weight, for example, we might consider their age, height, physical activity, and eating habits as the independent variables. Two or more *dependent* variables also may be of interest to the researcher. For example, suppose we wanted to compare the effectiveness of two methods of nursing care for children with cystic fibrosis. Several dependent variables could be designated as measures of treatment effectiveness, such as length of stay in the hospital, number of recurrent respiratory infections, presence of cough, and so forth. In short, it is common to design studies with multiple independent and dependent variables.

It is important to understand that variables are not inherently dependent or independent. A dependent variable in one study may be an independent variable in another study. For example, a study might examine the effect of nurses' contraceptive counseling (the independent variable) on unwanted births (the dependent variable). Another study might investigate the effect of unwanted births (the independent variable) on the incidence of child abuse (the dependent variable). In short, whether a variable is independent or dependent is a function of the role that the variable plays in a particular study.

CONSUMER TIP:

Almost no research report *explicitly* labels variables as dependent and independent, despite the importance of this distinction. Moreover, variables (especially independent variables) are sometimes not fully spelled out in research reports. Take the following research question: What is the effect of exercise on heart rate? In this example, heart rate is the dependent variable. Exercise, however, is not in itself a variable. Rather, exercise versus something else (*e.g.*, no exercise) is the variable; the "something else" is implied rather than stated in the research question. Note that, if exercise were not compared to something else, such as no exercise, then exercise would not be a variable. ∎

Example of independent and dependent variables:

Research question: What is the effect of the timing of an initial bath on temperature in newborns (Varda & Behnke, 2000)?
Independent variable: Timing of the initial bath (1 hour versus 2 hours after birth)
Dependent variable: Axillary temperature

Operational Definitions of Variables
In a quantitative study, the researcher clarifies and defines the research variables at the outset, indicating how the variable will be observed and measured in the actual research situation. Such a definition has a special name. An **operational definition** of a concept specifies the operations that the researcher must perform to collect the required information.

Variables differ in the ease with which they can be operationalized. The variable weight, for example, is easy to define and measure. We might operationally define weight as follows: the amount that an object weighs in terms of pounds, to the nearest full pound. Note that this definition designates that weight will be determined with one measuring system (pounds) rather than another (grams). The operational definition might also specify that the subjects' weight will be measured to the nearest pound using a spring scale with subjects fully undressed after 10 hours of fasting. This operational definition clearly indicates what is meant by the variable weight.

Unfortunately, few variables of interest in nursing research are operationalized as easily as weight. There are multiple methods of measuring most variables, and the researcher must choose the method that best captures the variables as he or she conceptualizes them. Take, for example, patient well-being, which can be defined in terms of either physiologic and psychological functioning. If the researcher chooses to emphasize the physiologic aspects of patient well-being, the operational definition might involve a measure such as heart rate, white blood cell count, blood pressure, or vital capacity. If, on the other hand, the researcher conceptualizes well-being as primarily a psychological phenomenon, the operational definition should identify the method by which emotional well-being will be assessed, such as the responses of the patient to certain questions or the behaviors of the patient as observed by the researcher. Readers of a research report may not agree with the way the investigator has conceptualized and operationalized the variables. Nevertheless, precision in defining the terms has the advantage of communicating exactly what the terms mean within the context of the study.

Example of an operational definition:

Research question: How can infants at highest risk for smoke-related health problems through environmental tobacco smoke best be identified (Stepans & Fuller, 1999)?
Operational definition of maternal smoking: The number of cigarette butts deposited by the mother into a designated container over a 24-hour period

---

Qualitative researchers do not define the concepts in which they are interested in operational terms. This is because they seek to have the meaning of concepts defined by those being studied rather than having *a priori* definitions. Nevertheless, in summarizing the results of a study, all researchers should be careful in describing to readers the conceptual and methodologic bases of key research concepts.

CONSUMER TIP:

A few research reports explicitly label the operational definitions, but most never use the term. Quantitative research reports do, however, provide information on how key variables were measured (*i.e.,* they specify the operational definitions even if they do not use this label). This information is generally included in a section of the research report called "Research Measures" or "Instruments." ■

Data

The research **data** (singular, datum) are the pieces of information obtained in a study. In a quantitative study, the researcher identifies the variables of interest, develops operational definitions of those variables, and then collects the relevant data from the subjects. The variables, because they vary, take on different values. The actual values of the study variables are the data for a research project.

In quantitative studies, the researcher collects primarily **quantitative data** (*i.e.,* numeric information). For example, suppose we were conducting a quantitative study in which the dependent variable was *depression.* In such a study, we would try to measure how depressed different study participants were. We might ask the question, "Thinking about the past week, how depressed would you say you have been on a scale from 0 to 10, where 0 means `not at all' and 10 means `the most possible'?" Box 2-1 presents some quantitative data from three fictitious respondents. The subjects have provided a number corresponding to their degree of depression: 9 for subject 1 (a high level of depression), 0 for subject 2 (no depression), and 4 for subject 3 (very mild depression). The numeric values for all subjects in the study, collectively, would comprise the data on the variable depression.

In qualitative studies, the researcher collects primarily **qualitative data,** which are narrative descriptions. Narrative information can be obtained by having conversations with the participants, by making detailed notes about how participants behave in naturalistic settings, or by obtaining narrative records, such as diaries. As an example, suppose we were studying depression qualitatively. Box 2-2 presents some qualitative data from three participants responding conversationally to the question, "Tell me about how you've been feeling lately. Have you felt sad or depressed at all, or have you generally been in good spirits?" Here, the data consist of narrative descriptions of the participants' emotional state.

BOX 2-1   **EXAMPLE OF QUANTITATIVE DATA**

Question

Thinking about the past week, how depressed would you say you have been on a scale from 0 to 10, where 0 means "not at all" and 10 means "the most possible"?

Data

Subject 1: 9

Subject 2: 0

Subject 3: 4

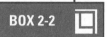

BOX 2-2

EXAMPLE OF QUALITATIVE DATA

Question

Tell me about how you've been feeling lately—have you felt sad or depressed at all, or have you generally been in good spirits?

Data

Participant 1: "I've been pretty depressed lately, to tell you the truth. I wake up each morning and I can't seem to think of anything to look forward to. I mope around the house all day, kind of in despair. I just can't seem to shake the blues, and I've begun to think I need to go see a shrink."

Participant 2: "I can't remember ever feeling better in my life. I just got promoted to a new job that makes me feel like I can really get ahead in my company. And I've just gotten engaged to a really great guy who is very special."

Participant 3: "I've had a few ups and downs the past week, but basically things are on a pretty even keel. I don't have too many complaints."

In both qualitative and quantitative research, the collection and analysis of the research data are typically the most time-consuming aspects of a study. The analysis of qualitative data is a particularly labor-intensive process.

Relationships

Researchers usually study phenomena in relation to other phenomena—they explore or test relationships. A **relationship** is a bond or connection between phenomena; for example, researchers repeatedly have found that there is a relationship between cigarette smoking and lung cancer. Both qualitative and quantitative studies examine relationships.

In a quantitative study, the researcher is primarily interested in the relationship between the independent variables and dependent variables. Variation in the dependent variable is presumed to be systematically related to variation in the independent variable. Relationships are usually expressed in quantitative terms, such as *more than, less than,* and so on. For example, let us consider as a possible dependent variable a person's body weight. What variables are related to (associated with) a person's weight? Some possibilities include height, caloric intake, and exercise. For each of these three independent variables, we can make a prediction about the nature of the relationship to the dependent variable:

Height: Taller people will weigh more than shorter people.
Caloric intake: People with higher caloric intake will be heavier than those with lower caloric intake.

Exercise: The lower the amount of exercise, the greater the person's weight.

Each of these statements expresses a presumed relationship between weight (the dependent variable) and a measurable independent variable. Most quantitative research is conducted to determine whether relationships do or do not exist among variables, and often to quantify how strong the relationship is.

Variables can be related to one another in different ways. One type of relationship is referred to as a **cause-and-effect** (or **causal**) **relationship.** Within the positivist paradigm, natural phenomena are assumed not to be haphazard; they have antecedent causes that are presumably discoverable. In our example about a person's weight, we might speculate that there is a causal relationship between caloric intake and weight: all else being equal, eating more calories causes weight gain.

Example of a study focusing on a causal relationship:

Dowling (1999) studied whether breastfeeding versus bottle feeding with an orthodontic nipple (the independent variable) caused differences in preterm infants' physiologic responses (sucking, breathing, and oxygen saturation).

Not all relationships between variables can be interpreted as cause-and-effect relationships. There is a relationship, for example, between a person's pulmonary artery and tympanic temperatures: people with high readings on one have high readings on the other. We cannot say, however, that pulmonary artery temperature caused tympanic temperature, nor that tympanic temperature caused pulmonary artery temperature, despite the relationship that exists between the two variables. This type of relationship is sometimes referred to as a **functional** (or **associative**) **relationship** rather than a causal one.

Example of a study focusing on a functional relationship:

King (2000) studied the relationship between gender and postsurgical outcomes (e.g., functional status, life quality) among patients recovering from cardiac surgery.

Qualitative researchers are not concerned with quantifying relationships, nor in testing and confirming causal relationships. Rather, qualitative researchers seek patterns of association as a way of illuminating the underlying meaning and dimensionality of phenomena of interest. Patterns of interconnected themes and processes are identified as a means of understanding the whole.

> **Example of a qualitative study of patterns:**
>
> Roberts (1999) studied drug use in the lives of urban African American women and discovered that patterns of loss resulting from separations of someone or something from the women's lives (e.g., death of a significant other, loss of child custody) were associated with drug use.

MAJOR STEPS IN A QUANTITATIVE STUDY

One of the first decisions a researcher makes is whether to conduct a quantitative or qualitative study. Researchers generally work within a paradigm consistent with their world view—the paradigm that gives rise to questions that excite their curiosity. The maturity of the concept of interest also may lead to one or the other paradigm; when little is known about a topic, a qualitative approach is often more fruitful than a quantitative one. After the appropriate paradigm is identified, the progression of activities differs for the qualitative and quantitative researcher.

In a quantitative study, a researcher moves from the beginning point of a study (the posing of a question) to the end point (the obtaining of an answer) in a logical sequence of steps that is similar across studies. This section describes the flow of activities that is typical in a quantitative study; the next section describes how qualitative studies differ.

Phase 1: The Conceptual Phase

The early steps in a quantitative study typically involve activities with a strong conceptual or intellectual element. These activities include thinking, reading, rethinking, theorizing, and reviewing ideas with colleagues or advisors. During this phase, the researcher calls on such skills as creativity, deductive reasoning, insight, and grounding in previous research on the study topic.

Step 1: Formulating and Delimiting the Problem
The first step is to develop a significant, interesting research problem. In developing a research problem, nurse researchers need to consider its substantive dimensions (Is this research question of clinical or theoretical importance?); its methodologic dimensions (How can this question best be studied?); its practical dimensions (Are adequate resources available to conduct a study?); and its ethical dimensions (Can this question be studied in a manner consistent with guidelines for protecting subjects?).

Step 2: Reviewing the Related Literature
Quantitative research is typically conducted within the context of previous knowledge. To build on existing theory or research, the quantitative

researcher strives to understand what is already known about a topic. A thorough **literature review** provides a foundation on which to base new knowledge and generally is conducted well before any data are collected.

Step 3: Defining the Theoretical Framework

Theory is the ultimate aim of science: it transcends the specifics of a particular time, place, and group of people and aims to identify regularities in the relationships among variables. When quantitative research is performed within the context of a theoretical framework (*i.e.,* when previous theory is used as a basis for generating predictions that can be tested), it is more likely that its findings will have broad significance and utility.

Step 4: Formulating Hypotheses

A **hypothesis** is the researcher's prediction of the relationship the researcher expects to find. The research question identifies the variables under investigation; a hypothesis predicts how those variables will be related. For example, the research question might be as follows: Is preeclamptic toxemia in pregnant women related to stress factors present during pregnancy? This might lead to the following hypothesis: Pregnant women with preeclamptic toxemia will report a higher incidence of stressful events during pregnancy than pregnant women who do not have symptoms. Most quantitative studies are designed to test research hypotheses.

Phase 2: The Design and Planning Phase

In the second major phase of a quantitative research project, the investigator makes decisions about the methods to be used to address the research question, and carefully plans for the collection of data. As a consumer, you should be aware that the methodologic decisions the researcher makes during this phase have implications for the integrity, interpretability, and clinical utility of the results. Thus, you must be able to evaluate the decisions so that you can determine how much faith can be put in the findings. A major objective of this book is to help you evaluate methodologic decisions.

Step 5: Selecting a Research Design

The **research design** is the overall plan for obtaining answers to the questions being studied. The design normally specifies which of the various research approaches will be adopted and how the researcher will implement controls to enhance the interpretability of the results. In quantitative studies, research designs tend to be highly structured and to include tight controls that reduce the effects of contaminating influences.

Step 6: Identifying the Population to Be Studied

During the design phase, quantitative researchers identify the population to be studied. A **population** is the aggregate of all the individuals or objects with some common, defining characteristic. For example, a researcher might specify that the study population consists of all licensed nurses residing in Canada. Quantitative researchers need to specify a population to indicate what characteristics the subjects should possess and to clarify the group to which the results of the study can be generalized.

Step 7: Designing the Sampling Plan

Research studies generally collect data from a **sample**, which is a subset of the population. Using a sample is more practical than collecting data from the population, but the risk is that the sample will not adequately reflect the population's traits. In a quantitative study, a sample's adequacy is assessed by the criterion of **representativeness;** that is, the quality of the sample is a function of how typical, or representative, the sample is of the population. The **sampling plan** specifies in advance *how* the sample will be selected and *how many* subjects there will be.

Step 8: Specifying Methods to Measure the Research Variables

Quantitative researchers develop or borrow methods to measure the research variables as accurately as possible. The first step is to clarify the conceptual meaning of the variables. The researcher then needs to select or design appropriate tools for operationalizing the variables (*i.e.,* for collecting the data). A variety of quantitative data collection approaches exist (*i.e.,* biophysiologic measurements, interviews, formal observations, and so on). The task of accurately measuring research variables is complex and challenging.

Step 9: Finalizing and Reviewing the Research Plan

Normally, researchers have their research plan reviewed before proceeding to the actual implementation of the plan. Students conducting a study as a requirement have their plans reviewed by faculty advisors. When a researcher needs financial support for the conduct of a study, the research plan is presented as a formal **research proposal** to a potential funder. Researchers also may need approval by a human subjects committee to ensure that the research plan does not violate ethical principles.

Step 10: Conducting a Pilot Study and Making Revisions

Unforeseen problems may arise in the course of a project. The effects of these problems may be sufficiently major that the study has to be stopped so that changes can be made. In a quantitative study, changes in the research design, the sampling plan, or the data collection instruments after the study is underway usually mean that data collected before the change must be discarded. Thus, some researchers carry out a **pilot study**—a small-scale trial run of the study—to obtain information for improving the project or assessing its feasibility.

Phase 3: The Empirical Phase

The empirical portion of a quantitative study involves the collection of research data and the preparation of those data for analysis. The empirical phase is usually the most time-consuming part of the investigation.

Step 11: Collecting the Data

The actual collection of data in a quantitative study normally proceeds according to a preestablished plan. The researcher's plan typically specifies procedures for recruiting the sample, describing the study to the subjects, obtaining the necessary consents, training those who will be involved in the collection of the data, and collecting the data (*e.g.,* specifying where, when, and how the data will be gathered).

Step 12: Preparing the Data for Analysis

The data collected in a quantitative study are rarely amenable to direct analysis. Preliminary steps are needed before the analysis can proceed. One such step is known as **coding**, which is the process of translating data into numeric form. For example, patients' responses to a question about their gender might be coded (1) for females and (2) for males. Another preliminary step involves transferring the data from written documents to computer files for analysis.

Phase 4: The Analytic Phase

The quantitative data gathered in the empirical phase are not reported in raw form. They are subjected to analysis and interpretation, which occurs in the fourth major phase of the project.

Step 13: Analyzing the Data

To answer the research questions, the data must be processed and analyzed in an orderly, coherent fashion so that patterns and relationships can be discerned. Quantitative data are analyzed through statistical procedures. **Statistical analyses** cover a broad range of techniques, including some simple procedures as well as complex and sophisticated methods.

Step 14: Interpreting the Results

Interpretation is the process of making sense of the results and examining the implications of the findings within a broader context. Interpretation in quantitative studies is the researcher's attempt to explain the findings in light of what is known about theory and previous findings in the area and in light of the adequacy of the methods used in the investigation. Interpretation also involves determining how the findings can best be used in clinical practice, or what further research is needed before utilization can be recommended.

Phase 5: The Dissemination Phase

In the analytic phase, the researcher comes full circle: the questions posed in the first phase of the project are answered. The researcher's job is not completed, however, until the results of the study are disseminated.

Step 15: Communicating the Findings

The results of a research investigation are of little use if they are not communicated to others. Another—and often final—task of a research project, therefore, is the preparation of a **research report** that can be shared with others. We discuss research reports in the next chapter.

Step 16: Utilizing the Findings

Many nursing studies have little effect on nursing practice. Ideally, the concluding step of a high-quality study is to plan for its utilization in the real world. Although nurse researchers are not always in a position to implement a plan for utilizing research findings in clinical settings, they can contribute to the process by including recommendations in their research reports regarding how the results of the study could be incorporated into the practice of nursing.

ACTIVITIES IN A QUALITATIVE STUDY

Quantitative research involves a fairly linear progression of tasks (*i.e.,* the researcher lays out in advance the steps to be taken to maximize the integrity of the study and then follows those steps as faithfully as possible). In a qualitative study, by contrast, the progression is closer to a circle than to a straight line—the qualitative researcher is continually examining and interpreting data and making decisions about how to proceed based on what has already been discovered.

Because the qualitative researcher has a flexible approach to the collection and analysis of data, it is impossible to define the flow of activities precisely; the flow varies from one study to another, and researchers do not know ahead of time exactly how the study will proceed. We try to provide a sense of how a qualitative study is conducted, however, by describing some major activities and indicating how and when they might be performed.

Conceptualizing and Planning a Qualitative Study

Qualitative researchers are usually interested in an aspect of a topic that is poorly understood and about which little is known, and thus they do not develop hypotheses or pose refined research questions before going into the field. The topic area may be clarified on the basis of self-reflection and discussion with colleagues or clients, but usually the researcher proceeds with a broad research question that is sharpened and more clearly delineated after the study is underway.

There are conflicting ideas among qualitative researchers regarding the performance of a literature review at the outset of the study. At one extreme are those who believe that researchers should not consult the literature at all before collecting data. Their concern is that prior studies might unduly influence the researcher's conceptualization of the phenomena under study. According to this view, the phenomena should be elucidated based on participants' viewpoints rather than on prior information. Others believe that the researcher should conduct at least a cursory up-front literature review to obtain guidance, including guidance in identifying biases in previous studies.

In any event, qualitative researchers typically find a relatively small body of relevant literature because of the type of questions they ask.

During the planning phase, the qualitative researcher must also identify a study **site** that is consistent with the research topic. For example, if the topic is the health care beliefs of the urban poor, an inner-city neighborhood with a concentration of low-income residents must be identified. The researcher may have to further identify the types of **setting** within the site where data collection will occur (*e.g.,* in homes, clinics, the workplace, and so on). In many cases, the researcher needs to make preliminary contacts with key actors in the selected site to ensure cooperation and access to informants (*i.e.,* the researcher needs to **gain entrée** into the setting).

Conducting the Qualitative Study

In a qualitative study, the activities of sampling, data collection, data analysis, and interpretation take place iteratively. The qualitative researcher begins by talking with or observing people who have first-hand experience with the phenomenon under study. The discussions and observations are loosely structured, allowing for the expression of a full range of beliefs, feelings, and behaviors. Analysis and interpretation are ongoing and concurrent activities, used to guide the people to sample next and the questions to ask or observations to make. The actual process of data analysis, which is an intensive and time-consuming activity, involves clustering together related types of narrative information into a coherent scheme.

As analysis and interpretation progress, the researcher begins to identify themes and categories, which are used to build a descriptive theory of the phenomenon. The kinds of data obtained become increasingly focused and purposeful as a theory emerges. Theory development and verification shape the sampling process—as the theory develops, the researcher seeks participants who can confirm and enrich the theoretical understandings as well as participants who can potentially challenge them and lead to further theoretical development.

A quantitative researcher decides in advance how many subjects to include in the study, but a qualitative researcher's sampling decisions are guided by the data. Many qualitative researchers use the principle of **saturation**, which occurs when themes and categories in the data become repetitive and redundant, such that no new information can be gleaned by further data collection.

Quantitative researchers seek to collect high-quality data by selecting measuring instruments that have been previously demonstrated to be accurate and rigorous. The qualitative researcher, by contrast, *is* the main data collection instrument and he or she takes steps to demonstrate the trustworthiness of the data while in the field. The central feature of these efforts is to confirm that the findings accurately reflect the experiences and viewpoints of the participants, rather than the perceptions of the researcher. For example, one confirmatory activity involves going back to participants and sharing preliminary interpretations with them so that they can evaluate whether the researcher's thematic analysis is consistent with their experiences.

Disseminating Qualitative Findings

Qualitative nursing researchers also strive to share their findings with other nurses and other health care specialists. Qualitative research reports are increasingly being published in the nursing literature.

Quantitative reports almost never contain any **raw data**—data exactly in the form they were collected, which are numeric values. Qualitative reports, by contrast, are generally filled with rich verbatim passages directly from the participants. The excerpts are used in an evidential fashion to support or illustrate the researcher's interpretations and theoretical formulations.

Example of raw data in a qualitative report:

Johnson, Noble, Matthews, and Aguilar (1999) studied how bilingual health care staff use their language skills in patient encounters. They found that social engagement was an important aspect of being bilingual and supported this with the following quote from a study participant:

> Even if you don't do anything to a patient you can say just a few sentences. . . . Just stop, one or two little sentences, speak to them, just ask them, "How are you today?" or "What is your wife's name?" because they feel that they're not alone. (p. 335)

Like quantitative researchers, qualitative nurse researchers want to see their findings used by other nurses. Qualitative findings often are used as the basis for the formulation of hypotheses that are tested by quantitative researchers. Qualitative findings are also useful in the development of assessment instruments used for both research and clinical purposes. Most importantly, qualitative studies can help to shape nurses' perceptions of a problem or situation, their conceptualization of potential solutions, and their understanding of patients' concerns and experiences.

GENERAL QUESTIONS IN REVIEWING A RESEARCH STUDY

The remaining chapters of this book contain guidelines to help you evaluate different aspects of a research report critically, focusing primarily on the methodologic decisions that the researcher made in conducting the study. Box 2-3 presents some further suggestions for performing a preliminary overview of a research report, drawing on the concepts explained in this chapter. These guidelines supplement those presented in Box 1-1, Chapter 1.

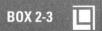

BOX 2-3 | **ADDITIONAL QUESTIONS FOR A PRELIMINARY OVERVIEW OF A STUDY**

1. What is the study all about? What are the main phenomena, concepts, or constructs under investigation?

2. If the study is quantitative, what are the independent and dependent variables?

3. Are the key concepts clearly explained? Are operational definitions provided?

4. What is the nature of the relationship (if any) under study?

RESEARCH EXAMPLES

This section presents brief overviews of a quantitative and a qualitative study. Our overviews deal primarily with the key concepts of the research. Use the questions in Box 2-3 as a guide to thinking about these studies. You may wish to consult the full research report in answering these questions and in thinking about the differences in style and content of qualitative and quantitative reports.

Research Example of a Quantitative Study

Depression has been identified as a major health concern among the elderly. McCurren, Dowe, Rattle, and Looney (1999) conducted a study that focused on the assessment and amelioration of depression among nursing home elders.

Research Summary

McCurren and her colleagues began their study by assessing the levels of depression of residents from three nursing home facilities. Depression was operationalized through scores on the 30-item Geriatric Depression Scale (GDS). Residents were classified as severely depressed if their scores were 21 or higher on the scale and as mildly depressed if their scores were between 11 and 20. The researchers found that the prevalence rate of depressive symptoms was 68%.

The researchers then proceeded to test the effectiveness of a low-cost intervention strategy among those with scores greater than 10 on the GDS. Half of those eligible for the study were selected, at random, to receive the intervention, which involved using a geropsychiatric nurse in conjunction with trained older adult volunteers in the role of mental health paraprofessionals. Although the specific intervention was individualized according to unique needs, the standardized aspects included weekly visits by the nurse and visits twice a week by the volunteer for a 24-week period. Depression was assessed both before and after the intervention. The dependent variable was changes in levels of depressive symptoms. The independent variable was whether or not the person received the special treatment.

The findings were encouraging. Among those who received the intervention, scores on the depression scale were significantly reduced during the 24-week period. By contrast, GDS scores for those who did not receive the intervention were virtually unchanged.

Clinical Relevance

As the population ages, dramatic increases in nursing home residency can be expected in the years ahead. High rates of depression among the institutionalized elderly have been documented. Depression among the elderly has been found to be associated with mortality and cognitive declines. Moreover, depression among the residents is likely to be stressful to their caregivers. Thus, McCurren and her colleagues addressed a problem that has great potential for clinical significance.

The study was also methodologically strong. Half of the residents, selected at random, received the special treatment, and the other half received routine care. This design permitted an equitable comparison of the two groups of women who, because selection into the groups was random, were presumably alike in most respects—except for the treatment. Although the number of nursing home residents was small—and therefore replications are clearly needed—it is noteworthy that the sample was drawn from three different nursing homes.

Importantly, the researchers designed a low-cost intervention that involved trained community volunteers as the primary delivery system. Although it would clearly be desirable to have professional psychological services available to nursing home residents, fiscal constraints make such services unfeasible in most nursing homes. Thus, the findings from this study suggest that it is possible to develop effective, but relatively inexpensive, methods for addressing the psychological needs of the elderly. Further research may determine that such strategies may, indeed, be cost-effective (*e.g.*, if they resulted in a lowered need for antidepressant drug therapy).

RESEARCH EXAMPLE OF A QUALITATIVE STUDY

Schaefer, Ladd, Lammers, and Echenberg (1999) studied what it was like to live with ovarian cancer during the childbearing years. Although earlier qualitative research had explored the experience of having ovarian cancer, Schaefer and her colleagues were the first to focus on having the disease during a period when childbearing could be affected.

Research Summary

Schaefer and her co-researchers conducted an in-depth study of five women with ovarian cancer. Three to four intensive interviews, lasting 60 to

90 minutes, were conducted with each of the five women living with ovarian cancer for 1- to 10-years. The women were asked to talk about the experience of having ovarian cancer, as they actually lived it. The interviews were tape-recorded and then transcribed for analysis. One researcher was primarily responsible for the analysis, but the other researchers collaborated in clarifying, validating, and expanding the themes.

The following 12 themes provide a window into the experience of women living with ovarian cancer: serendipitous diagnosis; managing treatment; horrible hair experience; hysterectomy violating one's sense of being; unfairness of menopause; body changes; intimate dreaming; being with others; being normal/different; being vigilant; being heard; and trying to make sense of it. The theme of "horrible hair experience" is illustrated by the following quote:

> I remember it was a Monday morning and . . . actually I woke up and I saw some hair on the bed. . . . I lost so much in my shower that it made the shower clog immediately. I couldn't even get the pick through my hair. The next day the same thing happened. I [didn't] wash my hair the next day. I got my hair cut again, and it lasted for two days. . . . I was lying in bed. He got up to get ready for work and I heard him go, "Oh." (p. 232).

Clinical Relevance

Although there had been prior studies about the experience of having ovarian cancer, this study was the first to focus on living with the disease during the childbearing years. The team of researchers carefully collaborated in doing a thorough, intensive inquiry about how the experience evolved over time.

The findings demonstrated how crucial it was to the survival and well-being of the women in the study to find meaning in their experiences with ovarian cancer. This suggests that nurses should provide support for these women while they search for meaning, so that they can make peace with having to live with the disease.

The themes that emerged from this study alert health care professionals to the complexity of the experience of living with ovarian cancer during the childbearing years, such as struggling with the inability to bear children and fear of recurrence. As various issues emerge over time, women with ovarian cancer are likely to benefit from continual reinforcement of information and from ongoing explanations of menopause and treatment effects. The abrupt and premature loss of childbearing ability calls for skilled nursing care as these women mourn this loss of a natural life process and struggle for a voice in their own health care.

• • • • • SUMMARY POINTS

- A research study (or investigation or research project) is undertaken by one or more **researchers** (or **investigators** or scientists). The people who provide information to the researchers are referred to as **subjects, study partici-pants,** or **respondents** (in quantitative research) or study participants or **informants** (in qualitative research).

- Researchers investigate **concepts** and phenomena (or **constructs**), which are abstractions or mental representations inferred from behavior or events.
- Concepts are the building blocks of **theories,** which are systematic expla-nations of some aspect of the real world.
- In quantitative studies, concepts are referred to as variables. A **variable** is a characteristic or quality that takes on different values (*i.e.,* a variable varies from one person or object to another).
- The **dependent variable** is the behavior, characteristic, or outcome the researcher is interested in understanding, explaining, predicting, or affect-ing. The independent variable is the presumed cause of, antecedent to, or influence on the dependent variable.
- An **operational definition** is the specification of the procedures and tools required to measure a variable.
- **Data**—the information collected during the course of a study—may take the form of narrative information (**qualitative data**) or numeric values (**quantitative data**).
- Researchers often focus on the relationship between two or more concepts. A **relationship** is a bond or connection (or pattern of association) between two phenomena.
- In a quantitative study, the steps involved in conducting a study are fairly standard, and the researcher progresses in a linear fashion from posing a research question to answering it.
- The main phases and steps in a quantitative study are as follows:
  - The conceptual phase: defining the problem to be studied, doing a **liter-ature review**, developing a theoretical framework, and formulating **hypotheses** to be tested.
  - The design and planning phase: selecting a **research design**, specifying the **population**, selecting a **sample**, specifying the methods to measure the research variables, finalizing the research plan, and, in some cases, conducting a **pilot study** and making revisions.
  - The empirical phase: collecting the data and preparing the data for analysis.
  - The analytic phase: analyzing the data through **statistical analysis** and interpreting the results.
  - The dissemination phase: communicating the findings and promoting their utilization.
- The flow of activities in a qualitative study is more flexible and less linear than in a quantitative study.
- Qualitative researchers begin with a broad question that is narrowed through the actual process of data collection and analysis. After selecting a **site** and **gaining entrée** into it, the researcher selects informants, collects data, and analyzes and interprets the data iteratively. Early analysis leads to refinements in sampling and data collection, until **saturation** (redundancy of information) is achieved.

➤ ➤ ➤ ➤ *CRITICAL THINKING ACTIVITIES*

Chapter 2 of the accompanying *Study Guide to Accompany Essentials of Nursing Research*, 5th edition offers various exercises and study suggestions for reinforcing the concepts presented in this chapter. In addition, you can address the following:

1. Read the abstracts and the introduction from one or both of the actual research studies in the Appendix of this book, and then answer the questions in Box 2-3.

2. In describing the study, do either of the reports in the Appendix actually use the terms *operational definition, independent variable,* or *dependent variable*?

*For additional review, see questions 16–27 on the study CD provided with Polit: Study Guide to Accompany Essentials of Nursing Research.

SUGGESTED READINGS

Methodologic References

Kerlinger, F. N. (1986). *Foundations of behavioral research* (3rd ed.). New York: Holt, Rinehart & Winston.

Morse, J. M., & Field, P. A. (1995). *Qualitative research methods for health professionals* (2nd ed.). Thousand Oaks, CA: Sage Publications.

Substantive References

Dowling, D. A. (1999). Physiological responses of preterm infants to breast-feeding and bottle-feeding with the orthodontic nipple. *Nursing Research, 48,* 78–85.

King, K. M. (2000). Gender and short-term recovery from cardiac surgery. *Nursing Research, 49,* 29–36.

Johnson, M., Noble, C., Matthews, C., & Aguilar, N. (1999). Bilingual communicators within the health care setting. *Qualitative Health Research, 9,* 329–343.

McCurren, C., Dowe, D., Rattle, D., & Looney, S. (1999). Depression among nursing home elders: Testing an intervention strategy. *Applied Nursing Research, 12,* 185–195.

Roberts, C. A. (1999). Drug use among inner-city African American women: The process of managing loss. *Qualitative Health Research, 9,* 620–638.

Schaefer, K. M., Ladd, E. C., Lammers, S. E., & Echenberg, R. J. (1999). In your skin you are different: Women living with ovarian cancer during childbearing years. *Qualitative Health Research, 9,* 227–242.

Stepans, M. F., & Fuller, S. G. (1999). Measuring infant exposure to environmental tobacco smoke. *Clinical Nursing Research, 8,* 198–221.

Varda, K. E., & Behnke, R. S. (2000). The effect of timing of initial bath on newborn's temperature. *Journal of Obstetric, Gynecologic, and Neonatal Nursing, 29,* 27–32.

Reading Research Reports

● ●

Student Objectives

On completion of this chapter, the student will be able to:

○ identify major types of research reports
○ identify and describe the major sections in a research journal article
○ characterize the style used in quantitative and qualitative research reports
○ describe tools for reading and comprehending research reports
○ distinguish research synopses and research critiques
○ define new terms presented in the chapter

● ●

New Terms

Abstract
Blind review
Journal article
Level of significance
Peer reviewer
Poster session

Research critique
Research findings
Research report
Statistical analysis
Statistical significance
Statistical test

TYPES OF RESEARCH REPORTS

Information about a nursing study is communicated to the nursing community through **research reports** that describe what was studied, how it was studied, and what was found. Research reports—especially reports for a quantitative study—are often daunting to those without research training. This chapter is designed to help make research reports more accessible even before you become familiar with research methods.

Researchers communicate information about their studies in various ways. The most common types of research reports are the following:

- *Theses and dissertations.* Most master's and doctoral degrees are granted on the successful completion of a study that is described in a thesis or dissertation.
- *Books.* Sometimes, research is reported in books or in a chapter in a book on a specific research topic.
- *Presentations at conferences.* Professional organizations (*e.g.,* Sigma Theta Tau) and institutions sponsor conferences that provide a forum for describing studies orally or in visual displays.
- *Journal articles.* Many nursing journals publish articles that summarize the results of a study.

Consumers of nursing research are most likely to encounter research results at professional conferences or in journals.

Presentations at Professional Conferences

There are two main formats for presenting research findings at a conference: oral presentations and poster sessions. Oral presentations follow a format similar to that used in journal articles, which we discuss later in this chapter. The presenter of an oral report is typically allotted 10 to 20 minutes to describe the most important aspects of the study. In a **poster session**, many researchers simultaneously present visual displays summarizing their studies, and conference attendees circulate around the room perusing these displays.

Conference presentations are an important avenue for communicating research information. One attractive feature is that there is less time elapsed between the completion of a study and the dissemination of the findings than is the case with journal articles. Conferences also offer an opportunity for dialogue between the researcher and conference attendees. The listeners at oral presentations and viewers of poster displays can ask questions to help them better understand how the study was conducted or what the findings mean; moreover, they can offer the researchers suggestions relating to the clinical implications of the study. Thus, professional conferences offer a particularly valuable forum for a clinical audience.

Research Journal Articles

Research **journal articles** are reports in professional journals that summarize an investigation. Because the competition for journal space is keen, the typical research article is brief—generally only 10 to 15 double-spaced pages. This means that the researcher must condense a lot of information about the study purpose, methods used, findings, interpretation, and clinical significance into a short report.

Journals accept research reports on a competitive basis. Usually, research articles are reviewed by several **peer reviewers** (other researchers doing work in the field) who make a recommendation about whether the article should be accepted, rejected, or revised and re-reviewed. These are usually **"blind" reviews**—the reviewers are not told the names of the researchers, and the researchers are not told the identity of the reviewers.

In major nursing research journals, the rate of acceptance is low—it can be as low as 5% of all submitted articles. Thus, consumers of research journal articles have some assurance that the reports have already been scrutinized for their merit and nursing relevance by other nurse researchers. Nevertheless, the publication of an article does not mean that the research findings can be uncritically accepted. The validity of the findings and their utility for clinical practice depend to a large degree on how the study was conducted. Research methods courses help consumers to understand the strengths and limitations of studies reported in professional journals.

THE CONTENT OF RESEARCH JOURNAL ARTICLES

Research reports in journals tend to follow a certain format and to be written in a particular style. Research reports begin with a title that succinctly conveys (typically in 15 or fewer words) the nature of the study. In qualitative studies, the title normally includes the central phenomenon and group under investigation; in quantitative studies, the title generally indicates the independent and dependent variables and the population under study. Research reports often consist of six major sections: an abstract, an introduction, a method section, a results section, a discussion, and references.

The Abstract

The **abstract** is a brief description of the study placed at the beginning of the journal article. The abstract answers, in about 100 to 200 words, the following questions: What were the research questions? What methods did the researcher use to address those questions? What did the researcher discover? and What are the implications for nursing practice? Readers can readily review an abstract to assess whether the entire report is of interest.

Some journals have moved from having traditional abstracts—which are single paragraphs summarizing the main features of the study—to slightly longer and more informative abstracts with specific headings. For example, abstracts in *Nursing Research* after 1997 present information about the study organized under the following headings: Background, Objectives, Method, Results, Conclusions, and Key Words.

Box 3-1 presents abstracts from two actual studies. The first is a "new style" abstract for a quantitative study entitled "The effects of crossed leg on blood pressure measurement" (Foster-Fitzpatrick, Ortiz, Sibilano, Marcantonio, & Braun, 1999). The second is a more traditional abstract for a qualitative study entitled "Functional status from the patient's perspective: The challenge of preserving personal integrity" (Leidy & Haase, 1999). These two studies are used as illustrations throughout this chapter.

The Introduction

The introduction acquaints readers with the research problem and with the context within which it was formulated. The introduction may or may not be specifically labeled "Introduction," but it nevertheless follows immediately after the abstract. The introduction usually describes the following:

- *The central phenomena, concepts, or variables under study.* The key topic under investigation is identified.

BOX 3-1 **EXAMPLES OF ABSTRACTS FROM JOURNAL ARTICLES**

Quantitative Study

Background: It is clear that numerous factors influence an individual's blood pressure measurement. However, guidelines for accurately measuring blood pressure inconsistently specify that the patient should keep feet flat on the floor.

Objective: To determine if the crossing of a leg at the knee during blood pressure measurement has an effect on the patient's blood pressure reading

Methods: A convenience sample of 100 hypertensive male subjects was selected from various outpatient clinics in an inner-city acute-care veteran's hospital. The first 50 subjects positioned their feet flat on the floor while their blood pressure was measured. After 3 minutes, the blood pressure was measured again with the subject's leg crossed at the knee. The procedure was reversed for the second 50 subjects.

Results: The results indicated that both systolic and diastolic blood pressure increased significantly ($p < .0001$) with the crossed leg position.

Conclusion: When blood pressure is measured, patients should be instructed to have feet flat on the floor to eliminate a potential source of error. (Foster-Fitzpatrick et al., 1999, p. 105)

Qualitative Study

The purpose of this naturalistic, qualitative study was to describe the meaning of functional performance from the perspective of patients themselves. Twelve men and women with moderate to severe chronic obstructive pulmonary disease (COPD) participated in unstructured, tape-recorded interviews. The essential structure of the experience of finding purpose and meaning through activity was derived through an adaptation of Colaizzi's phenomenological method and the consensus dialogue approach to concept clarification. Results suggest people who are ill face an ongoing challenge of preserving their personal integrity, defined as a satisfying sense of wholeness, as they encounter a variety of physical changes that can interfere with day-to-day activity. Qualities most salient to integrity are a sense of effectiveness, or "being able," and of connectedness, or "being with." Identifying personal integrity as a motivating and explanatory factor in day-to-day activity performance may be an important consideration in designing effective intervention programs to improve capacity, strengthen performance, and enhance quality of life. Leidy, N.K., & Haase, J.E. (1999). Functional status from the patient's perspective: The challenge of preserving personal integrity. *Research in Nursing & Health*, 22, 67–77. Reprinted by permission of Wiley-Liss, Inc., a subsidiary of John Wiley & Sons, Inc.

- *The statement of purpose, research questions, and/or hypotheses to be tested.* The reader is told what the researcher set out to accomplish by conducting the study.
- *A review of the related literature.* Current knowledge relating to the study problem is briefly described so that readers can understand how the

study fits in with previous findings and can assess the contribution of the new study.

- *The theoretical framework.* In theoretically driven studies, the framework is usually presented in the introduction.
- *The significance of and need for the study.* The introduction to most research reports includes an explanation of why the study is important to nursing.

Thus, the introduction sets the stage for a description of what the researcher did and what was discovered.

Example of an introductory paragraph:

Some guidelines for accurately measuring blood pressure specify that the patient should keep feet flat on the floor. However, research is lacking on the effect of crossing the leg at the knee during blood pressure measurement. The current study was initiated to determine if blood pressure measurement is affected by the leg crossed at the knee as compared with feet flat on the floor (Foster-Fitzpatrick et al., 1999).

In this paragraph, the researchers indicated the independent variable (feet/leg position), the dependent variable (blood pressure), the study purpose (to determine whether blood pressure measurements are affected by foot and leg position), and the need for the study ("research is lacking").

The Method Section

The method section communicates to readers what methods the researcher used to answer the research questions. The method section tells readers about major methodologic decisions and may offer rationales for those decisions. For example, a report for a qualitative study often explains why a qualitative approach was considered to be especially appropriate and fruitful.

In a quantitative study, the method section usually describes the following, which may be presented as labeled subsections:

- *The subjects.* Quantitative research reports generally describe the population under study, specifying the criteria by which the researcher decided whether a person would be eligible for the study. The method section also describes the actual sample, indicating how people were selected and the number of subjects in the sample.
- *The research design.* A description of the research design focuses on the overall plan for the collection data, often including the steps the researcher took to minimize biases and enhance the interpretability of the results by instituting various controls.

- *Measures and data collection.* In the method section, researchers describe the methods and procedures used to collect the data, including how the critical research variables were operationalized; they may also present information concerning the quality of the measuring tools.
- *Study procedures.* The method section contains a description of the procedures used to conduct the study, including a description of any intervention. The researcher's efforts to protect the rights of human subjects may also be documented in the method section.

Table 3-1 presents excerpts from the method section of the quantitative study by Foster-Fitzpatrick and her colleagues (1999).

Qualitative researchers discuss many of the same issues, but with different emphases. For example, a qualitative study often provides more information about the research setting and the context of the study and less information on sampling. Also, because formal instruments are not used to collect qualitative data, there is little discussion about data collection methods, but there may be more information on data collection procedures. Increasingly, reports of qualitative studies are including descriptions of the researchers' efforts to ensure high-quality data. Many qualitative reports also have a subsection on data analysis. There are fairly standard ways of analyzing quantitative data, but such standardization does not exist for qualitative data, so that qualitative researchers may describe their analytic approach. Table 3-2 presents excerpts from the method section of the qualitative study by Leidy and Haase (1999).

TABLE 3-1. Excerpts from Method Section, Quantitative Report

METHODOLOGIC ELEMENT	EXCERPT FROM FOSTER-FITZPATRICK ET AL., 1999
Research design	In the first 50 subjects, the initial blood pressure was measured with the subject's feet positioned flat on the floor. In the second 50 subjects, the initial blood pressure was measured with the leg crossed over the knee. For the second blood pressure measurement, the leg position was the reverse of the initial leg position (p. 107).
Sample	Subjects were recruited from the outpatient clinics of a midwestern Veteran's Administration medical center. A convenience sample of 100 male patients, ages 31 to 81 years, participated in the study. All subjects had a medical diagnosis of hypertension (p. 106).
Measurement	Blood pressure measurements were monitored and recorded by two clinical nurses, who followed a written protocol to ensure identical technique. To exclude observer bias, the blood pressures were measured with the IVAC Vital.Check® Vital Signs Measurement System, Model 4200 (p. 106).
Procedure	Potential subjects were identified and verbal consent was obtained. The subjects were placed in a room with a temperature of 73°F away from the noise of the clinic to control environmental stress. Each subject was instructed to remove constricting clothes (p. 106).

TABLE 3-2.   Excerpts from Method Section, Qualitative Report

METHODOLOGIC ELEMENT	EXCERPT FROM LEIDY & HAASE, 1999
Sample	The purposive sample of 12 persons with COPD was recruited through a pulmonary outpatient clinic in the southeastern United States. . . . To maximize transferability of results, the sample included people of varying sociodemographic background (p. 68).
Data collection	The tape-recorded interviews, conducted by the first author, took place in a private room in the clinic. To begin the interview, participants again were told the nature of the study and asked to describe a typical day. Following this initial data-generating question, respondents were encouraged to self-direct the content of the interview (p. 69).
Data analysis	The essential structure of the experience of finding purpose and meaning through activity within the context of COPD was derived through a combination of two research methods previously used and adapted by the authors: (a) an adaptation of Colaizzi's phenomenological method; and (b) an adaptation of the consensus dialogue approach that was part of the Simultaneous Concept Analysis method of concept clarification (p. 69).

Leidy, N.K., & Haase, J.E. (1999). Functional status from the patient's perspective: The challenge of preserving personal integrity. *Research in Nursing and Health, 22,* 67–77. Reprinted by permission of Wiley-Liss, Inc., a subsidiary of John Wiley & Sons, Inc.

The Results Section

The results section presents the **research findings** (*i.e.,* the results obtained in the analyses of the data). The text summarizes the findings, often accompanied by tables or figures that highlight the most noteworthy results.

Virtually all results sections contain basic descriptive information, including a description of the study participants (*e.g.,* their average age). In quantitative studies, the researcher provides basic descriptive information for the key variables, using simple statistics. For example, in a study of the effect of prenatal drug exposure on the birth outcomes of infants, the results section might begin by describing the average birth weights and Apgar scores of the infants, or the percentage who were of low birth weight (less than 2500 g).

In quantitative studies, the results section also reports the following information relating to the **statistical analyses** performed:

- *The name of statistical tests used.* A **statistical test** is a procedure for testing hypotheses and evaluating the believability of the findings. For example, if the percentage of low-birth-weight infants in the sample of drug-exposed infants is computed, how probable is it that the percentage is accurate? If the researcher finds that the average birth weight of drug-exposed infants in the sample is lower than the birth weight of infants who were not exposed to drugs, how probable is it that the same would be true for other infants not in the sample? That is, is the relationship between prenatal drug exposure and infant birth weight real and likely to be replicated with a new sample of infants? Statistical tests answer such questions. Dozens of statistical tests exist, but they are all based on common principles; readers do not have to know the names of all statistical tests to comprehend the findings.

- *The value of the calculated statistic.* Computers are used to compute a numeric value for the particular statistical test used. The value allows the researchers to draw conclusions about the meaning of the results. The actual numeric value of the statistic, however, is not inherently meaningful and need not concern readers of research reports.
- *The significance.* The most important information is whether the results of the statistical tests were significant (not to be confused with important or clinically relevant). If a researcher reports that the results have **statistical significance**, it means that, based on the statistical test, the findings are probably valid and replicable with a new sample of subjects. Research reports also indicate the **level of significance**, which is an index of how probable it is that the findings are reliable. For example, if a report indicates that a finding was significant at the .05 level, this means that only 5 times out of 100 (5 / 100 = .05) would the obtained result be spurious or haphazard. In other words, 95 times out of 100, similar results would be obtained. Both the researcher and readers can therefore have a high degree of confidence—but not total assurance—that the findings are reliable.

Example from the results section of a quantitative study:

The main effect for leg crossing indicated that systolic and diastolic blood pressure, considered together, increased significantly when the leg was crossed ($F = 66.78$, $p < .0001$). (Foster-Fitzpatrick et al., 1999, p. 107).

In this excerpt, the authors indicate that blood pressure measurements are higher when legs are crossed than when feet are flat on the floor, and that the probability (*p*) that this finding is spurious is less than 1 in 10,000 (1 / 10,000 = .0001). Thus, the findings are highly reliable. Note that to comprehend this finding, it is not necessary for you to understand what the *F* statistic is, nor to concern yourself with the value of the statistic, 66.78.

In qualitative reports, the researcher often organizes findings according to the major themes or processes that were identified in the data. The results section of qualitative reports sometimes has several subsections, the headings of which correspond to the researcher's labels for the themes. Excerpts from the raw data are presented to support and provide a rich description of the thematic analysis. The results section of qualitative studies may also present the researcher's emerging theory about the phenomenon under study, although this may appear in the concluding section of the report.

> **EE**   *Example from the results section of a qualitative study:*
>
> Two characteristics are central to a sense of personal integrity: effectiveness, or "being able," and connectedness, or "being with," each of which are expressed through daily activities and challenged through limitations to physical capacity. . . . Fatigue and lack of energy were an important challenge to effectiveness, particularly for those describing themselves as energetic people.
>
> > (Mrs. G. T.): "I don't have as much energy. . . . I'm sort of like a little loose noodle . . . where I always was a very energetic person, I always thought. I'm not a very energetic person anymore" (Leidy & Haase, 1999, p. 71).

In this excerpt, the researchers illustrate their finding that lack of energy impinged on patients' perception of effectiveness with a direct quote from a study participant.

The Discussion

In the discussion, the researcher draws conclusions about the meaning and implications of the findings. This section tries to unravel what the results mean, why things turned out the way they did, and how the results can be used in practice. The discussion in both qualitative and quantitative reports may incorporate the following elements:

- *An interpretation of the results.* The interpretation involves the translation of findings into practical, conceptual, and/or theoretical meaning.
- *Implications.* Researchers often offer suggestions for how their findings could be used to improve nursing, and they may also make recommendations on how best to advance knowledge in the area through additional research.
- *Study limitations.* The researcher is in the best position possible to discuss study limitations, such as sample deficiencies, design problems, weaknesses in data collection, and so forth. A discussion section that presents these limitations demonstrates to readers that the author was aware of these limitations and probably took them into account in interpreting the findings.

> **EE**   *Example from a discussion section of a qualitative report.*
>
> The results of this study suggest that people with an illness such as COPD experience declines in functional performance as a challenge to their personal integrity, as a potential threat to their sense of effectiveness and connectedness with the world. Viewing performance from this perspective places emphasis on the meaning of activity, providing insight into the factors that motivate performance, the psychosocial responses people can exhibit in response to the innumerable challenges they face, and the approaches health care providers might take to help people maintain their performance and enhance the quality of their lives (Leidy & Haase, 1999, p. 75).

The References

Research journal articles conclude with a list of the books, reports, and journal articles that were referenced in the text of the report. For those interested in pursuing additional reading on a substantive topic, the reference list of a current research study is an excellent place to begin.

THE STYLE OF RESEARCH JOURNAL ARTICLES

Research reports tell a story. However, the style in which many research journal articles are written—especially reports of quantitative studies—makes it difficult for beginning research consumers to become interested in the story. To unaccustomed audiences, research reports may seem stuffy, pedantic, and bewildering. Four factors contribute to this impression:

- *Compactness.* Journal space is limited; hence, authors try to compress many ideas and concepts into a short space. Interesting, personalized aspects of the investigation often cannot be reported. And, in qualitative studies, only a handful of supporting quotes can be included.
- *Jargon.* The authors of both qualitative and quantitative reports use research terms that are assumed to be part of the reader's vocabulary but that may seem esoteric.
- *Objectivity.* Quantitative researchers normally avoid any impression of subjectivity; thus, research stories are told in a way that makes them sound impersonal. For example, most quantitative research reports are written in the passive voice (*i.e.,* personal pronouns are avoided). Use of the passive voice tends to make a report less inviting and lively than use of the active voice, and it tends to give the impression that the researcher did not play an active role in conducting the study. (Qualitative reports, by contrast, are more subjective and personal and are written in a more conversational style.)
- *Statistical information.* In quantitative reports, numbers and statistical symbols may intimidate readers who do not have strong mathematic interest or training. Most nursing studies are quantitative; thus, most research reports summarize the results of statistical analyses.

A major goal of this textbook is to assist nurses in understanding the content of research reports and in overcoming anxieties about their jargon, style, and statistical information.

READING, SUMMARIZING, AND CRITIQUING RESEARCH REPORTS

Nurses who seek to base their practice on research evidence must be able to read and critically appraise research reports. This section offers some general guidance on reading and evaluating nursing research reports.

Reading and Summarizing Research Reports

Beginning consumers of nursing research cannot be expected to critically appraise research immediately. The skills involved in critical appraisal must be developed over time. The first step in being able to use research findings in clinical practice is to read and comprehend research reports. In all likelihood, your first few attempts to read a research report will seem overwhelming, and you may wonder whether being able to comprehend, let alone appraise, research reports is a realistic goal. As you progress through this textbook, you will acquire skills to help you evaluate various aspects of research reports. Some preliminary tips on digesting research reports follow.

- Grow accustomed to the style of research reports by reading them frequently, even though you may not yet understand all the technical points. Try to keep the underlying rationale for the style of research reports in mind as you read.
- Read from a report that has been photocopied so that you can use a highlighter, underline portions of the article, write questions or notes in the margins, and so on.
- Read journal articles slowly. It may be useful to skim the article first to get the major points and then to read the article more carefully a second time.
- On the second or later reading of a journal article, train yourself to become an active reader. Reading actively involves constantly monitoring yourself to determine whether you understand what you are reading. If you are having comprehension problems, go back and re-read difficult passages or make notes about your confusion so that you can ask someone for clarification. In most cases, that "someone" will be your research instructor or another faculty member, but also consider contacting the researchers themselves. The postal and e-mail addresses of the researchers are usually included in the journal article, and researchers are generally more than willing to discuss their research with others.
- Keep this textbook with you as a reference while you are reading articles initially. This will enable you to look up unfamiliar terms in the glossary at the end of the book or in the index.
- Try not to get bogged down in (or scared away by) the statistical information. Try to grasp the gist of the story without letting formulas and numbers frustrate you.
- Until you become more accustomed to the style and jargon of research journal articles, you may want to translate, mentally or in writing, research articles. You can do this by translating compact paragraphs into looser constructions, by translating jargon into more familiar terms, by recasting the report into an active voice, and by summarizing the findings with words rather than with numbers. As an example, Box 3-2 presents a summary of a fictitious study, written in the style

typically found in research journal articles. Terms that can be looked up in the glossary of this book are underlined, and the notes in the margins indicate the type of information the author is communicating. Box 3-3 presents a "translation" of this summary, recasting the research information into language that is more digestible. Note that it is not just the jargon specific to research methods that makes the original version complicated (*e.g.*, "sequelae" is more obscure than "consequences"). Thus, a dictionary may also be needed when reading research reports.

When you attain a reasonable level of comprehension of a research report, a useful next step is to write a brief (one- to two-page) synopsis of the study. A synopsis summarizes the study's purpose, research questions, methods, findings, interpretation of the findings, and implications for practice. You do not need to be concerned at this point about critiquing the study's strengths and weaknesses, but rather about succinctly and objectively presenting a summary of what was done and what was learned. By preparing a synopsis, you will become more aware of aspects of the study that you did not comprehend.

Critiquing Research Reports

A written **research critique** is different from a research summary or synopsis. A research critique is a careful, critical appraisal of the strengths and limitations of a study. Critiques usually conclude with the reviewer's summary of the study's merits, recommendations regarding the utilization of the findings, and suggestions about improving the study or the report itself.

Research critiques of individual studies are prepared for various reasons, and they differ in scope, depending on their purpose. Peer reviewers who are asked to prepare a written critique for a journal considering publication of the report generally critique the following aspects of the study:

- *Substantive*—Was the research problem significant to nursing? Can the study make an important contribution?
- *Theoretical*—Were the theoretical underpinnings sound?
- *Methodologic*—Were the methods appropriate? Are the resulting findings believable?
- *Interpretive*—Did the researcher properly interpret data and develop reasonable conclusions?
- *Ethical*—Were the rights of the study participants protected?
- *Stylistic*—Is the report clearly written, grammatical, and well organized?

In short, the peer reviewer does a comprehensive review with the aim of providing feedback to the researchers and to journal editors about the merit of both the study and the report.

By contrast, a critique of a study that is designed to inform decisions about nursing practice need not be as comprehensive. For example, it is of

BOX 3-2

SUMMARY OF A FICTITIOUS STUDY FOR TRANSLATION

Purpose of the study	The potentially negative sequelae of having an abortion on the psycho- logical adjustment of adolescents have not been adequately studied. The present study sought to determine whether alternative pregnancy resolution decisions have different long-term effects on the psychological functioning of young women.	Need for the study
Research design	Three groups of low-income pregnant teenagers attending an inner-city clinic were the <u>subjects</u> in this study: those who delivered and kept the baby; those who delivered and relinquished the baby for adoption; and those who had an abortion. There were 25 subjects in each group.	Study population
Research instruments	The study <u>instruments</u> included a self-administered <u>questionnaire</u> and a battery of psychological tests measuring depression, anxiety, and psychosomatic symptoms. The instruments were administered upon entry into the study (when the subjects first came to the clinic) and then 1 year after termination of the pregnancy.	Research sample Research design & data collection procedures
Data analysis procedure	The <u>data</u> were analyzed using <u>analysis of variance (ANOVA)</u>.The ANOVA tests indicated that the three groups did not differ significantly in terms of depression, anxiety, or psychosomatic symptoms at the initial testing. At the <u>posttest</u>, however, the abortion group had significantly higher scores on the depression scale, and these girls were significantly more likely than the two delivery groups to report severe tension headaches. There were no <u>significant</u> differences on any of the <u>dependent variables</u> for the two delivery groups.	Results
Implications	The results of this study suggest that young women who elect to have an abortion may experience a number of long-term negative consequences. It would appear that appropriate efforts should be made to follow-up abortion patients to determine their need for suitable treatment.	Interpretation

| BOX 3-3 | **TRANSLATED VERSION OF FICTITIOUS RESEARCH STUDY** |

As researchers, we wondered whether young women who had an abortion had any emotional problems in the long run. It seemed to us that not enough research had been done to know whether any psychological harm resulted from an abortion.

We decided to study this question ourselves by comparing the experiences of three types of teenagers who became pregnant—first, girls who delivered and kept their babies; second, those who delivered the babies but gave them up for adoption; and third, those who elected to have an abortion. All teenagers in the sample were poor, and all were patients at an inner-city clinic. Altogether, we studied 75 girls—25 in each of the three groups. We evaluated the teenagers' emotional states by asking them to fill out a questionnaire and to take several psychological tests. These tests allowed us to assess things such as the girls' degree of depression and anxiety and whether they had any complaints of a psychosomatic nature. We asked them to fill out the forms twice: once when they came into the clinic, and then again a year after the abortion or the delivery.

We learned that the three groups of teenagers looked pretty much alike in terms of their emotional states when they first filled out the forms. But when we compared how the three groups looked a year later, we found that the teenagers who had abortions were more depressed and were more likely to say they had severe tension headaches than teenagers in the other two groups. The teenagers who kept their babies and those who gave their babies up for adoption looked pretty similar one year after their babies were born, at least in terms of depression, anxiety, and psychosomatic complaints.

Thus, it seems that we might be right in having some concerns about the emotional effects of having an abortion. Nurses should be aware of these long-term emotional effects, and it even may be advisable to institute some type of follow-up procedure to find out if these young women need additional help.

little significance to practicing nurses that a research report is ungrammatical. A critique on the clinical utility of a study focuses on whether the findings are accurate, believable, and clinically meaningful. If the findings cannot be trusted, it makes little sense to incorporate them into nursing practice.

By understanding research methods, you will be in a position to critique the scientific merit of studies, and this is a primary aim of this book. Each chapter in this book offers guidelines for evaluating various research decisions that will help you come to an overall appraisal of a research study.

Nurses who are intelligent consumers of nursing research must be able to critique not only single, independent studies, but also a body of studies on a topic of clinical interest. We discuss literature reviews in Chapter 6, and we further explore the role of critical reviews in the final chapter of this book.

RESEARCH EXAMPLES

In this section, we present researchers' abstracts from two additional research studies. As we did in Box 3-2, we underline terms that can be looked up in the glossary of this book to help you read the original abstract more readily. We also provide a "translated" version of the abstract.

RESEARCH EXAMPLE OF A QUANTITATIVE STUDY

White-Traut and colleagues (1999) conducted a study to evaluate a developmentally appropriate intervention for preterm infants:

Research Summary (Abstract)
Preterm infants with periventrical leukomalacia (PVL) were evaluated to determine whether multi-sensory stimulation is safe and to assess whether it improved neurobehavior and neurodevelopment. Thirty preterm infants with documented PVL were randomly assigned to control ($n = 15$) or experimental (Group E) ($n = 15$) groups at 33 weeks post-conceptual age. Group E infants received 15 minutes of auditory, tactile, visual, and vestibular (ATVV) intervention twice a day, five days a week, for four weeks during hospitalization. Repeated-measures ANOVA demonstrated that Group E infants experienced significant increases in heart and respiratory rate and a 0.72% drop in hemoglobin saturation, coinciding with a significant behavioral state shift from sleep to alertness during intervention. No differences were identified in neurobehavioral function and neurodevelopment, indicating that Group E suffered no injury. Group E had an average hospital stay nine days shorter than that of controls, with the associated cost savings of $213,840. The earlier hospital discharge indicates that ATVV intervention promotes alertness without compromising physiologic status in vulnerable infants (White-Traut et al., 1999, p. 131).

Translated Version
We wanted to evaluate a special nursing intervention for preterm infants who had the condition of periventricular leukomalacia (PVL). The special treatment involved stimulation of the infants along several sensory dimensions, including auditory, tactile, visual, and vestibular stimulation (abbreviated as ATVV). We wondered whether this special treatment was safe, and whether it would lead to improvements in the behavior and development of the infants. A total of 30 preterm infants with PVL who

were 33 weeks' postconception were the subjects in the study. Half of them (15) were in a group that did not receive the special treatment. The other 15 infants, selected at random, were in the special treatment group, Group E. Group E infants received 15 minutes of the ATVV stimulation twice a day, 5 days a week, for 4 weeks while they were in the hospital. The statistical analysis indicated that the infants in the special treatment group had increases in heart and respiratory rate compared with the other infants and also had a drop in hemoglobin saturation. Those in Group E also showed greater alertness during the course of the treatment. We found that the two groups were comparable in terms of neurobehavioral function and neurodevelopment, indicating that the treatment had no harmful effects. We also learned that the infants in the treatment group spent 9 fewer days in the hospital than the other infants, on average, resulting in a cost savings of $213,840. Thus, it appears that the ATVV treatment promoted alertness and led to earlier hospital discharge, with no negative side effects.

Clinical Relevance

Periventricular leukomalacia is a common injury to premature infants and is associated with elevated risks for cerebral palsy. In addition to compromising infant development, PVL is a major issue for cost-containment. Thus, interventions that can improve neurodevelopment in infants with PVL have both clinical and practical significance.

White-Traut and her colleagues designed their study as an extension of earlier studies that had demonstrated the efficacy of multimodal sensory interventions with preterm infants. There is increasing research evidence that multiple modalities provide a more protective effect against negative autonomic nervous system responses than a single type of stimulation. By building on a base of solid prior research, the researchers ensured that their study would have considerable potential to lead to improvements in practice. This potential was strengthened by their use of a strong research design. By assigning infants to the special intervention at random, the researchers had greater assurance that the two groups of infants were comparable in all respects, except for the treatment itself; thus, any differences could be attributed to that treatment.

The findings were uniformly favorable. The intervention was not associated with any neurologic damage and therefore appears to be safe for infants with PVL. Moreover, the intervention promoted alertness and led to substantially shorter hospital stays. The earlier hospital discharge of the intervention group infants not only provides evidence of the cost-effectiveness of this intervention but also has implications for promoting earlier mother–infant bonding. Mothers of these infants were able to take their infants home a full 9 days earlier, on average, than mothers of the other infants.

RESEARCH EXAMPLE OF A QUALITATIVE STUDY

Kahn (1999) conducted a qualitative study of older people's adaptation to the ambivalence of a nursing home. The author's abstract is presented next.

Research Summary (Abstract)

This article is based on a 9-month <u>ethnographic study</u> of a nursing home for older Jewish people. In this article, the process that 21 key <u>informants</u> went through in adapting to the dual nature of the nursing home as institution and as home is examined. A widely used phrase, "Making the best of it," was used by informants and other residents of the nursing home to describe this process. Interpretive analysis of this <u>emic</u> phrase revealed four dimensions: (a) recognizing the ambivalence of their living environment and situation; (b) downplaying negative aspects of it, (c) having no other options, and (d) using their will to transcend and create a home (Kahn, 1999).

Translated Version

I conducted an in-depth study of older Jewish people's adaptation to a nursing home environment. In the article, I describe how 21 nursing home residents with whom I spoke adapted to the fact that the nursing home was an institution yet was also their home. The process of adjusting to the dual nature of the nursing home was captured by the phrase, "making the best of it." This phrase, which was widely expressed by the "insiders" in the nursing home, encompasses four aspects. First, it indicates the ambivalence that the elders felt about their environment and their situation. Second, the phrase downplays the negative aspects of their arrangement. Third, it reflects the fact that the residents had no other options for their living arrangement. Finally, the phrase suggests that the elders made deliberate efforts to create a home for themselves.

Clinical Relevance

Kahn recognized the dual nature of the nursing home environment for its residents and was curious about how this duality might pose challenges for those trying to adapt to the environment. To learn about the shared meanings of the residents as they evolved through complex social interactions, Kahn spent 9 months in the field, interviewing the informants on numerous separate occasions (from 5 to 18 times). With such an intensive and lengthy scrutiny, Kahn was able to describe the residents' process of adaptation thoroughly.

The findings from this qualitative study provide nurses with a valuable, insiders' view of life in a nursing home. Helping seniors to adapt to this institution as their "home" for the remainder of their lives is a challenging one for nurses. As revealed in this study, everyday life in a nursing home is filled with fixed schedules, loss of choices, and loss of privacy. The elderly residents who successfully adapted to nursing home life engaged in an active process of making the best of their situations—which entailed concerted and continual efforts to reframe and reconstruct their social environment. Seniors were aware that they were unable to change the reality of their situations but were able to reconstruct different aspects of their situation cognitively and emotionally. Based on this insider's view of nursing home life, nurses can focus on helping seniors achieve this adaptation.

• • • • • SUMMARY POINTS

- The most common types of research reports are theses and dissertations, books, conference presentations (including oral reports and **poster sessions**), and, especially, journal articles.
- Research **journal articles** provide brief descriptions of research studies and are designed to communicate the contribution the study has made to knowledge.
- Journal articles often consist of six major sections: the **abstract** (a brief synopsis of the study); introduction (explanation of the study problem and its context); method section (the strategies used to address the research problem); results (the actual study findings); discussion (the interpretation of the findings); and references.
- Research reports are often difficult to read because they are dense, concise, and contain a lot of jargon.
- Qualitative research reports are written in a more inviting and conversational style than quantitative ones, which are more impersonal and include information on statistical tests.
- **Statistical tests** are procedures for testing research hypotheses and evaluating the believability of the findings. Findings that are **statistically significant** are ones that have a high probability of being valid.
- The ultimate goal of this book is to help students to prepare a **research critique**, which is a careful, critical appraisal of the strengths and limitations of a piece of research, often for the purpose of considering its utility for nursing practice.

➤ ➤ ➤ ➤ CRITICAL THINKING ACTIVITIES

Chapter 3 of the accompanying *Study Guide to Accompany Essentials of Nursing Research,* 5th edition offers various exercises and study suggestions for reinforcing the concepts presented in this chapter. In addition, you can address the following:

1. Read the abstracts from one or both of the actual research studies in the Appendix of this book. Underline technical terms and look them up in the glossary. Then write a translated version of the abstract.

2. Make an outline of the major sections and subsections of one or both of the research studies in the Appendix. Compare this outline to the outline of sections described in this chapter.

3. Skim both of the research studies in the Appendix. Which story is more difficult to grasp? Why? Which parts of these research reports were especially problematic?

For additional review, see questions 28–35 on the study CD provided with Polit: Study Guide to Accompany Essentials of Nursing Research.

SUGGESTED READINGS

Methodologic References

Downs, F. S. (1999). How to cozy up to a research report. *Applied Nursing Research, 12,* 215–216.

Rankin, M., & Esteves, M. D. (1996). How to assess a research study. *American Journal of Nursing, 96,* 32–37.

Tornquist, E. M., Funk, S. G., Champagne, M. T., & Wiese, R. A. (1993). Advice on reading research: Overcoming the barriers. *Applied Nursing Research, 6,* 177–183.

Substantive References

Foster-Fitzpatrick, L., Ortiz, A., Sibilano, H., Marcantonio, R., & Braun, L. T. (1999). The effects of crossed leg on blood pressure measurement. *Nursing Research, 48,* 105–108.

Kahn, D. L. (1999). Making the best of it: Adapting to the ambivalence of a nursing home environment. *Qualitative Health Research, 9,* 119–132.

Leidy, N. K., & Haase, J. E. (1999). Functional status from the patient's perspective: The challenge of preserving personal integrity. *Research in Nursing & Health, 22,* 67–77.

White-Traut, R. C., Nelson, M. N., Silvestri, J. M., Patel, M., Vasan, U., Han, B. K., Cunningham, N., Burns, K., Kopishchke, K., & Bradford, L. (1999). Developmental intervention for preterm infants diagnosed with periventricular leukomalacia. *Research in Nursing & Health, 22,* 131–143.

CHAPTER 4

Understanding the Ethics of Nursing Research

Student Objectives

On completion of this chapter, the student will be able to:

○ discuss the historical background that led to the creation of various codes of ethics

○ understand the nature of the conflict, in certain situations, between ethics and research demands

○ identify the three primary ethical principles articulated in the *Belmont Report* and the important dimensions encompassed by each

○ describe the concept of vulnerable subjects and identify several relevant groups

○ describe the role of Institutional Review Boards in the review of research plans

○ given sufficient information, evaluate the ethical dimensions of a research report

○ define new terms in the chapter

New Terms

Anonymity	Human subjects committees
Belmont Report	Identification number
Beneficence	Implied consent
Code of ethics	Informed consent
Confidentiality	Institutional Review Board
Consent form	Process consent
Covert data collection	Risk/benefit ratio
Debriefing	Stipend
Full disclosure	Vulnerable subjects

THE NEED FOR ETHICAL GUIDELINES

Nurses face many ethical dilemmas in their practice; the prolongation of life by artificial means, the institution of tube feedings when patients are unable to sustain oral nourishment, and the testing of new products to monitor care are but a few examples. Dilemmas such as these have led to numerous discussions and debates concerning ethical issues in nursing practice. Similarly, the increase of research with humans has led to ethical concerns about the rights of study participants. This chapter discusses some of the major ethical principles that should be considered in reviewing studies.

The requirement for ethical conduct in research may strike you as so self-evident as to require no further comment, but the fact is that ethical considerations have not always been given adequate attention.

Historical Background

As modern, civilized people, we might like to think that systematic violations of moral principles within a research context occurred centuries ago rather than in recent times, but this is not the case. The Nazi medical experiments of the 1930s and 1940s are the most famous example of recent disregard for ethical conduct. The Nazi program of research involved the use of prisoners of war and racial "enemies" in experiments designed to test the limits of human endurance and human reaction to diseases and untested drugs. The studies were unethical not only because they exposed these people to permanent physical harm and even death but also because the participants could not refuse participation.

Some recent examples come from the United States. For instance, between 1932 and 1972, a study known as the Tuskegee Syphilis Study, sponsored by the U. S. Public Health Service, investigated the effects of syphilis on 400 men from a poor black community. Medical treatment was deliberately withheld to study the course of the untreated disease. Another well-known case of unethical research involved the injection of live cancer cells into elderly patients at the Jewish Chronic Disease Hospital in Brooklyn without the consent of those patients. Even more recently, it was revealed in 1993 that U. S. federal agencies had sponsored radiation experiments since the 1940s on hundreds of people, many of them prisoners or elderly hospital patients. Many other examples of studies with ethical transgressions—often much more subtle than these examples—have emerged to give ethical concerns the high visibility they have today.

Ethical Dilemmas in Conducting Research

Research that violates ethical principles is rarely done to be cruel but more typically occurs out of a conviction that knowledge is important and potentially beneficial in the long run. There are situations in which the rights of participants and the demands of the research project are put in direct conflict. Here are some examples of research problems in which the desire for rigor conflicts with ethical considerations:

1. *Research question:* How empathic are nurses in their treatment of patients in intensive care units?
   Ethical dilemma: Ethics require that participants be cognizant of their role in a study. Yet if the researcher informs the nurses participating in this study that their degree of empathy in treating patients will be scrutinized, will their behavior be "normal"? If the nurses' behavior is altered because of the known presence of research observers, the findings will not be valid.
2. *Research question:* What are the coping mechanisms of parents whose children have a terminal illness?
   Ethical dilemma: To answer this question, the researcher may need to probe into the psychological state of the parents at a vulnerable time

in their lives; such probing could be painful and even traumatic. Yet knowledge of the parents' coping mechanisms might help to design more effective ways of dealing with parents' grief and anger.

3. *Research question:* Does a new medication prolong life in cancer patients?
   Ethical dilemma: The best way to test the effectiveness of an intervention is to administer the intervention to some participants but withhold it from others to see whether differences between the groups emerge. However, if the intervention is untested (*e.g.*, a new drug), the group receiving the intervention may be exposed to potentially hazardous side effects. On the other hand, the group not receiving the drug may be denied a beneficial treatment.

4. *Research question:* What is the process by which adult children adapt to the day-to-day stresses of caring for a terminally ill parent?
   Ethical dilemma: In a qualitative study, which would be appropriate for this research question, the researcher sometimes becomes so closely involved with the study participants that they become willing to share "secrets" and privileged information. Interviews can become confessions—sometimes of unseemly or even illegal or immoral behavior. In this example, suppose a participant admitted to abusing their adult parent physically—how does the researcher respond to that information without undermining a pledge of confidentiality? And, if the researcher divulges the information to appropriate authorities, how can a pledge of confidentiality be given in good faith to other participants?

As these examples suggest, researchers are sometimes in a bind: their goal is to advance knowledge, using the best methods possible, but they must also adhere to the dictates of ethical rules that have been developed to protect the rights of study participants. It is precisely because of such conflicts that codes of ethics have been developed to guide the efforts of researchers and to help others evaluate their actions.

Codes of Ethics

Since the 1950s, largely in response to the human rights violations described earlier, various codes of ethics have been developed. One of the first internationally recognized set of ethical standards is referred to as the **Nuremberg Code,** developed after the Nazi atrocities were made public in the Nuremberg trials. Several other international standards have followed, the most notable of which is the **Declaration of Helsinki,** which was adopted in 1964 by the World Medical Assembly and then later revised in 1975.

Most disciplines have established their own **code of ethics.** The American Nurses Association (1975) has put forth a document entitled *Human Rights Guidelines for Nurses in Clinical and Other Research.* The American Sociological Association published its *Code of Ethics* in 1984. Guidelines for psychologists were published by the American Psychological Association (1982) in *Ethical Principles in the Conduct of Research With Human Participants.* There is considerable overlap in the principles articulated in these documents, but each deals with problems of particular concern to their respective disciplines.

In the United States, an especially important code of ethics was adopted by the National Commission for the Protection of Human Subjects of Biomedical and Behavioral Research (1978). The Commission, established by the National Research Act (Public Law 93-348), issued a report in 1978 that served as the basis for regulations affecting research sponsored by the federal government. The report, sometimes referred to as the ***Belmont Report,*** served as a model for many of the guidelines adopted by specific disciplines.

The *Belmont Report* articulated three primary ethical principles on which standards of ethical conduct in research are based: beneficence, respect for human dignity, and justice.

PRINCIPLE OF BENEFICENCE

One of the most fundamental ethical principles in research is that of **beneficence,** which encompasses the maxim: Above all, do no harm. This principle contains multiple dimensions.

Freedom From Harm

Clearly, exposing study participants to experiences that result in serious or permanent harm is unacceptable. An ethical researcher must be prepared to terminate the research if there is reason to suspect that continuation would result in injury, death, disability, or undue distress to study participants. When a new medical procedure or drug is being tested, experimentation with animals or tissue cultures usually precedes tests with humans.

The psychological consequences of participating in a study are generally subtle and thus require close attention and sensitivity. For example, participants may be asked questions about their personal views, weaknesses, or fears. Such queries might lead people to reveal sensitive personal information. The point is not that researchers should refrain from asking questions but rather that they need to analyze the nature of the intrusion on people's psyches. Researchers strive to avoid inflicting psychological harm by tactfully phrasing questions, by providing **debriefing** sessions after the data collection is completed to permit participants to ask questions or air complaints, and, in some situations, by making referrals to appropriate health, social, or psychological services.

> **Example of risk reduction:**
>
> Varda and Behnke (2000) studied the effect of the timing of an initial bath (1 hour versus 2 hours after birth) on newborn temperature. To minimize risks, the researchers excluded all infants with conditions (e.g., infection, fetal distress, hypoglycemia) that could predispose them to temperature instability.

Freedom From Exploitation

Involvement in a study should not place participants at a disadvantage or expose them to situations for which they have not been explicitly prepared. Participants need to be assured that their participation, or the information they might provide to the researcher, will not be used against them. For example, a person describing his or her economic circumstances to a researcher should not be exposed to the risk of losing Medicaid benefits; the person reporting drug abuse should not fear exposure to criminal authorities.

Study participants enter into a special relationship with researchers, and it is crucial that this relationship not be exploited. Exploitation might be overt and malicious (*e.g.,* sexual exploitation, use of participants' identifying information to create a mailing list, and use of donated blood for the development of a commercial product), but it might also be more subtle. For example, suppose subjects have agreed to participate in a study requiring 30 minutes of their time and that the researcher decided 1 year later to go back to them, to follow their progress or circumstances. Unless the researcher had previously explained to the participants that there might be a follow-up study, the researcher could be accused of not adhering to the agreement previously reached with participants and of exploiting the researcher–participant relationship.

Because nurse researchers may have a nurse–client (in addition to a researcher–participant) relationship, special care may be needed to avoid exploiting that bond. Patients' consent to participate in a study may result from their understanding of the researcher's role as *nurse,* not as *researcher.*

In qualitative research, the risk of exploitation may be especially acute because the psychological distance between the investigator and the participant typically declines as the study progresses. The emergence of a pseudotherapeutic relationship between the researcher and participant is not uncommon, and this imposes additional responsibilities on the researcher—and additional risks that exploitation could inadvertently occur. On the other hand, qualitative researchers are typically in a better position than quantitative researchers to do good, rather than just to avoid doing any harm, because of the close relationships they often develop with participants. Munhall (1988) has argued that qualitative nurse researchers have the responsibility of ensuring that the "therapeutic imperative of nursing (advocacy) takes precedent over the research imperative (advancing knowledge) if conflict develops" (p. 151).

Risk/Benefit Ratio

Box 4-1 summarizes major costs and benefits of research participation. Researchers can perhaps best evaluate the **risk/benefit ratio** by considering how comfortable they would feel having family members participate in the study. In your evaluation of the risk/benefit ratio of a study, you might consider whether you would have felt comfortable being a study participant.

BOX 4-1

POTENTIAL BENEFITS AND COSTS OF RESEARCH TO PARTICIPANTS

Major Potential Benefits to Participants

Access to an intervention to which they otherwise may not have access

Gratification in being able to discuss their situation or problem with a nonjudgmental and friendly person

Increased knowledge about themselves or their conditions, either through opportunity for introspection and self-reflection or through direct interaction with the researcher

Escape from normal routine and excitement of being part of a study

Satisfaction that the information they provide may help others with similar problems or conditions

Direct monetary or material gains through stipends or other incentives

Major Potential Costs to Participants

Physical harm, including unanticipated side effects

Physical discomfort, fatigue, or boredom

Psychological or emotional distress resulting from self-disclosure, introspection, fear of the unknown or interacting with strangers, fear of eventual repercussions, anger or embarrassment at the type of questions being asked

Loss of privacy

Loss of time

Monetary costs (*e.g.,* for transportation, child care, or time lost from work)

The risk/benefit ratio should also be considered in terms of whether the risks to research participants are commensurate with the benefit to society and the nursing profession. The degree of risk to be taken by those participating in the research should never exceed the potential humanitarian benefits of the knowledge to be gained. Thus, an important question in assessing the overall risk/benefit ratio is whether the study focuses on a significant topic that has the potential to improve patient care.

PRINCIPLE OF RESPECT FOR HUMAN DIGNITY

Respect for the human dignity of participants is the second ethical principle articulated in the *Belmont Report.* This principle includes the right to self-determination and the right to full disclosure.

Right to Self-Determination

Humans should be treated as autonomous agents, capable of controlling their own activities. The principle of **self-determination** means that prospective participants have the right to decide voluntarily whether to participate in a study, without the risk of incurring any penalty or prejudicial treatment. It also means that participants have the right to ask questions, to refuse to give information, or to terminate their participation.

A person's right to self-determination includes freedom from coercion of any type. **Coercion** involves explicit or implicit threats of penalty for failing to participate in a study or excessive rewards from agreeing to participate. The obligation to protect potential participants from coercion requires careful consideration when the researcher is in a position of authority, control, or influence over potential participants, as might be the case in a nurse–patient relationship. The issue of coercion may also require scrutiny even when there is not a preestablished relationship. For example, a generous monetary incentive (or **stipend**) offered to encourage the participation of an economically disadvantaged group (*e.g.*, the homeless) might be mildly coercive because such incentives could place undue pressure on prospective participants.

Right to Full Disclosure

The principle of respect for human dignity includes people's right to make informed, voluntary decisions about study participation, which requires full disclosure. **Full disclosure** means that the researcher has fully described the nature of the study, the person's right to refuse participation, the researcher's responsibilities, and the likely risks and benefits that would be incurred. The right to self-determination and the right to full disclosure are the two major elements on which informed consent is based.

Informed Consent

Informed consent means that participants have adequate information regarding the research; comprehend the information; and have the power of free choice, enabling them to consent voluntarily to participate in the research or decline participation. Researchers may document the informed consent process by having participants sign a **consent form**, an example of which is presented in Figure 4-1. This form includes information about the study purpose, the specific expectations regarding participation (*e.g.*, how much time will be involved), the voluntary nature of participation, and the potential costs and benefits.

Researchers rarely obtain written informed consent when the primary means of data collection is through a self-administered questionnaire. The researcher generally assumes **implied consent** (*i.e.*, that the return of the completed questionnaire reflects the respondent's voluntary consent to participate). This assumption, however, is not always warranted (*e.g.*, if patients

In signing this document, I am giving my consent to be interviewed by an employee of Human-alysis, Inc., a nonprofit research organization based in Saratoga Springs, New York. I understand that I will be part of a research study that will focus on the experiences and needs of mothers of young children in the United States. This study, supported by a grant from the U.S. Department of Health and Human Services, will provide some guidance to people who are trying to help mothers and their children.

I understand that I will be interviewed in my home at a time convenient to me. I will be asked some questions about my experiences as a parent, my feelings about how to raise children, the health and characteristics of my oldest child, and my use of community services. I also understand that the interviewer will ask to have my oldest child present during at least some portion of the interview. The interview will take about 1½ to 2 hours to complete. I also understand that the researcher may contact me for more information in the future.

I understand that I was selected to participate in this study because I was involved in a study of young mothers at the time of my oldest child's birth. At that time, I was recruited into the study, along with about 500 other young mothers, through a hospital or service agency.

This interview was granted freely. I have been informed that the interview is entirely voluntary, and that even after the interview begins I can refuse to answer any specific questions or decide to terminate the interview at any point. I have been told that my answers to questions will not be given to anyone else and no reports of this study will ever identify me in any way. I have also been informed that my participation or nonparticipation or my refusal to answer questions will have no effect on services that I or any member of my family may receive from health or social services providers.

This study will help develop a better understanding of the experiences of young mothers and the services that can be most helpful to them and their children. However, I will receive no direct benefit as a result of participation. As a means of compensating for any fatigue, inconvenience or monetary costs associated with participating in the study, I have received $25 for granting this interview.

I understand that the results of this research will be given to me if I ask for them and that Dr. Denise Polit is the person to contact if I have any questions about the study or about my rights as a study participant. Dr. Polit can be reached through a collect call at (518) 587-3994.

_____	_____
Date	Respondent's Signature
	_____
	Interviewer's Signature

FIGURE 4-1. Sample consent form.

feel that their treatment might be affected by failure to cooperate with the researcher).

In some qualitative studies, especially those requiring repeated contact with participants, it is difficult to obtain a meaningful informed consent at the outset. A qualitative researcher does not always know in advance how the study will evolve. Because the research design emerges during the data collection and analysis process, the researcher may not know the exact nature of the data to be collected, what the risks and benefits to participants will be, nor how much of a time commitment they will be expected to make. Thus, in a qualitative study, consent is often viewed as an ongoing, transactional process, referred to as **process consent.** In process consent, the researcher continuously renegotiates the consent, allowing participants to play a collaborative role in the decision-making process regarding their ongoing participation.

Example of informed consent:

Menzel (1999) studied whether patients' self-esteem differed during intubation and after extubation. Prospective subjects were given an explanation of the study and told that the risks of participating might involve fatigue and emotions related to their feelings about themselves. They were advised that they could withdraw at any time and that their responses were confidential. Alert patients who could communicate were asked for consent.

Issues Relating to the Principle of Respect

Certain circumstances make participants' right to self-determination and full disclosure problematic. One issue concerns some people's inability to make well-informed judgments about the costs and benefits of participation. Children, for example, may be unable to give truly informed consent. The issue of groups that are vulnerable within a research context is discussed later in this chapter.

Another issue is that full disclosure can sometimes result in two types of biases: (1) the bias resulting from distorted information and (2) the bias resulting from failure to recruit a good sample. Suppose a researcher were studying the relationship between high school students' substance abuse and their absenteeism from school; the researcher hypothesizes that students with a high rate of absenteeism are more likely to be substance abusers than students with a good attendance record. If the researcher approached potential participants and explained the purpose of the study, some students might refuse to participate, and nonparticipation would be selective; we would expect, in fact, that those least likely to volunteer for such a study would be students who are substance abusers—the very group of primary interest in the research. Moreover, by knowing the specific research question, those who do participate might be less inclined to give candid responses. The researcher in such a situation might argue that full disclosure would totally undermine the study.

One technique that researchers sometimes use in such situations is **covert data collection,** or *concealment*—the collection of information without the participants' knowledge and thus without their consent. This might happen, for example, if a researcher wanted to observe people's behavior in a real-world setting and was concerned that doing so openly would result in changes in the very behavior of interest. The researcher might choose to obtain the information through concealed methods, such as by observing through a one-way mirror, videotaping participants through hidden equipment, or observing while pretending to be engaged in other activities.

A second, and more controversial, technique is the researcher's use of deception. **Deception** can involve either deliberately withholding information about the study or providing participants with false information. For example, the researcher studying high school students' use of drugs might describe the research as a study of students' health practices, which is a mild form of misinformation.

Deception and concealment are problematic from an ethical standpoint because they interfere with the participants' right to make a truly informed decision regarding the personal costs and benefits of participation. Some people argue that the use of deception and concealment are never justified. Others, however, believe that, if the study involves minimal risk to participants and if there are anticipated benefits to science and society, deception or concealment may be justified to enhance the validity of the findings. Covert data collection and deception are least likely to be ethically acceptable if the research is focused on sensitive aspects of the participants' behavior, such as drug use, sexual conduct, or illegal acts.

PRINCIPLE OF JUSTICE

The third broad principle articulated in the *Belmont Report* concerns justice. This principle includes the participants' right to fair treatment and their right to privacy.

Right to Fair Treatment

Participants have the right to fair and equitable treatment before, during, and after their participation in the study. Fair treatment includes the following:

- The fair and nondiscriminatory selection of participants such that any risks or benefits will be equitably shared; selection should be based on research requirements and not on the vulnerability or compromised position of certain people
- The nonprejudicial treatment of people who decline to participate or who withdraw from the study after agreeing to participate
- The honoring of all agreements between the researcher and the participant, including adherence to the procedures described in advance and the payment of any promised stipends
- Participants' access to research personnel at any point in the study to clarify information
- Participants' access to appropriate professional assistance if there is physical or psychological damage

- Debriefing, if necessary, to divulge information withheld before the study or to clarify issues that arose during the study
- Sensitivity to and respect for the beliefs, habits, and lifestyles of people from different cultures
- Courteous and tactful treatment at all times

Right to Privacy

Virtually all research with humans constitutes an intrusion into personal lives. Researchers should ensure that their research is not more intrusive than it needs to be and that the participants' privacy is maintained throughout the study.

Participants have the right to expect that any data they provide will be kept in strictest confidence. This can occur either through anonymity or through other confidentiality procedures. **Anonymity** occurs when even the researcher cannot link a participant with his or her data. For example, if questionnaires were distributed to a group of nursing home residents and were returned without any identifying information on them, the responses would be anonymous. As another example, if a researcher reviewed hospital records from which all identifying information (*e.g.*, name, address, Social Security number, and so forth) had been expunged, anonymity would again protect people's right to privacy.

> **Example of anonymity:**
>
> Thurmond (1999) studied perceptions of the use of chemical restraint among nurses working in long-term care. Data were collected by having a person at each long-term care facility attach a questionnaire to the nurse's paycheck, along with a cover letter describing the purposes of the study. Subjects were assured anonymity: the researcher did not know who received the questionnaires, and they were returned to her by mail. No identifying information was collected.

In situations in which anonymity is impossible, researchers implement other confidentiality procedures. A promise of **confidentiality** to participants is a pledge that any information the participant provides will not be publicly reported or made accessible to parties not involved in the research.

Researchers generally develop elaborate confidentiality procedures. These include securing individual confidentiality assurances from everyone involved in collecting or analyzing research data; maintaining identifying information in a locked file to which few people have access; substituting **identification numbers** for participants' names on study records and computer files to prevent any accidental breach of confidentiality; and reporting only aggregate data for groups of participants or taking steps to disguise a person's identity in a research report.

Extra precautions are often needed to safeguard the privacy of participants in qualitative studies. Anonymity is almost never possible in qualitative research because the researcher becomes thoroughly involved with participants. Moreover, because of the in-depth nature of many qualitative studies, there may be a greater invasion of privacy than is true in quantitative research. Researchers who spend time in the home of a study participant may, for example, have difficulty segregating the public behaviors the study participant is willing to share from the private behaviors that unfold unwittingly during the course of data collection. A final thorny issue many qualitative researchers face is adequately disguising study participants in their research reports. Because the number of respondents is small and because rich descriptive information is presented in a research report, qualitative researchers need to take extra precautions to safeguard participants' identity. This may mean more than simply using a fictitious name—it may also mean withholding information about the characteristics of the informant, such as age and occupation.

> **CONSUMER TIP:**
>
> As a means of enhancing both personal and institutional privacy, research reports frequently avoid giving explicit information about the locale of the study. For example, the report might state that data were collected in a 200-bed, private, for-profit nursing home, without mentioning its name or location. ■

VULNERABLE GROUPS

Adherence to ethical standards is often straightforward. The rights of special vulnerable groups, however, may need to be protected through additional procedures and heightened sensitivity on the part of the researcher. **Vulnerable subjects** may be incapable of giving informed consent (*e.g.,* people in a coma) or may be at high risk of unintended side effects because of their circumstances (*e.g.,* pregnant women). You should pay particular attention to the ethical dimensions of a study when people who are vulnerable are involved. Vulnerable groups include the following:

- *Children.* Legally and ethically, children do not have the competence to give their informed consent; therefore, the informed consent of children's parents or legal guardians is obtained. If the child is developmentally mature enough to understand the basic information involved in informed consent (*e.g.,* a 12-year-old child), the researcher should also obtain consent from the child as evidence of respect for the child's right to self-determination. With younger children, the study should be explained in simple terms, and informal assent obtained.
- *Mentally or emotionally disabled people.* People whose disability makes it impossible for them to weigh the risks and benefits of participation and

make an informed decision (*e.g.,* people affected by mental retardation, senility, mental illness, unconsciousness, and so on) also cannot legally or ethically provide informed consent. In such cases, the researcher obtains the written consent of the person's legal guardian. To the extent possible, informed consent from prospective participants should be sought as a supplement to consent from the guardian.

Example of research with a vulnerable group:

Mate-Kole, Danquah, Twum, and Danquah (1999) tested the effectiveness of three alternative behavior interventions for improving self-care behavior in moderately intellectually impaired individuals. The researchers sought to recruit 20 residents of a rehabilitation center. The guardians of 15 residents gave informed consent.

Physically disabled people. For certain physical disabilities, special procedures for obtaining consent may be required. For example, with deaf people, the entire consent process may need to be in writing. For people who cannot read or write or who have a physical impairment preventing them from writing, alternative procedures for documenting informed consent (*e.g.,* videotaping the consent proceedings) can be used.

Institutionalized people. Nurses often conduct studies with hospitalized or institutionalized people, and such people may feel pressured into participating or may believe that their treatment would be jeopardized by failure to cooperate. Inmates of prisons and other correctional facilities, who have lost their autonomy in many spheres of activity, may similarly feel constrained in their ability to give free consent. Researchers studying institutionalized groups need to emphasize the voluntary nature of participation.

Pregnant women. The U.S. government has issued stringent requirements governing research with pregnant women. These requirements reflect a desire to safeguard both the pregnant woman, who may be at heightened physical and psychological risk, and the fetus, who cannot give informed consent. The regulations stipulate that a pregnant woman cannot be involved in a study unless the purpose of the research is to meet the health needs of the pregnant woman and unless risks to her and the fetus will be minimized.

CONSUMER TIP:

Many of the terms introduced in this chapter are rarely used explicitly in a research report. For example, a report almost never calls to the readers' attention that the participants in the study were vulnerable subjects. Consumers need to be sensitive to the special needs of groups that may be unable to act as their own advocates or to assess adequately the costs and benefits of participating in a study. ■

INSTITUTIONAL REVIEW BOARDS AND EXTERNAL REVIEWS

It is sometimes difficult for researchers to be objective in their assessment of the risk/benefit ratio or in the development of procedures to protect participants' rights. Biases may arise as a result of researchers' commitment to an area of knowledge and their desire to conduct a valid study. Because of the risk of a biased evaluation, the ethical dimensions of a study are usually subjected to external review.

Most hospitals, universities, and other institutions where research is conducted have established formal committees and protocols for reviewing research plans. These committees are sometimes called **human subjects committees.** In the United States, if the institution receives federal funds to pay for the research, it is likely that the committee will be an **Institutional Review Board** (IRB). Studies supported with federal funds are subject to strict guidelines regarding the treatment of humans (and animals) used in research, and the IRB's duty is to ensure that proposed plans adhere to these guidelines.

Example of IRB approval:

Coyne and her colleagues (1999) studies nurses' knowledge of pain assessment and pain management among medical and surgical nurses in three hospitals. Approval of the study plans was obtained from the Human Subjects Protection Review Committee at the University of Southern Mississippi (the researchers' affiliation) and from the IRBs of the three hospitals.

Not all research is subject to federal guidelines, and thus not all studies are reviewed by IRBs or other formal committees. Nevertheless, researchers have a responsibility to ensure that their research plans are ethically acceptable, and it is a good practice for researchers to solicit external advice even when they are not required to do so.

CONSUMER TIP:

Research reports do not always provide readers with information regarding adherence to ethical principles because space limitations in professional journals make it impossible to document all aspects of the study. The absence of any mention of procedures to safeguard participants' rights does not necessarily imply that no precautions were taken. When information about ethical considerations is presented, it almost always appears in the method section, typically in the subsection devoted to data collection procedures but sometimes in the subsection describing the sample. ■

CRITIQUING THE ETHICS OF RESEARCH STUDIES

Guidelines for critiquing the ethical aspects of a study are presented in Box 4-2. A person serving on an IRB or human subjects committee should be provided with sufficient information to answer all these questions. As noted earlier, however, it may not always be possible to critique the ethical aspects of a study based on a published research report. Nevertheless, we offer a few suggestions for considering the ethical aspects of a study.

Many research reports do acknowledge that the study procedures were reviewed by an IRB or human subjects committee of the institution with which the researchers are affiliated. When a research report specifically mentions a formal external review, it is generally safe to assume that a panel of concerned people thoroughly reviewed the ethical issues raised by the study.

You can also come to some conclusions based on a description of the study methods. There is usually sufficient information to judge, for example, whether the study participants were subjected to any physical or psychological harm or discomfort. Reports do not always specifically state whether informed consent was secured, but you should be alert to situations in which the data could not have been gathered as described if participation were purely voluntary.

It is often especially difficult to determine by reading research reports whether the privacy of the participants was safeguarded unless the researcher specifically mentions pledges of confidentiality or anonymity. A situation requiring special scrutiny arises when data are collected from two people simultaneously (*e.g.*, a husband and wife who are jointly interviewed); in such

---

BOX 4-2

GUIDELINES FOR CRITIQUING THE ETHICAL ASPECTS OF A STUDY

1. Were the study participants subjected to any physical harm, discomfort, or psychological distress? Did the researchers take appropriate steps to remove or prevent the harm?

2. Did the benefits to participants outweigh any potential risks or actual discomfort they experienced? Did the benefits to society outweigh the costs to participants?

3. Was any type of coercion or undue influence used in recruiting participants? Were vulnerable subjects used?

4. Were participants deceived in any way? Were they fully aware of participating in a study, and did they understand the purpose of the research? Were appropriate consent procedures implemented?

5. Were appropriate steps taken to safeguard the privacy of participants?

6. Was the research approved and monitored by an Institutional Review Board or other similar ethics review committee?

situations, the absence of privacy raises not only ethical concerns but also questions regarding the participants' candor.

RESEARCH EXAMPLES

Two research examples that highlight ethical issues are presented below. Use the guidelines in Box 4-2 to evaluate the ethical aspects of the studies. You may need to review the actual research reports (cited at the end of the chapter) to assess more fully the adequacy of the steps the researchers took to safeguard the participants.

RESEARCH EXAMPLE OF A QUANTITATIVE STUDY

Mikhail (1999) conducted a study to describe the prenatal care experiences of low-income African American women and to identify their perceived impediments to prenatal care.

Research Summary

Mikhail recruited a sample of 126 women who had given birth in the previous year from three community agencies that offer services to low-income women. The data were collected at the study sites through a face-to-face interview and a self-administered questionnaire.

The study design was approved by the researcher's IRB and by all agencies in which data were collected. The study was described to potential participants, who were also provided with a consent form. Those who agreed to participate were asked to sign the form. The study participants were recruited and interviewed by an African American woman, who obtained data on the women's experiences with their last pregnancy. The women were then asked to complete a questionnaire on the perceived impediments to prenatal care.

The findings indicated that, despite the fact that 90% of the women were receiving Medicaid benefits and thus could access prenatal care services at no or nominal cost, only about one third of the women had adequate prenatal care. The impediments to care that were cited most frequently were transportation, long waiting time, and having too many other problems. Four of the impediments distinguished between those who did and did not have adequate prenatal care: substance abuse, fear of medical examination, the belief that prenatal care is not necessary, and lack of child care for other children.

Clinical Relevance

Early and regular prenatal care is widely accepted as an important determinant of maternal health during the pregnancy and of birth outcomes. There is also substantial evidence that African American women are more likely than other women to obtain inadequate or no prenatal care and that

African American infants are at substantially higher risk for prematurity and low birth weight than other infants. Consequently, studies that shed light on factors influencing the use of prenatal care can play an important role in addressing these problems.

Although Mikhail's sample was relatively small, the study had many strengths, including a solid conceptual and theoretical foundation, the recruitment of participants from several agencies, the use of well-established data collection instruments, and careful data collection procedures. The research also appears to have adhered to ethical principles.

The study has a number of important implications for health care professionals, which were thoughtfully delineated by the researcher herself. Mikhail recommended a number of strategies to meet the women's psychosocial and practical needs, including arranging for on-site child care; offering transportation assistance; providing counseling services regarding family conflict, single parenting, and substance use; and making greater efforts in communicating with pregnant women to reduce their anxiety about the medical examination. The findings also suggest that nurses ought to make efforts to gain women's trust and to convey a caring presence so that the women are more receptive to advice about the importance of early and regular prenatal care. Finally, the findings indicate that strategies are needed to decrease long waiting times at obstetrical clinics and offices to make it more attractive for women to obtain prenatal care.

RESEARCH EXAMPLE OF A QUALITATIVE STUDY

Wackerbarth (1999) undertook an in-depth study designed to describe the dynamics of caregiver decision-making.

Research Summary

Wackerbarth's study focused on understanding the decision process among family caregivers of people with dementia. A local chapter of the Alzheimer's Association mailed 100 preinterview questionnaires with an introductory letter from the director of the chapter. Caregivers interested in participating in the study mailed back a completed consent form and the preinterview questionnaire. From the pool of 80 caregivers who returned the questionnaire, 28 were selected to be interviewed. The sample was carefully selected to represent a broad viewpoint for developing a decision-making model.

Wackerbarth's article carefully explained the attention that was paid to participants' rights in this study: (1) the study objectives and methods were described orally and in writing to ensure that they were understood; (2) an informed consent form, which highlighted the voluntary nature of participation and indicated the safeguards that would be taken to protect their confidentiality, was signed before data collection began; (3) all preinterview questionnaires, tape recordings, and interview transcripts were kept in a locked file cabinet; (4) no identifying information was appended to study materials; and (5) participants were asked to review written materials and to give permission before publication of quotes and study findings.

On the basis of the interviews, Wackerbarth developed a model charting the caregiving experience over time and documented decisions made to maintain tolerable situations. The model captured the intrapersonal struggle driving the decision-making efforts of caregivers who care for family members with dementia.

Clinical Relevance

Family members often care for loved ones with dementia for 10 years or more before institutionalization or the death of these people occurs. The stress of day-to-day decisions regarding all aspects of the loved ones' lives contributes to caregivers' burden. To understand the decisions confronting caregivers as the disease progresses, Wackerbarth viewed decision making as a process and not as an individual event.

Wackerbarth appropriately chose a qualitative design to gain insight into the dynamics of caregivers' decision making and was careful in her handling of ethical considerations. Her study was strengthened by having used multiple sources of data (preinterview questionnaires, individual interviews, and group interviews). Wackerbarth verified her preliminary decision-making model with three groups of caregivers who had not participated in the interviews and solicited feedback from the caregivers who had been interviewed, thereby strengthening the credibility of the findings.

Wackerbarth's decision-making model provides clinicians with an insider's perspective of the interpersonal struggle that characterizes the decision making of family members who care for loved ones with dementia. This model can be used as a first step in designing strategies to provide much-needed support for caregivers confronted with difficult decisions as the disease progresses and their ability to provide care diminishes. Five decision-making styles were identified in this study: caregivers who (1) plan ahead, (2) take one day at a time, (3) have difficulty implementing decisions, (4) receive support from service providers, and (5) feel that caregiving decisions are made by others or the disease itself. Health care providers can match specific interventions with the type of decision-making style of the caregiver to increase the efficacy of their support. Wackerbarth's model can also be used by clinicians for education of the caregivers and as a long-term planning model.

• • • • SUMMARY POINTS

- Because research has not always been conducted ethically, and because of the genuine ethical dilemmas researchers often face in designing studies that are both ethical and methodologically rigorous, **codes of ethics** have been developed to guide researchers.

- The three major ethical principles incorporated into most guidelines are beneficence, respect for human dignity, and justice.
- **Beneficence** involves the protection of participants from physical and psychological harm, protection of participants from exploitation, and the performance of some good.
- In evaluating the **risk/benefit ratio** of a study, consumers should weigh the benefits of participation against the costs to individual participants as well as the risks to participants against the potential benefits to society.
- Respect for human dignity includes the participants' right to self-determination, which means participants have the freedom to control their own activities, including their voluntary participation in the study.
- **Full disclosure** means the researcher has fully described to prospective participants their rights and the full nature of the study. When full disclosure poses the risk of biased results, researchers sometimes use **covert data collection** or concealment (the collection of information without the participants' knowledge or consent) or deception (either withholding information from participants or providing false information).
- **Informed consent** procedures, which provide prospective participants with information needed to make a reasoned decision about participation, normally involve the signing of a **consent form** to document voluntary and informed participation. In qualitative studies, consent may need to be continually renegotiated with participants as the study evolves, through **process consent** procedures.
- Justice includes the right to fair treatment and to privacy. Privacy can be maintained through **anonymity** (wherein not even the researcher knows the identity of the participants) or through formal **confidentiality** procedures that safeguard the information participants provide.
- **Vulnerable subjects** require additional protection as study participants. These people may be vulnerable because they are not able to make a truly informed decision about study participation (*e.g.*, children); because their circumstances make them believe free choice is constrained (*e.g.*, prisoners); or because their circumstances heighten the risk of physical or psychological harm (*e.g.*, pregnant women).
- External review of the ethical aspects of a study by a human subjects committee or **Institutional Review Board (IRB)** is highly desirable and may be required by either the agency funding the research or the organization from which participants are recruited.

➤ ➤ ➤ ➤ *CRITICAL THINKING ACTIVITIES*

Chapter 4 of the accompanying *Study Guide to Accompany Essentials of Nursing Research*, 5th edition offers various exercises and study suggestions for reinforcing the concepts presented in this chapter. In addition, you can address the following:

1. Read the introduction and method section from one or both of the actual research studies in the Appendix of this book, and then answer the questions in Box 4-2.

2. How comfortable would you have felt as a participant in the studies described in the Appendix? How likely is it that some of the participants in the study might have felt uncomfortable or anxious?

For additional review, see questions 36–47 on the study CD provided with Polit: Study Guide to Accompany Essentials of Nursing Research.

SUGGESTED READINGS

References on Research Ethics

American Nurses Association. (1975). *Human rights guidelines for nurses in clinical and other research.* Kansas City, MO: Author.

American Nurses Association. (1985). *Code for nurses with interpretive statements.* Kansas City, MO: Author.

American Psychological Association. (1982). *Ethical principles in the conduct of research with human participants.* Washington, DC: Author.

American Sociological Association. (1984). *Code of ethics.* Washington, DC: Author.

Munhall, P. L. (1988). Ethical considerations in qualitative research. *Western Journal of Nursing Research, 10,* 150–162.

National Commission for the Protection of Human Subjects of Biomedical and Behavioral Research. (1978). *Belmont Report: Ethical principles and guidelines for research involving human subjects.* Washington, DC: U. S. Government Printing Office.

Substantive References

Coyne, M. L., Reinert, B., Cater, K., Dubuisson, W., Smith, J., Parker, M., & Chatham, C. (1999). Nurses' knowledge of pain assessment, pharmacologic and nonpharmacologic interventions. *Clinical Nursing Research, 8,* 153–165.

Mate-Kole, C., Danquah, S., Twum, M., & Danquah, A. (1999). Outcomes of a nonaversive behavior intervention in intellectually impaired individuals using goal attainment scaling. *Nursing Research, 48,* 220–225.

Menzel, L. K. (1999). Ventilated patients' self-esteem during intubation and after extubation. *Clinical Nursing Research, 8,* 51–68.

Mikhail, B. I. (1999). Perceived impediments to prenatal care among low-income women. *Western Journal of Nursing Research, 21,* 335–355.

Thurmond, J. A. (1999). Nurses' perceptions of chemical restraint use in long-term care. *Applied Nursing Research, 12,* 159–162.

Varda, K. E., & Behnke, R. S. (2000). The effect of timing of initial bath on newborn's temperature. *Journal of Obstetric, Gynecologic, and Neonatal Nursing, 29,* 27–32.

Wackerbarth, S. (1999). Modeling a dynamic decision process: Supporting the decisions of caregivers of family members with dementia. *Qualitative Health Research, 9,* 294–314.

PART II

PRELIMINARY STEPS IN THE RESEARCH PROCESS

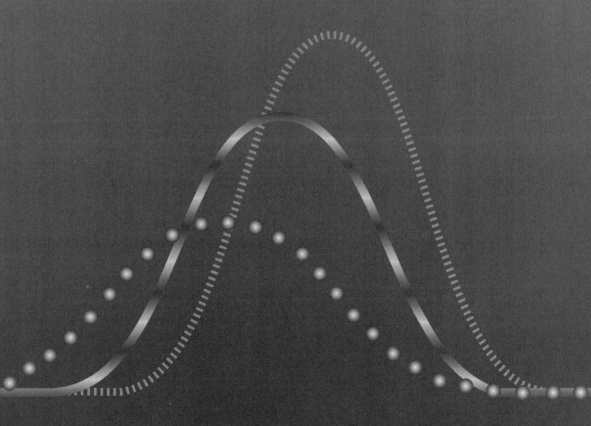

Scrutinizing Research Problems, Research Questions, and Hypotheses

● ●

Student Objectives

On completion of this chapter, the student will be able to:

○ evaluate the compatibility of a research problem and a paradigm

○ describe the process of developing and refining a research problem

○ distinguish the functions and forms of statements of purpose and research questions for quantitative and qualitative studies

○ describe the function and characteristics of research hypotheses and distinguish different types of hypotheses (*e.g.,* directional versus nondirectional, research versus null)

○ critique statements of purpose, research questions, and hypotheses in research reports with respect to their placement, clarity, wording, and significance to nursing

○ define new terms in the chapter

● ●

New Terms

Directional hypothesis	Research aim
Hypothesis	Research hypothesis
Nondirectional hypothesis	Research problem
Null hypothesis	Research question
Problem statement	Statement of purpose
	Statistical hypothesis

RESEARCH PROBLEMS AND RESEARCH QUESTIONS

A research study begins as a problem that a researcher would like to solve or as a question that a researcher would like to answer. This chapter discusses the formulation and evaluation of research problems, research questions, and hypotheses. We begin by clarifying some related terms.

Basic Terms Relating to Research Problems

At the most general level, a researcher is interested in a topic, which is sometimes referred to as the **focus** of the research. Patient compliance, coping with disability, and pain management are examples of research topics. Within these broad topic areas are many potential research questions or research problems. In this section, we illustrate various terms using the topic *side effects in chemotherapy patients.*

A **research problem** involves an enigmatic, perplexing, or troubling condition. The purpose of disciplined research is to "solve" the problem—or to contribute to its solution—by accumulating relevant information. A **problem**

statement articulates the problem to be addressed. Table 5-1 presents a problem statement related to the topic of side effects in chemotherapy patients.

A **research question** is a statement of the specific query the researcher wants to answer, to address the research problem. The research question or questions guide the types of data to be collected in the study. A researcher who makes a prediction regarding answers to the research question poses a **hypothesis** that is tested empirically. Examples of both research questions and hypotheses are presented in Table 5-1.

In a research report, consumers might also encounter other related terms. For example, many reports include a **statement of purpose** (or purpose statement), which is the researcher's summary of the overall study goal. A researcher might also identify several specific **research aims** or *objectives*—the specific accomplishments the researcher hopes to achieve by conducting the study. The objectives include obtaining answers to the research questions but may also encompass some broader aims (*e.g.,* to develop recommendations

---

TABLE 5-1. Example of Terms Relating to Research Problems

TERM	EXAMPLE
Topic/focus	Side effects in chemotherapy patients
Problem statement	Nausea and vomiting are common side effects among chemotherapy patients, and interventions to date have been only moderately successful in reducing these effects. New interventions that can reduce or prevent these side effects need to be identified.
Research question	What is the relative effectiveness of patient-controlled antiemetic therapy versus nurse-controlled antiemetic therapy with regard to (1) medication consumption and (2) control of nausea and vomiting in chemotherapy patients?
Hypotheses	(1) Subjects receiving antiemetic therapy by way of a patient-controlled pump will report less nausea than subjects receiving the therapy by way of nurse administration. (2) Subjects receiving antiemetic therapy by way of a patient-controlled pump will vomit less than subjects receiving the therapy by way of nurse administration. (3) Subjects receiving antiemetic therapy by way of a patient-controlled pump will consume less medication than subjects receiving the therapy by way of nurse administration.
Statement of purpose	The purpose of the study is to test an intervention to reduce chemotherapy-induced side effects—specifically, to compare the effectiveness of patient-controlled and nurse-administered antiemetic therapy for controlling nausea and vomiting in chemotherapy patients.
Aims/objectives	This study seeks to accomplish the following objectives: (1) to develop and implement two alternative procedures for administering antiemetic therapy for patients receiving moderate emetogenic chemotherapy (patient controlled versus nurse controlled); (2) to test three hypotheses concerning the relative effectiveness of the alternative procedures on medication consumption and control of side effects; and (3) to use the findings to develop recommendations for possible changes to therapeutic procedures.

for changes to nursing practice based on the study results), as illustrated in Table 5-1.

Research Problems and Paradigms

Some research problems are better suited for studies using qualitative versus quantitative methods. Quantitative studies usually involve concepts that are well developed and for which reliable measurement methods have been developed. For example, a quantitative study might be undertaken to determine whether postpartum depression is higher among women who return to work 6 months after delivery than among those who stay home with their babies. There are relatively accurate measures of depression that would yield quantitative information about the level of depression in a sample of employed and nonemployed postpartum women.

Qualitative studies are often undertaken because some aspect of a concept is poorly understood, and the researcher wants to develop a rich, comprehensive, and context-bound understanding of a phenomenon. In the example of postpartum depression, qualitative methods would not be well suited to comparing levels of depression among the two groups of women, but they would be ideal for exploring, for example, the *meaning* of postpartum depression among new mothers. In evaluating a research report, an important consideration is whether the research problem fits the chosen paradigm and its associated methods.

Sources of Research Problems

Where do ideas for research problems come from? At the most basic level, research topics originate with the researcher's interests. Because research is a time-consuming enterprise, curiosity about and interest in a topic are essential to the success of the project. Explicit sources that might fuel the researcher's curiosity include the following:

- *Clinical experience.* The nurse's everyday experience provides a rich supply of problems for investigation. Problems that are in need of immediate solution have high potential for clinical significance.
- *Nursing literature.* Ideas for studies often come from reading the nursing literature, including research reports, opinion articles, and summaries of clinical issues. Research reports may suggest problem areas indirectly by stimulating the reader's imagination and directly by explicitly stating what additional research is needed.
- *Social issues.* Topics are sometimes suggested by global social issues of relevance to the health care community. For example, the feminist movement has raised questions about such topics as gender equity and domestic violence.
- *Theories.* Another source of problems lies in theories from nursing and other related disciplines. Beginning with a theory, the researcher asks,

If this theory is correct, what would I predict about people's behaviors, states, or feelings? The predictions can then be tested through research.

• *Ideas from external sources.* External sources can sometimes provide the impetus for a research idea. For example, ideas for studies may emerge from reviewing research priorities or as a result of a brainstorming session with other nurses, researchers, or nursing faculty.

Development and Refinement of Research Problems

The development of a research problem is a creative process. Researchers often begin with an interest in a topic area, and then develop the topic into a more specific researchable problem. As an example, suppose a nurse working on a medical unit observed that some patients complained about having to wait for pain medication when certain nurses were assigned to them. The nurse wonders why this occurs. The general research problem is discrepancy in complaints from patients regarding pain medications administered by different nurses. The nurse might ask, What accounts for this discrepancy? or, How could this situation be altered? These questions are too broad to be research questions, but they may lead to other questions, such as, How do the two groups of nurses differ? or What characteristics do the complaining patients share? At this point, the nurse may observe that the cultural background of the patients and nurses appears to be a relevant factor. This may direct the nurse to a review of the literature for studies concerning ethnic groups and their relationship to nursing behaviors, or it may provoke a discussion of these observations with peers. These efforts may result in several research questions, such as the following:

• What is the essence of patient complaints among patients of different ethnic backgrounds?
• How do complaints by patients of different ethnic backgrounds get expressed by patients and perceived by nurses?
• Is the ethnic background of nurses related to the frequency with which they dispense pain medication?
• Is the ethnic background of patients related to the frequency and intensity of their complaints of having to wait for pain medication?
• Does the number of patient complaints increase when the patients are of dissimilar ethnic backgrounds as opposed to when they are of the same ethnic background as the nurse?
• Do nurses' dispensing behaviors change as a function of the similarity between their own ethnic background and that of the patients?

These questions stem from the same general problem, yet each would be studied differently; for example, some suggest a qualitative approach, and others suggest a quantitative one. A quantitative researcher might become curious about nurses' dispensing behaviors, based on some evidence in the literature regarding ethnic differences. Both ethnicity and nurses' dispensing behaviors are variables that can be reliably measured. A qualitative researcher who noticed differences in patient complaints would likely be more interested in understanding the essence of the complaints, the patients' experience of frustration, the process by which the problem got resolved, or the full nature of the nurse–patient interactions regarding the dispensing of medications. These are aspects of the research problem that would be difficult to measure quantitatively. Researchers choose the final problem to be studied based on several factors, including its inherent interest to them and its compatibility with a paradigm of preference.

COMMUNICATING THE RESEARCH PROBLEM, PURPOSE, AND QUESTIONS

Researchers communicate their research problems in various ways in research reports. This section discusses the wording and placement of problem statements, statements of purpose, and research questions, and the following major section discusses hypotheses.

Problem Statements

A problem statement is an expression of the dilemma or disturbing situation that needs investigation. A problem statement identifies the nature of the problem that is being addressed in the study and, typically, its context and significance. Generally, the problem statement should be broad enough to include central concerns but narrow enough in scope to serve as a guide to study design.

**▣▣   *Example of a problem statement from a quantitative study:*

Hazardous noise is an important occupational health problem because it leads to hearing loss and may lead to increased stress and other deleterious physiological effects. . . . More than 30 million workers are exposed to hazardous noise on the job. . . . Use of hearing protection devices, specifically ear plugs and/or ear muffs, is known to reduce noise exposure and prevent noise-induced hearing loss. . . . There are, however, relatively few investigators who have examined factors related to the low use of hearing protection by workers (Lusk, Ronis, & Hogan, 1997).

In this example, the general topic is hazardous on-the-job noise, but the investigators narrowed the scope of their inquiry to factors affecting the low use of hearing protection by workers. This problem statement asserted the nature of the health problem and indicated its breadth (30 million workers). It also provided a rationale and justification for conducting a new study: the dearth of existing studies on the topic.

The problem statement for a qualitative study similarly expresses the nature of the problem, its context, and its significance.

> 🔳 **Example of a problem statement from a qualitative study:**
>
> Members of cultural minority groups may find themselves surrounded by people whose values, beliefs, and interpretations differ from their own during hospitalization. This is often the case for Canada's aboriginal population, as many live in culturally distinct communities . . . . To promote healing among clients from minority cultural communities, it is important for nurses to understand the phenomenon of receiving care in an unfamiliar culture. This exploratory study examined how members of the Big Cove Mi'kmaq First Nation Community . . . subjectively experienced being cared for in a nonaboriginal institution (Baker & Daigle, 2000).

As in the previous example, the researchers clearly articulated the nature of the problem and the justification for conducting a new study.

> 🔳 **CONSUMER TIP:**
>
> Problem statements generally appear in the introduction to a research report and are often interwoven with a review of the literature, which provides context by documenting knowledge gaps. They are rarely labeled "problem statement" and must therefore be ferreted out. ■

Statements of Purpose

Many researchers first articulate their goals as a broad statement of purpose, worded in the declarative form. The purpose statement captures, in one or two sentences, the essence of the study and establishes the general direction of the inquiry. The words *purpose* or *goal* usually appear in a purpose statement (*e.g.,* "The purpose of this study was. . ." or "The goal of this study was. . ."), but sometimes the words *intent, aim,* or *objective* are used instead.

In a quantitative study, a well-worded statement of purpose identifies the key study variables and their possible interrelationships as well as the nature of the population of interest.

> 🔳 **Example of a statement of purpose from a quantitative study:**
>
> The purpose of this study was to examine the relationship between nursing care and the development of sleep–wake states in high-risk preterm infants (Brandon, Holditch-Davis, & Beylea, 1999).

This statement identifies the population of interest (preterm infants), the independent variable (nursing care), and the dependent variable (the infants' sleep–wake states).

In qualitative studies, the statement of purpose indicates the nature of the inquiry, the key concept or phenomenon under investigation, and the group, community, or setting under study.

> **Example of a statement of purpose from a qualitative study:**
>
> The purpose of this study was to describe end-of-life care in intensive care units as perceived by critical care nurses who have taken care of dying patients (Kirchhoff, Spuhler, Walker, Hutton, Cole, & Clemmer, 2000).

This statement indicates that the central phenomenon of interest is end-of-life care and that the group under study is dying patients and critical care nurses caring for them.

The statement of purpose communicates more than just the nature of the problem. Through the researcher's selection of verbs, a purpose statement suggests the state of knowledge on the topic or the manner in which the researcher sought to solve the problem. A study whose purpose is to *explore* or *describe* a phenomenon is likely to focus on a little-researched topic; such a study often involves a qualitative approach. A statement of purpose for a qualitative study may also imply a flexible design through the use of verbs such as *understand, discover,* and *develop.* By contrast, a purpose statement indicating that the purpose is to *test* the effectiveness of some intervention or to *compare* two alternative nursing strategies suggests a study with a more established knowledge base, using a quantitative approach and perhaps a design with tight controls. Note that the researcher's choice of verbs in a statement of purpose should connote a certain degree of objectivity. A statement of purpose indicating that the intent of the study was to *prove, demonstrate,* or *show* something suggests a bias on the part of the researcher.

Research Questions

Research questions are, in some cases, direct rewordings of statements of purpose, phrased interrogatively rather than declaratively. The research questions for the examples cited earlier might be as follows:

- What is the relationship between nursing care and the development of sleep–wake states in high-risk preterm infants?
- What influence does chronic and potentially fatal illness have on the caregiving process over time among family caregivers?

Questions that are simple and direct invite an answer and help to focus attention on the kinds of data needed to provide that answer. Some research reports thus omit a statement of purpose and state only the research question. Other researchers use a set of research questions to clarify or amplify the purpose statement.

> **Example of research questions clarifying a statement of purpose:**
>
> *Statement of purpose:* The purpose of this study was to explore the relationship between method of pain management during labor and specific labor and birth outcomes.

Research questions: Are nonepidural and epidural methods of pain relief associated with augmentation during the first stage of labor? Is the length of second stage labor associated with epidural and nonepidural methods of pain relief? Are newborn Apgar scores at 1 minute and 5 minutes associated with method of pain relief? Does epidural anesthesia affect maternal temperature? (Walker & O'Brien, 1999)

In this example, the statement of purpose provides a global message about the researchers' goal. The research questions delineated the two methods of pain management being compared, and the labor and birth outcomes of interest.

In a quantitative study, research questions identify the key variables (most often, the independent and dependent variable), the relationships among them, and the population under study.

Example of a research question from a quantitative study:

Are there group differences in the perceived levels of stress, social support, and immune responses between healthy and asthmatic adolescents (Kang, Coe, Karaszewski, & McCarthy, 1998)?

In this example, the independent variable is whether or not the person has asthma; the dependent variables are perceived levels of stress, social support, and immune responses; and the population under study is adolescents.

In qualitative studies, the research question may evolve over the course of the study. The researcher begins with a focus that defines the general boundaries of the inquiry. However, in a qualitative study the boundaries are not cast in stone; the boundaries "can be altered and, in the typical naturalistic inquiry, will be" (Lincoln & Guba, p. 228). The naturalist thus begins with a research question in mind but is sufficiently flexible that the question can be modified as new information makes it relevant to do so. As we will discuss in Chapter 9, several disciplines provide alternative traditions for qualitative research, and these traditions vary in their conceptualization of what types of questions are important and what type of methods should be used to answer them.

Example of a research question from a qualitative study:

What are the fears, concerns, or questions of women who have experienced a hysterectomy (Wade, Pletsch, Morgan, & Menting, 2000)?

CONSUMER TIP:

Researchers most often state their purpose or research questions at the end of the introduction or immediately after the review of the literature. Sometimes, a separate section of a research report—typically located just before the method section—is devoted to stating the research problem formally and might be labeled "Purpose," "Statement of Purpose," or "Research Questions." ■

RESEARCH HYPOTHESES

In quantitative studies, researchers often present a statement of purpose and then one or more hypotheses. A hypothesis is a tentative prediction about the relationship between two or more variables in the population under study. In a qualitative study, the researcher does not begin with a hypothesis, in part because there is generally too little known about the topic to justify a hypothesis and in part because qualitative researchers want their inquiry to be guided by participants' viewpoints rather than by their own (although some qualitative studies may lead to the formulation of hypotheses). Thus, our discussion here focuses on hypotheses in quantitative research.

Function of Hypotheses in Quantitative Research

A hypothesis translates a research question into a prediction of expected outcomes. For instance, the research question might ask: Does the temperature of normal saline used in endotracheal suctioning affect heart rate alterations? The researcher might hypothesize as follows: Room-temperature normal saline used in endotracheal suctioning results in a greater decline in heart rate alterations than body temperature normal saline.

Hypotheses sometimes emerge from a theoretical framework. The scientist reasons from theories to hypotheses and tests those hypotheses in the real world. The validity of a theory is never examined directly, but the worth of a theory can be evaluated through hypothesis testing. For example, the theory of reinforcement maintains that behavior or activity that is positively reinforced (rewarded) tends to be learned or repeated. The theory is too abstract to test, but predictions (hypotheses) based on the theory can be tested. For instance, the following hypotheses have been deduced from reinforcement theory:

- Elderly patients who are praised (reinforced) by nursing personnel for self-feeding require less assistance in feeding than patients who are not praised.
- Pediatric patients who are given a reward (*e.g.,* a snack treat or permission to watch television) when they cooperate during nursing procedures are more compliant during those procedures than nonrewarded peers.

Both of these propositions can be tested in the real world. The theory gains support if the hypotheses are confirmed.

Even in the absence of a theoretical underpinning, well-conceived hypotheses can offer direction and suggest explanations. For example, suppose we hypothesized that nurses with a baccalaureate education are more likely to experience stress in their first nursing job than nurses with a diploma-school education. This prediction could be based on theory (*e.g.,* role conflict theory), earlier studies, or personal observations.

The development of predictions in and of itself forces the researcher to think logically, to exercise critical judgment, and to tie together earlier research findings.

Now let us suppose the above hypothesis is not confirmed by the evidence collected; that is, we find that baccalaureate and diploma nurses experience comparable stress in their first nursing assignment.

The failure of data to support a prediction forces the investigator to analyze theory or previous research critically, to review the limitations of the study's methods carefully, and to explore alternative explanations for the findings.

The use of hypotheses in quantitative studies tends to induce critical thinking and, hence, to facilitate interpretation of the data.

To further illustrate the utility of hypotheses, suppose the researcher conducted the study guided only by the research question, Is there a relationship between a nurse's educational preparation and the degree of stress experienced on the first job? The investigator without a hypothesis is, apparently, prepared to accept any results. The problem is that it is almost always possible to explain something superficially after the fact, no matter what the findings are. Hypotheses guard against superficiality and minimize the possibility that spurious results will be misconstrued.

 CONSUMER TIP:

Some quantitative research reports explicitly state the research hypotheses that guided the investigation, but most do not. In some cases, the absence of a hypothesis is appropriate, but often, the absence of a hypothesis is an indication that the researcher has failed to consider critically the implications of theory or the existing knowledge base or has failed to disclose the hunches that may have influenced the design of the study. ■

Characteristics of Testable Hypotheses

Testable research hypothesis state the expected relationship between the independent variable (the presumed cause or antecedent) and the dependent variable (the presumed effect) within a population.

 Example of a research hypothesis:

Women diagnosed with preterm labor who receive relaxation therapy will have longer pregnancies than will women who do not receive relaxation therapy (Janke, 1999).

In this example, the independent variable is whether or not a woman with preterm labor received relaxation therapy, and the dependent variable is length of pregnancy. The hypothesis predicts that these two variables are related—longer pregnancies are expected among women who receive the therapy.

Unfortunately, researchers occasionally present hypotheses that fail to make a relational statement. For example, the following prediction is not a testable research hypothesis: Pregnant women who receive prenatal instruction by a nurse regarding the postpartum experience are not likely to experience postpartum depression. This statement expresses no anticipated relationship; in fact, there is only one variable (postpartum depression), and a relationship by definition requires at least two variables. This prediction, however, can be altered to make it a suitable hypothesis with an independent variable and dependent variable: Pregnant women who receive prenatal instruction are less likely to experience postpartum depression than pregnant women with no prenatal instruction. Here, the dependent variable is the women's depression and the independent variable is their receipt or nonreceipt of prenatal instruction.

The relational aspect of the prediction is embodied in the phrase "less . . . than." If a hypothesis lacks a phrase such as *more than, less than, greater than, different from, related to,* or something similar, it is not amenable to testing. As an example of why this is so, consider the original prediction: Pregnant women who receive prenatal instruction are not likely to experience postpartum depression. How would we know whether this hypothesis was supported—what absolute standard could be used to decide whether to accept or reject the hypothesis? To illustrate the problem more concretely, suppose we asked a group of mothers who received prenatal instructional the following question 1 month after delivery: On the whole, how depressed have you been since you gave birth? Would you say:

1. Extremely depressed
2. Moderately depressed
3. Somewhat depressed
4. Not at all depressed

Based on this question, how could we compare the actual outcome with the predicted outcome? Would all the women in the sample have to say they were not at all depressed? Would the prediction be supported if 51% of the women said they were not at all depressed or only somewhat depressed? There is no adequate way of testing the accuracy of the prediction. A test is simple, however, if we modify the prediction, as suggested previously, to "Pregnant women who receive prenatal instruction are less likely to experience postpartum depression than those with no prenatal instruction." We would ask two groups of women with different prenatal instruction experiences to respond to the question and then compare the responses. The absolute degree of depression of either group would not be at issue.

Hypotheses, ideally, should be based on sound, justifiable rationales. The most defensible hypotheses follow from previous research findings or are deduced from a theory. When a relatively new area is being investigated, the researcher may have to turn to logical reasoning or personal experience to justify the predictions.

 CONSUMER TIP:

If a research report includes the researcher's hypotheses, they usually appear at the end of the introduction, just before the method section. Hypotheses are typically fairly easy to find and identify because the researcher makes a statement such as, "The study tested the following hypotheses . . ." or, "It was hypothesized that. . . ." ■

Wording of the Hypothesis

Hypotheses state the expected relationship between the independent variables and dependent variables. A hypothesis can predict the relationship between a single independent variable and a single dependent variable (a *simple hypothesis*), or it can predict a relationship between two or more independent variables or two or more dependent variables (a *complex hypothesis*). In the following examples, independent variables are indicated as IVs and dependent variables are identified as DVs:

Example of a simple hypothesis:

Lower levels of exercise postpartum (IV) will be associated with greater weight retention (DV) (Sampselle, Seng, Yeo, Killion, & Oakley, 1999).

Example of a complex hypothesis—multiple independent variables:

Low-risk pregnant women who (1) value health highly, (2) believe that engaging in health-promoting behaviors will result in positive outcomes, and (3) perceive fewer barriers to health-promoting activities (IVs) are more likely than other women to attend pregnancy-related educational programs (DV) (Serafine & Broom, 1999).

Example of a complex hypothesis—multiple dependent variables:

The implementation of an evidence-based protocol for urinary incontinence (IV) will result in (1) decreased frequency of urinary incontinence episodes, (2) decreased urine loss per episode, and (3) decreased avoidance of activities (DVs) among women in ambulatory care settings (Sampselle, Wyman, Thomas, Newman, Gray, Dougherty, & Burns, 2000).

Hypotheses can be stated in various ways as long as the researcher specifies or implies the relationship that will be tested. Here is an example:

1. Lower levels of exercise postpartum are associated with greater weight retention.

2. There is a relationship between level of exercise postpartum and weight retention.
3. The greater the level of exercise postpartum, the lower the weight retention.
4. Women with different levels of exercise postpartum differ with regard to weight retention.
5. Weight retention postpartum decreases as the woman's level of exercise increases.
6. Women who exercise vigorously postpartum have lower weight retention than women who do not.

Other variations are also possible. The important point to remember is that the hypothesis specifies the independent variable (here, level of exercise), the dependent variable (weight retention), and the anticipated relationship between them.

Hypotheses, ideally, are worded in the present tense. The researcher makes a prediction about a relationship in the population—not just about a relationship that will be revealed in a particular sample of study participants.

Hypotheses can be either directional or nondirectional. A **directional hypothesis** is one that specifies the expected direction of the relationship between variables. That is, the researcher predicts not only the existence of a relationship but also its nature. In the six versions of the same hypothesis above, versions 1, 3, 5, and 6 are directional because there is an explicit prediction that women who do not exercise postpartum are at greater risk of weight retention than women who do. A **nondirectional hypothesis,** by contrast, does not stipulate the direction of the relationship, as illustrated in versions 2 and 4. These hypotheses predict that a woman's level of exercise and weight retention are related, but they do not stipulate whether the researcher thinks that exercise is related to more or less weight retention.

Hypotheses derived from theory are usually directional because theories provide a rationale for expecting variables to relate in certain ways. Existing studies also offer a basis for specifying directional hypotheses. When there is no theory or related research, when the findings of prior studies are contradictory, or when the researcher's own experience results in ambivalent expectations, the investigator may use nondirectional hypotheses. Some people argue, in fact, that nondirectional hypotheses are preferable because they connote a degree of impartiality. Directional hypotheses, it is said, imply that the researcher is intellectually committed to a certain outcome, and such a commitment might lead to bias. This argument fails to recognize that researchers typically do have hunches about the outcomes, whether they state those expectations explicitly or not. We prefer directional hypotheses—when there is a reasonable basis for them—because they demonstrate that the researcher has thought critically about the phenomena under investigation and because they clarify the study's framework.

Another distinction is the difference between research and null hypotheses. **Research hypotheses** (also referred to as *substantive, declarative,* or *scien-*

tific hypotheses) are statements of expected relationships between variables. Such hypotheses indicate what the researcher expects to find as a result of conducting a study.

The logic of statistical inference, which is used in hypothesis testing, dictates that, for the purposes of the statistical analysis, hypotheses be expressed as though no relationship were expected. **Null hypotheses** (or **statistical hypotheses**) state that there is no relationship between the independent variables and dependent variables. The null form of the hypothesis used in our preceding examples would be: Weight retention is unrelated to exercise levels postpartum. The null hypothesis might be compared to the assumption of innocence of an accused criminal in the U.S. system of justice; the variables are assumed to be "innocent" of any relationship until they can be shown to be "guilty" through statistical procedures. The null hypothesis is the formal statement of this presumed innocence.

Research reports typically present research rather than null hypotheses. When statistical tests are performed, the underlying null hypotheses are assumed without being explicitly stated. If the researcher's actual research hypothesis is that no relationship among variables exists, the hypothesis cannot be adequately tested using traditional statistical procedures. This issue is explained in Chapter 13.

 CONSUMER TIP:

If the researcher used any statistical tests (and most quantitative studies do use them), it means that there are underlying hypotheses—whether the researcher explicitly stated them or not—because statistical tests are designed to test hypotheses. ■

Hypothesis Testing and Proof

Hypotheses are never *proved* through hypothesis testing; rather, they are *accepted* or *supported*. Findings are always tentative. Certainly, if the same results are replicated in numerous investigations, greater confidence can be placed in the conclusions. Hypotheses come to be increasingly supported with mounting evidence.

Let us look more closely at why this is so. Suppose we hypothesized that height and weight are related. We predict that, on average, tall people weigh more than short people. We would then obtain height and weight measurements from a sample and analyze the data. Now suppose we happened by chance to choose a sample that consisted of short, fat people, and tall, thin people. Our results might indicate that there is no relationship between a person's height and weight. Would we then be justified in stating that this study *proved* or *demonstrated* that height and weight in humans are unrelated?

As another example, suppose we hypothesize that tall people are better nurses than short people. This hypothesis is used here only to illustrate a point because, in reality, we would expect no relationship between height and a nurse's job performance. Now suppose that, by chance again, we draw a sample of nurses in which tall nurses received better job evaluations than short ones. Could we conclude definitively that height is related to a nurse's performance? These two examples illustrate the difficulty of using observations from a sample to generalize to the population from which the sample has been taken. Other problems, such as the accuracy of the measures, the validity of underlying assumptions, and the reasonableness of the logical deductions, prohibit researchers from concluding with finality that hypotheses are proved.

CRITIQUING RESEARCH PROBLEMS, RESEARCH QUESTIONS, AND HYPOTHESES

In critiquing research reports, you will need to evaluate the extent to which the researcher has adequately communicated the research problem. The researcher's description of the problem, the statement of the study purpose, the research questions, and the hypotheses set the stage for the description of what was done and what was learned by the researcher. Ideally, you should not have to dig too deeply to decipher the research problem or to discover the questions.

Critiquing the Significance of a Research Problem

A critique of the research problem involves multiple dimensions, including a substantive dimension. That is, you need to consider whether the problem has significance for nursing. The following issues are relevant in considering the significance of a study problem:

1. *Implications for nursing practice.* A primary consideration in evaluating the significance of a research problem for a nursing study is whether it has the potential to produce findings that can improve nursing practice. The following questions should be posed: Are there practical applications that might stem from research on the problem? Will more knowledge about the problem make a difference that matters to practicing nurses? Will the findings challenge (or lend support to) untested assumptions about nursing or health status? If the answer to such questions is no, the significance of the problem is bound to be low. Numerous studies have focused on problems with strong implications for nursing practice. For example, researchers have studied (1) the effects of body posture on the pressure of seat surfaces, as a way to prevent pressure ulcers (Defloor & Grypdonck, 1999); (2) the effects of a structured protocol for identifying delirium in elderly patients (Lacko, Bryan, Dellasega, & Salerno, 1999); and (3) the effects of a nurse-delivered smoking cessation intervention for hospitalized cardiac patients (Johnson, Budz, Mackay, & Miller, 1999). These studies yielded information that can be used to improve patient care.

2. *Extension of knowledge base.* A study that extends, refines, or corroborates previous knowledge has a better chance of being significant than a study on an isolated research problem. Studies that build in a meaningful way on the existing knowledge base are most likely to be immediately useful to nursing practice. For example, Grey and colleagues (1999) tested a behavioral intervention for improving metabolic control in diabetic adolescents using a rigorous research design. Their study corroborated earlier positive findings that had been less conclusive because of their weaker designs. Researchers who develop a systematic program of research, building on their own earlier findings, are especially likely to make significant contributions. For example, Beck's series of studies relating to postpartum depression (*e.g.,* Beck & Gable, in press; Beck, 1995, 1996, 1998, 1999) have influenced women's health care worldwide.

3. *Promotion of theory development.* Studies that either test or develop a theory have a better chance of making a lasting contribution to knowledge than studies that do not have a conceptual context. For example, Durham (1999) conducted an in-depth study of the management of preterm labor and developed a theory that suggested improvements for clinical practice.

4. *Correspondence to research priorities.* Research priorities have been established by research scholars, agencies that fund nursing research (such as the National Institute of Nursing Research, and professional nursing organizations. Clearly, research problems stemming from such priorities have a high likelihood of yielding knowledge of importance to the nursing profession because they reflect expert opinion about areas of needed research. A research report typically indicates whether a study was based on a priority area. As an example, the Agency for Healthcare Research and Quality (AHRQ), formerly the Agency for Health Care Policy and Research (AHCPR), funds health services research on patient outcomes and the effectiveness of clinical practice and has also issued clinical practice guidelines in several areas. Devine and her colleagues (1999) conducted a study that specifically examined patient outcomes following AHRQ's guidelines on surgical pain management.

When critiquing a study, you need to consider whether the research problem was meaningfully based on prior research; has a relationship to a theoretical context; addresses a current research priority; and, most importantly, can improve nursing practice.

Critiquing Other Aspects of Research Problems

Another dimension in critiquing the research problem concerns methodologic issues—in particular, whether the research problem is compatible with the chosen research paradigm and its associated methods. You should also evaluate whether the statement of purpose or research questions have been properly worded and lend themselves to empirical inquiry.

In a quantitative study, if the research report does not contain explicit hypotheses, you need to consider whether their absence is justified. If there are hypotheses, you should evaluate whether the hypotheses are logically connected to the research problem and whether they are consistent with available knowledge or relevant theory. The wording of the hypothesis should also be assessed. The hypothesis is a valid guidepost to scientific inquiry only if it is testable. To be testable, the hypothesis must contain a prediction about the relationship between two or more variables that can be measured. The hypothesis must imply the criteria by which it could be rejected or accepted through the collection of empirical data.

Specific guidelines for critiquing research problems, research questions, and hypotheses are presented in Box 5-1.

BOX 5-1

GUIDELINES FOR CRITIQUING RESEARCH PROBLEMS, RESEARCH QUESTIONS, AND HYPOTHESES

1. What is the research problem? Has the researcher appropriately delimited the scope of the problem?

2. Does the problem have significance for the nursing profession? How will the research contribute to nursing practice, nursing administration, or nursing education?

3. Is there a good match between the research problem and the paradigm within which the research was conducted?

4. Is the problem to be addressed formally stated as a statement of purpose, research question, or hypothesis to be tested? Is this information communicated clearly and concisely?

5. Are the purpose statements and research questions worded appropriately (*e.g.,* are key concepts or variables identified and the study group or population of interest specified)?

6. If the report does not formally state any hypotheses, is their absence justifiable?

7. Do the hypotheses (if any) flow from a theory or from previous research? If not, what is the basis for the researcher's predictions?

8. Are hypotheses (if any) properly worded (*i.e.,* do they state a predicted relationship between two or more variables?)

9. Are hypotheses directional or nondirectional? Is there a rationale for the manner in which they were stated?

10. Are hypotheses stated as research hypotheses or null hypotheses?

RESEARCH EXAMPLES

This section describes how the research problem and research questions were communicated in two nursing studies, one quantitative and one qualitative. The guidelines in Box 5-1 may be useful in evaluating these aspects of the study.

RESEARCH EXAMPLE OF A QUANTITATIVE STUDY

Lindgren, Connelly, and Gaspar (1999) studied grief among the spouse and children caregivers of dementia patients. Their research appeared in the *Western Journal of Nursing Research*.

Research Summary

Lindgren and her colleagues noted that family caregivers of patients with dementia experience numerous losses arising directly and indirectly from the deteriorating health of their loved ones. Grief as a reaction to nondeath losses had previously been found to be part of their experience. However, the researchers noted that no prior study had actually measured grief during the caregiving of a patient.

As stated by the researchers, the purpose of their study "was to determine the patterns of grief of caregivers of family members with dementia and the relationship of those patterns to the losses and experiences of the caregivers" (p. 521).

Based on the overall study purpose, the researchers articulated six specific research questions:

1. What are the relationships between caregivers' expressions of grief and their levels of emotional health?
2. What are the relationship among caregivers' expressions of grief, impact of diagnosis, and length of time of caregiving?
3. What is the relationship between the afflicted individuals' deterioration and expressions of grief of caregivers?
4. What is the relationship between caregivers' previous affective relationships with afflicted individuals and expressions of grief?
5. What are the relationships between caregivers' losses of personal relationships with the afflicted individual and the expression of grief?
6. What are the relationships between the caregivers' losses of expectations of the future and their expressions of grief?

The data for the study were collected from 22 spouse caregivers and 11 adult children caregivers of family members with dementia. The study yielded a number of interesting results. For example, it was found that the higher the level of the caretaker's grief symptoms, the less emotionally healthy they saw themselves. However, grief symptoms were not related to the length of time of caregiving, nor to the ill family members' deterioration.

Clinical Relevance

It is estimated that 10% of the population older than 65 years of age suffers from Alzheimer's disease. This devastating chronic degenerative disease has powerful repercussions not only for the affected person but also for the entire family.

Lindgren and colleagues' study adds to nursing's body of knowledge regarding patterns of nondeath-related grief of caregivers whose loved ones struggle with dementia. Even though the generalizability of this study is constrained by its small sample size and other methodologic features, this research indicates that caregiver grief from chronic, nondeath losses is not uncommon and needs to be addressed by clinicians. Moreover, the findings indicate that the chronic grief or sorrow of caregivers of Alzheimer's victims remains at a relatively constant level through the caregiving experiences. On the basis of this information about the pattern of emotional hardship, nursing interventions can be designed to provide support for these caregivers who live in the "land of the living dead."

RESEARCH EXAMPLE OF A QUALITATIVE STUDY

Sherman and Kirton studied unsafe sexual behavior among men who previously tested positive for human immunodeficiency virus (HIV).

Research Summary

Sherman & Kirton (1999) examined the experience of relapse to unsafe sexual behavior among HIV-positive, heterosexual men. In describing their research problem, the researchers said that, despite numerous attempts to provide health education on HIV transmission and on the dangerous consequences of unsafe sexual behaviors, many HIV-infected adults relapse into unsafe practices. The overall purpose of their descriptive qualitative study was to investigate individual perceptions, modifying variables, and factors that influence health, beliefs, and sexual behavior in HIV-infected men who have reported they had relapsed into unsafe sexual behavior after practicing safer sex.

Sherman and Kirton identified five specific research objectives for their study (pp. 91–92):

1. Identify the individual's perceived susceptibility and perceived seriousness of the HIV health threat regarding progression to acquired immunodeficiency syndrome (AIDS).
2. Describe the nature and extent of the relapse event.
3. Identify modifying factors, internal or external cues, HIV knowledge, and social pressures that may influence sexual behaviors.

4. Explore personal attitudes toward sexual relapse.
5. Identify the perceived benefits and barriers and perceived sense of control related to safer sexual behaviors.

A sample of 18 heterosexual minority men participated in in-depth interviews. The researchers' analysis revealed nine themes that related to relapse to unsafe sexual practices: drug and alcohol use, state of mind, beliefs, weighing the risks, sexual preparation, influence of others, male–female relationship issues, uncontrollable sexual urges, and the symbolic meaning of condoms.

Clinical Relevance

Relapse to unsafe sexual behaviors in HIV-positive men is an important health problem because it not only places sexual partners at risk for acquiring HIV but also may increase the virulence of HIV and hasten its progression. Information about why HIV-positive men may engage in unsafe sexual practices has clear relevance for health professionals. Sherman and Kirton enhanced the utility of their study findings by taking a number of steps to ensure the trustworthiness of their data.

The researchers offered some specific implications for nursing practice based on the study findings. They suggested a two-tiered approach to sexual education. The first step would involve discussing human sexuality, variations in behaviors/needs, and approaches to promoting sexual health. The second step would then address HIV infections or acquired immunodeficiency syndrome (AIDS), other sexually transmitted diseases, and methods to protect against transmission. The study findings suggest that knowledge and availability of condoms are only two components of relapse prevention. The symbolic meaning of condoms is also a crucial factor in increasing safer sexual practices. Thus, one nursing intervention could focus on having open discussions with the HIV-positive adults about their perceptions and feelings associated with condom use.

• • • • • SUMMARY POINTS

- A **research problem** is a perplexing or enigmatic situation that a researcher wants to address through disciplined inquiry. The most common sources of ideas for nursing research problems are experience, relevant literature, social issues, theory, and external sources.
- The researcher usually identifies a broad topic or focus, and then narrows the scope of the problem and identifies questions consistent with a paradigm of choice.
- A **statement of purpose** summarizes the overall goal of the study; in both qualitative and quantitative studies, the purpose statement identifies the key concepts (variables) and the study group or population.
- A **research question** states the specific query the researcher wants to answer to address the research problem.

- A **hypothesis** is a statement of a predicted relationship between two or more variables. A testable hypothesis states the anticipated association between one or more independent and one or more dependent variables.
- A **directional hypothesis** specifies the expected direction or nature of a hypothesized relationship; **nondirectional hypotheses** predict a relationship but do not stipulate the form that the relationship will take.
- **Research hypotheses** predict the existence of relationships; **statistical**, or **null**, **hypotheses** express the absence of any relationship.
- Hypotheses are never proved or disproved in an ultimate sense—they are accepted or rejected, supported or not supported by the data.

➤ ➤ ➤ ➤ *CRITICAL THINKING ACTIVITIES*

Chapter 5 of the accompanying *Study Guide to Accompany Essentials of Nursing Research,* 5th edition offers various exercises and study suggestions for reinforcing the concepts presented in this chapter. In addition, you can address the following:

1. Read the introduction from one or both of the actual research studies in the Appendix of this book. Which of the following are explicitly stated in the research report: problem statement; statement of purpose; research questions; hypotheses; aim/objective? Where in the research report were these elements presented?

2. Respond to the questions in Box 5-1 with regard to one or both of the research reports in the Appendix.

For additional review, see questions 48–61 on the study CD provided with Polit: Study Guide to Accompany Essentials of Nursing Research.

SUGGESTED READINGS

Methodologic References

Kerlinger, F. N. (1986). *Foundations of behavioral research* (3rd ed.). New York: Holt, Rinehart and Winston.

Lincoln, Y. S., & Guba, E. G. (1985). *Naturalistic inquiry.* Newbury Park, CA: Sage Publications.

Moody, L., Vera, H., Blanks, C., & Visscher, M. (1989). Developing questions of substance for nursing science. *Western Journal of Nursing Research, 11,* 393–505.

Polit, D. F., & Hungler, B. P. (1999). *Nursing research: Principles and methods* (6th ed.). Philadelphia: Lippincott, Williams & Wilkins.

Substantive References

Baker, C., & Daigle, M. C. (2000). Cross-cultural hospital care as experienced by Mi'kmaq clients. *Western Journal of Nursing Research, 22,* 8–28.

Beck, C. T. (1995). Perceptions of nurses' caring by mothers experiencing postpartum depression. *Journal of Obstetric, Gynecologic, and Neonatal Nursing, 24,* 819–825.

Beck, C. T. (1996). Postpartum depressed mothers' experiences interacting with their children. *Nursing Research, 45,* 98–104.

Beck, C. T. (1998). Effects of postpartum depression on child development: A meta-analysis. *Archives of Psychiatric Nursing, 12,* 12–20.

Beck, C. T. (1999). Maternal depression and child behavioral problems: A meta-analysis. *Journal of Advanced Nursing, 29,* 623–629.

Beck, C. T., & Gable, R. K. (in press). Postpartum Depression Screening Scale: Development and psychometric testing. *Nursing Research,* forthcoming.

Brandon, D. H., Holditch-Davis, D., & Beylea, M. (1999). Nursing care and the development of sleeping and waking behaviors in preterm infants. *Research in Nursing & Health, 22,* 217–229.

Defloor, T., & Grypdonck, M. H. F. (1999). Sitting posture and prevention of pressure ulcers. *Applied Nursing Research, 12,* 136–142.

Devine, E. C., Bevsek, S. A., Brubakken, K., Johnson, B. P., Ryan, P., Sliefert, M. K., & Rodgers, B. (1999). AHCPR clinical practice guideline on surgical pain management: Adoption and outcomes. *Research in Nursing & Health, 22,* 119–130.

Durham, R. F. (1999). Negotiating activity restriction: A grounded theory of home management of preterm labor. *Qualitative Health Research, 9,* 493–503.

Grey, M., Boland, E. A., Davidson, M., Yu, C., & Tamborlane, W. V. (1999). Coping skills training for youths with diabetes on intensive therapy. *Applied Nursing Research, 12,* 3–12.

Janke, J. (1999). The effect of relaxation therapy on preterm labor outcomes. *Journal of Obstetric, Gynecologic, and Neonatal Nursing, 28,* 255–263.

Johnson, J. L., Budz, B., Mackay, M., & Miller, C. (1999). Evaluation of a nurse-delivered smoking cessation intervention for hospitalized patients with cardiac disease. *Heart & Lung, 28,* 55–63.

Kang, D., Coe, C., Karaszewski, J., & McCarthy, D.O. (1998). Relationship of social support to stress responses and immune function in healthy and asthmatic adolescents. *Research in Nursing & Health, 21,* 117–128.

Kirchhoff, K. T., Spuhler, V., Walker, L., Hutton, A., Cole, B.V., & Clemmer, T. (2000). Intensive care nurses' experiences with end-of-life care. *American Journal of Critical Care, 9,* 36–42.

Lacko, L., Bryan, Y., Dellasega, C., & Salerno, F. (1999). Changing clinical practice through research: The case of delirium. *Clinical Nursing Research, 8,* 235–250.

Lindgren, C. L. , Connelly, C. T., & Gaspar, H. L. (1999). Grief in spouse and children caregivers of dementia patients. *Western Journal of Nursing Research, 21,* 521–537.

Lusk, S. L., Ronis, D. L., & Hogan, M. M. (1997). Test of the Health Promotion Model as a causal model of construction workers' use of hearing protection. *Research in Nursing & Health, 20,* 183–194.

Sampselle, C. M., Seng, J., Yeo, A., Killion, C., & Oakley, D. (1999). Physical activity and postpartum well-being. *Journal of Obstetric, Gynecologic, and Neonatal Nursing, 28,* 41–49.

Sampselle, C. M., Wyman, J., Thomas, K., Newman, D. K., Gray, M., Dougherty, M., & Burns, P. A. (2000). Continence for women: A test of AWHONN's evidence-based protocol in clinical practice. *Journal of Obstetric, Gynecologic, and Neonatal Nursing, 29,* 18–26.

Serafine, M., & Broom, B. L. (1999). Predicting low-risk women's attendance at a preterm birth prevention class. *Journal of Obstetric, Gynecologic, and Neonatal Nursing, 28,* 279–287.

Sherman, D., & Kirton, C. (1999). Experience of relapse to unsafe sexual behavior among HIV-positive, heterosexual, minority men. *Applied Nursing Research, 12,* 91–100.

Wade, J., Pletsch, P. K., Morgan, S. W., & Menting, S. A. (2000). Hysterectomy: What do women need and want to know? *Journal of Obstetric, Gynecologic, and Neonatal Nursing, 29,* 33–42.

Walker, N.C., & O'Brien, B. (1999). The relationship between method of pain management during labor and birth outcomes. *Clinical Nursing Research, 8,* 119–134.

Reviewing the Research Literature

• •

Student Objectives

On completion of this chapter, the student will be able to:

○ describe several purposes of a literature review
○ identify bibliographic aids for retrieving nursing research reports and locate references for a research topic
○ identify appropriate information to include in a review of the literature
○ understand the steps involved in writing a literature review
○ evaluate the adequacy of the types of information (*e.g.*, research findings versus anecdotes; primary versus secondary sources) included in a written literature review, and evaluate its organization and style
○ define new terms in the chapter

• •

New Terms

Abstract journal	Online catalog system
Author search	Online search
CINAHL database	Primary source
Electronic database	Print index
Key words	Secondary source
Literature review	Subject search
Mapping	Textword search
Meta-analysis	Unit of analysis
Metasynthesis	

PURPOSES AND USES OF LITERATURE REVIEWS

This chapter is different from other chapters in this book, which are aimed at helping nurses critically evaluate nursing research studies, rather than teaching them how to conduct research. The skills involved in reviewing the research literature and preparing a written review paper, however, are needed by both producers and consumers of nursing research. Thus, this chapter presents information on locating research reports, critiquing written literature reviews, and actually preparing a written research literature review.

The overall purpose of a research literature review is to assemble knowledge on a topic. The uses to which that knowledge are put are varied.

Researchers and Literature Reviews

For researchers, acquaintance with relevant research literature can help with the following:

- Identification of a research problem and development or refinement of research questions
- Orientation to what is known and not known about an area of inquiry, to ascertain what research can best make a contribution to knowledge
- Determination of any gaps or inconsistencies in a body of research
- Determination of a need to replicate a prior study in a different setting or with a different study population
- Identification or development of new or refined clinical interventions to test through empirical research
- Identification of relevant theoretical or conceptual frameworks for a research problem
- Development of hypotheses to be tested in a study
- Identification of suitable designs and data collection methods for a study
- Assistance in interpreting study findings and in developing implications and recommendations

Thus, a literature review helps to lay the foundation for a study with significance to nursing. A literature review is a crucial early task for most quantitative researchers. As previously noted, however, qualitative researchers sometimes deliberately avoid an in-depth literature search before entering the field to avoid having their inquiries guided by prior thought on the topic.

Researchers usually summarize relevant literature in the introduction to research reports, regardless of when they perform the literature search. The literature review provides readers with a background for understanding current knowledge on a topic and illuminates the significance of the new study. Written literature reviews thus serve an integrative function and facilitate the accumulation of knowledge. Written research reviews are also included in research proposals, documents that describe what a researcher is planning to study, how the study will be conducted, and, if funding is being sought, how much the study will cost to complete.

Nonresearchers and Literature Reviews

Research reviews are not prepared solely in the context of doing a research study. Nursing students, nursing faculty, clinical nurses, nurse administrators, and nurses involved in policy-making organizations also need to review and synthesize evidence-based information. The specific purpose of the review varies depending on the reviewer's role. Here are a few examples:

- Acquisition of knowledge on a topic (students, faculty, clinical nurses, administrators)
- Preparation of critiques of existing nursing practices, and recommendations for innovations (faculty, clinical nurses, administrators, policy-oriented nurses)

- Development of research-based clinical protocols and interventions to improve clinical practice (clinical nurses, administrators, graduate students)
- Development of a theory or conceptual framework (faculty)
- Development of and revisions to nursing curricula (faculty)
- Development of policy statements and practice guidelines (policy-oriented nurses)

Thus, both consumers and producers of nursing research need to acquire skills for preparing and reviewing written summaries of knowledge on a given problem.

LOCATING RELEVANT LITERATURE FOR A RESEARCH REVIEW

The ability to identify and locate documents on a research topic is an important skill. It is also a skill that requires adaptability; rapid technological changes, such as the expanding use of the Internet, are making manual methods of finding information from print resources obsolete, and more sophisticated methods of searching the literature are being introduced continuously. We urge you to consult with librarians at your institution or to search the Internet for updated information.

 CONSUMER TIP:

Locating all relevant information on a research question is a bit like being a detective. The various electronic and print literature retrieval tools are a tremendous aid, but there inevitably needs to be some digging for, and a lot of sifting and sorting of, the clues to knowledge on a topic. Be prepared for sleuthing! And don't hesitate to ask your reference librarians for help in your detective work. ■

Electronic Literature Searches

Most college and university libraries offer students the capability of performing their own searches of **electronic databases**—huge bibliographic files that can be accessed by computer. Most of the electronic databases of interest to nurses can be accessed either through an **online search** (*i.e.* by directly communicating with a host computer over telephone lines or the Internet) or by **CD-ROM** (compact disks that store the bibliographic information). Several competing commercial vendors (*e.g.*, Aries Knowledge Finder, Ovid, Paper-Chase, SilverPlatter) offer information retrieval services for bibliographic databases. Their programs are user-friendly—they are menu driven with on-screen support, so that retrieval usually can proceed with minimal instruction. Most of these service providers offer free trial services that allow you to test an online or CD-ROM system before subscribing.

The electronic databases that contain references on nursing research include the following:

- CINAHL (Cumulative Index to Nursing and Allied Health Literature)
- MEDLINE (**Med**ical Literature On-**Line**)
- PsycINFO (**Psyc**hology **Info**rmation)
- AIDSLINE (**AIDS** Information On-**Line**)
- CancerLit (**Cancer Lit**erature)
- HealthSTAR (**Health S**ervices, Technology, Administration, and **R**esearch)
- CHID (Combined Health Information Database)

Most libraries at institutions with nursing schools subscribe to CINAHL, one of the most useful databases for nurses. The CINAHL database is described more fully in the next section.

Several other types of electronic resources should be mentioned. First, the books and other holdings of libraries can almost always be scanned electronically using **online catalog systems.** Moreover, through the Internet, the catalog holdings of libraries across the country can be reviewed. Finally, it may be useful to search through Sigma Theta Tau International's Registry of Nursing Research on the Internet. This registry is an electronic research database with more than 11,000 studies that can be searched by key words, variables, and researchers' names. The registry provides access to studies that have not yet been published, which cuts down the publication lag time; however, caution is needed because these studies have not been subjected to peer review. Electronic publishing in general is expanding at a rapid pace; librarians and faculty should be consulted for the most useful web sites.

 CONSUMER TIP:

It is rarely possible to identify all relevant studies exclusively through literature retrieval mechanisms. An excellent method of identifying additional references is to find recently published studies and examine their bibliography. Researchers are usually knowledgeable about other relevant studies and cite them to provide context for their own investigations. ■

The CINAHL Database

This section illustrates some of the features of an electronic search, through the use of the CINAHL database, the most important electronic database for nurses. Our illustrated example relied on the Ovid Search Software for CD-ROM, but similar features are available through other software programs or through direct online access.

The CINAHL database covers references to all English-language and many foreign-language nursing journals as well as to books, book chapters, nursing dissertations, and selected conference proceedings in nursing and allied health fields. The database covers materials dating from 1982 to the present.

In addition to providing bibliographic information (*i.e.,* the author, title, journal, year of publication, volume, and page numbers of a reference), abstracts are available for more than 300 journals.

Most searches are likely to begin with a **subject search**—a search for references relating to a specific topic. After selecting the search command from the main menu, you would type in a word or phrase that captures the essence of the topic, and the computer would then proceed with the search. Fortunately, through **mapping** capabilities, the software translates (maps) the topic you type in to the most plausible CINAHL subject heading. An important alternative to a subject search is a **textword search** that looks for your specific words in text fields of each record, including the title and the abstract. (If you know the name of a researcher who has worked on a specific research topic, an **author search** might be productive.)

CONSUMER TIP:

If you want to identify all major research reports on a topic, you need to be flexible and to think broadly about the key words and subject headings that could be related to your topic. For example, if you are interested in anorexia nervosa, you should look under anorexia, eating disorders, and weight loss, and perhaps under appetite, eating behavior, nutrition, bulimia, body weight changes, and body image. ∎

After you have typed in your topic, the computer will tell you how many "hits" there are in the database (*i.e.,* matches against your topic). In most cases, the number of hits initially will be large, and you will want to constrain the search to ensure that you retrieve only the most relevant references. You can limit your search in a number of ways. For example, you can restrict the search to those entries for which your topic is the main focus of the document. You might also want only references published in nursing journals; only those that are for research studies; only those published in certain years (*e.g.,* after 1995); or only those dealing with study participants in certain age groups (*e.g.,* infants).

To illustrate with a concrete example, suppose we were interested in recent research on treatments for postoperative pain, and we began our subject search by typing in "postoperative pain." In the CINAHL database, there are 11 subheadings for this topic, three of which (diet therapy, drug therapy, and therapy) relate to treatments. Here is an example of how many hits there were on successive restrictions to the search, using the CINAHL database current to February 2000:

Search Topic	*Restriction Hits*
Postoperative pain	1,086
Restrict to main focus	818
Restrict to therapy subheadings	489
Limit to core nursing journals	210
Limit to research reports	69
Limit to 1996 to 2000 publications	18

This narrowing of the search—from 1,086 initial references on postoperative pain to 18 references for recent nursing research reports on treatments for postoperative pain—took less than a minute to perform. Next, we would review the 18 references on the monitor, and those references of interest could be printed or downloaded onto a disk. An example of one of the CINAHL record entries for a study identified through this search on postoperative pain treatments is presented in Figure 6-1. Each entry shows an accession number, which is the unique identifier for each record in the database. Then the authors and title of the study are displayed, followed by source information. The source indicates the following:

Name of the journal (*Clinical Nursing Research*)
Volume (8)
Issue (3)
Page numbers (267–282)
Year and month of publication (1999 Aug.)
Number of cited references (23 ref.)

The printout shows all the CINAHL subject headings for this entry, any one of which could have been used to retrieve this reference through a subject search. Note that the subject headings include both substantive/topical ones (*e.g.,* patient-controlled analgesia, length of stay) and methodologic ones (*e.g.,* purposive sample, retrospective design). Next, when formal, named instruments are used in the study, these are printed under Instrumentation. Finally, the abstract for the study is presented. Based on the abstract, you would decide whether this study was pertinent to your literature review; if so, the full research reports could be obtained and read. The reports in the CINAHL database can be ordered by mail or facsimile (fax); therefore, it is not necessary for your library to subscribe to the referenced journal.

 CONSUMER TIP:

If your topic includes independent and dependent variables, you may need to do separate searches for each. For example, if you were interested in learning about the effect of stress on the health beliefs of acquired immunodeficiency syndrome (AIDS) patients, you might want to read about the effects of stress (in general) and about people's health beliefs (in general). Moreover, you might also want to learn something generally about AIDS patients and their problems. If you are searching for references electronically, you can also combine searches, so that the references for two independent searches can be linked (*e.g.,* the computer can identify those references that have both stress and health beliefs as subject headings). ■

Print Resources

Print-based resources that must be manually searched are being overshadowed by electronic databases, but their availability should not be ignored. Smaller libraries (such as hospital libraries) sometimes rely on these print resources. Moreover, it may be necessary to refer to print resources for early

Accession Number
1999059764

Special Fields Contained
Fields available in this record: abstract, cited references

Authors
Cheever KH

Institution
Marquette University College of Nursing, Milwaukee

Title
Pain, analgesic use, and morbidity in appendectomy patients

Source
Clinical Nursing Research. 8(3): 267-82, 1999 Aug. (23 ref)

Abbreviated Source
CLIN NURS RES. 8(3):267-82, 1999 Aug. (23 ref)

CINAHL Subject Headings

Adolescence
Adult
Analgesics, Nonnarcotic/ad
  [Administration and Dosage]
Analgesics, Opioid/ad [Administration
  and Dosage]
*Appendectomy
Appendicitis/cl [Classification]
Chi Square Test
Clinical Assessment Tools
Clinical Nursing Research
Data Analysis Software
Descriptive Statistics
Female
Inpatients

Length of Stay
Male
Medical Records
Middle Age
*Morbidity
Pain Measurement
Patient-Controlled Analgesia
*Postoperative Complications
*Postoperative Pain/co [Complications]
*Postoperative Pain/dt [Drug Therapy]
Postoperative Period
Purposive Sample
Record Review
Retrospective Design

Instrumentation
Numeric Pain Intensity Scale (NPS).

Abstract
Pain has immunosuppressive effects among the critically and chronically ill and opioids may immunomodulate pain's deleterious effects. However, little is known about the relations between acute pain, acute illness, and morbidity among previously healthy surgical patients. This study retrospectively examined these relations in appendectomy patients (N = 61). Eleven patients (18%) had morbidity, with atelectasis (11.5%) the most frequent complication. There were no differences between those patients with and without morbidity and pain intensity, method of opioid admininstration, and total opioid dose. Patients who received nonopioid analgesics received fewer opioids, less preemptive analgesia, and had less morbidity, whereas patients whose appendixes perforated received higher opioid doses and received more preemptive analgesia. Although the relations between acute pain, opioid use, and morbidity among previously healthy surgical patients are unclear findings infer that clinical practice does not follow guidelines advocated by analgesic experts. (23 ref)

FIGURE 6-1. Example of a printout from a CINAHL search.

literature on a topic. For example, the CINAHL database does not include references to research reports published before 1982.

CONSUMER TIP:

For students learning to do literature reviews, it may be useful to begin with a manual search of print resources and card catalogs before proceeding with a computer search. Manual searches can help to clarify and narrow the research topic and to identify key terms. ■

Print indexes are books used to locate research reports in journals and other documents. Indexes that are particularly useful to nurses are the *International Nursing Index, Cumulative Index to Nursing and Allied Health Literature* (the "red books"), *Nursing Studies Index, Index Medicus,* and *Hospital Literature Index*. Indexes are published periodically throughout the year (*e.g.,* quarterly), with an annual cumulative index. When using a print index, you need to first identify the appropriate subject heading. Subject headings can be located in the index's thesaurus, which lists commonly used terms, or **key words.** After the proper subject heading is determined, you can proceed to the subject section, which lists the actual references.

Abstract journals summarize articles that have appeared in other journals. Abstracting services are generally more useful than indexes because they provide a summary of a study rather than just a title. Two important abstract sources for the nursing literature are *Nursing Abstracts* and *Psychological Abstracts.*

CONSUMER TIP:

If you are doing a completely manual search, it is a wise practice to begin the search for relevant references with the most recent issue of the index or abstract journal and then to proceed backward. (Most electronic databases are organized chronologically, with the most recent references appearing at the beginning of a listing.) ■

PREPARING WRITTEN LITERATURE REVIEWS

The task of identifying references for the literature review, using the guidelines and tools described in the previous section, is the first step in preparing a written review of research literature. Subsequent steps are summarized in Figure 6-2.

Screening References

As Figure 6-2 shows, after identifying potential references, you need to locate and screen them for relevance and appropriateness. In addition to obtaining reports through your library or through CINAHL and other electronic data-

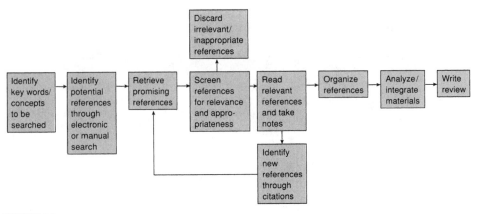

FIGURE 6-2. Flow of tasks in preparing a written research review.

bases, many nursing journals (including *Nursing Research* and *Research in Nursing & Health*) are now available online.

The relevance of the references, which concerns whether the reference bears on the research topic, usually can be judged quickly by reading the report's abstract or introduction. Appropriateness concerns the nature of the information in the reference. The most important information for a research review comes from research reports that describe study findings. You should rely primarily on **primary source** research reports, which are descriptions of studies written by the researchers who conducted them. **Secondary source** research articles are descriptions of studies prepared by someone other than the original researcher. Literature review articles are secondary sources. Review articles, if they are recent, are an especially good place to begin a literature search because they summarize what is known and because the reference lists are helpful. However, secondary descriptions of studies should not be considered substitutes for primary sources.

Examples of primary and secondary sources relating to neonatal skin care:

Secondary source—a review of the literature: Lund, C., Kuller, J., Lane, A., Lott, J. W., & Raines, D. A. (1999). Neonatal skin care: The scientific basis for practice. *Journal of Obstetric, Gynecologic, and Neonatal Nursing, 28,* 241–254.
Primary source—an original empirical study: Peters, K. L. (1999). Bathing premature infants: Physiological and behavioral consequences. *American Journal of Critical Care, 7,* 90–100.

For some topics, it is also important to include references from the conceptual literature (*i.e.,* references on a theory or conceptual model) in a literature review. In the conceptual literature, a primary source is a description of a theory written by the developer of the theory, and a secondary source is a discussion or critique of the theory.

In addition to empirical and conceptual references, two other types of references may be identified through a literature search: opinion articles, and articles describing anecdotes or clinical impressions. Opinion articles and anecdotal or other nonresearch articles may serve to broaden understanding of a research problem, illustrate a point, or demonstrate a need for research. They may thus play important roles in formulating research ideas, but they generally have limited utility in written research reviews because they are subjective and do not address the central question of written reviews: What is the current state of knowledge on this research problem?

Abstracting and Recording Notes

After a reference is judged to be relevant, the entire report should be read critically, using guidelines that are provided throughout this book. It is useful to photocopy an article, so that you can highlight or underline crucial information. Even with a copied article, taking notes or writing a summary of the report and its strengths and limitations is a good idea. A formal protocol is sometimes helpful for recording information in a systematic fashion. An example of such a protocol is presented in Figure 6-3. Although many of the terms on this protocol are probably unfamiliar to you at this point, you will learn their meaning as you progress through this book.

Organizing the Review

Organization of information is a crucial task in preparing a written review. When the literature on a topic is extensive, it is useful to prepare a summary table. The table could include columns with headings such as Author, Type of Study (Qualitative versus Quantitative), Sample, Design, Data Collection Approach, and Key Findings. Such a table provides a quick overview that allows the reviewer to make sense of a large mass of information.

Example of tabular organization:

Frazier (1999) reviewed research related to neurohormonal responses during positive-pressure mechanical ventilation. Her article included six tables that summarized research in different areas. For example, her first table summarized 12 human studies of atrial natriuretic peptide and positive-pressure mechanical ventilation. The headings in her column were: Authors, Purpose, Sample, Methods, and Results/Conclusions.

Most writers find it helpful to work from an outline—a written one if the review is lengthy and complex, a mental one for short reviews. The important point is to sit back and work out a structure before writing so that the presentation has a meaningful flow. Lack of organization is a common weakness in early attempts to write a research review. Although the specifics of the organization differ from topic to topic, the overall goal is to structure the

Citation: _____

_____

Type of Study: _____ Quantitative _____ Qualitative _____ Both

Location/setting: _____

Key concepts/ Concepts: _____
Variables: Intervention/
Indep. Variable: _____

Dependent Variable:

_____

Controlled
Variables: _____

Design Type: ___Experimental ___Quasi-experimental ___Pre-experimental ___Nonexperimental
Specific Design: _____

Sample: Size:_____ Type of sampling used: _____
Sample characteristics:_____

Measures: Type: ___ Self-report ___ Observational ___Biophysiologic ___Other
Description of measures:_____

_____

_____

Statistical Tests: Bivariate: _____
Multivariate: _____

Findings: _____

_____

_____

Recommendations: _____

Strengths: _____

_____

Weaknesses: _____

_____

FIGURE 6-3. Example of a literature review protocol.

review in such a way that the presentation is logical, demonstrates meaningful integration, and leads to a conclusion of what is known and not known about the topic.

After organization of topics has been determined, a review of the notes (or the summary table) is in order. This not only helps refresh your memory about material read earlier but also lays the groundwork for decisions about where a particular reference fits in the outline. If certain references do not seem to fit anywhere, they may need to discarded; the number of references is much less important than their relevance and the overall organization and quality of the review.

Content of a Written Review

A written research review should provide readers with an objective and thorough summary of the current state of knowledge on a topic. A literature review should be neither a series of quotes nor a series of abstracts. The central tasks are to summarize and evaluate the evidence in order to reveal the current state of knowledge on a topic. The review should point out both consistencies and contradictions in the literature, and offer possible explanations for inconsistencies (*e.g.*, different conceptualizations or data collection methods).

Although important studies should be described in some detail, it is not necessary to provide extensive coverage for every reference. Reports of lesser significance that result in comparable findings can be summarized together.

Example of grouped studies:

Smyer and Chang (1999) summarized several studies as follows: "Research has shown only modest benefits to caregivers from respite interventions, with nonsignificant differences on standardized measures of depression, social support, burden, and stress (Bourgeois et al., 1996; Haley et al., 1987; Lundervold & Levin, 1987)."

The literature should be summarized in your own words. The review should demonstrate that consideration has been given to the cumulative significance of the body of research. Stringing together quotes from various documents fails to show that previous research on the topic has been assimilated and understood.

Another point to bear in mind is that the review should be as objective as possible. Studies that conflict with personal values or hunches should not be omitted. In addition, the review should not deliberately ignore a study because its findings contradict other studies. Inconsistent results should be analyzed and the supporting evidence evaluated objectively.

The literature review should conclude with a summary of the state-of-the-art knowledge on the topic. The summary should recap study findings and indicate how credible they are; it should also make note of gaps or areas of research inactivity. The summary thus requires critical judgment about the extensiveness and dependability of the evidence on a topic.

As you progress through this book, you will become increasingly proficient in critically evaluating the research literature. We hope you will understand the mechanics of writing a research review when you have completed this chapter, but we do not expect that you will be in a position to write a state-of-the-art review until you have acquired more skills in research methods.

Style of a Research Review

Students preparing their first written research review often have trouble adjusting to the style of research reviews. Some students accept research results without criticism or reservation, reflecting a common misunderstanding about the conclusiveness of empirical research. You should keep in mind that no hypothesis or theory can be proved or disproved by empirical testing, and no research question can be definitely answered in a single study. The problem is partly a semantic one: hypotheses are not proved, they are supported by research findings; theories are not verified, but they may be tentatively accepted if a substantial body of evidence demonstrates their legitimacy. You should learn to adopt this language of tentativeness in writing a review of the literature.

A related stylistic problem is an inclination of novice reviewers to intersperse opinions (their own or someone else's) with the findings of research investigations. The review should include opinions sparingly and should be explicit about their source. The researcher's own opinions do not belong in a review, with the exception of an assessment of the studies' quality.

The left-hand column of Table 6-1 presents several examples of stylistic flaws. The right-hand column offers recommendations for rewording the sen-

---

TABLE 6-1.   **Examples of Stylistic Difficulties for Research Reviews**

INAPPROPRIATE STYLE OR WORDING	RECOMMENDED CHANGE*
1. It is known that unmet expectations engender anxiety.	1. Several experts (Abraham, 1999; Lawrence, 2000) have asserted that unmet expectations engender anxiety
2. The woman who does not participate in childbirth preparation classes tends to manifest high degree of stress during labor.	2. Previous studies indicate that women who participate in preparation for childbirth classes manifest less stress during labor than those who do not (Klotz, 2000; McTygue, 1998).
3. Studies have proved that doctors and nurses do not fully understand the psychobiologic dynamics of recovery from a myocardial infarction.	3. The studies by Singleton (1999) and Fortune (2000) suggest that doctors and nurses do not fully understand the psychobiologic dynamics of recovery from a myocardial infarction.
4. Attitudes cannot be changed overnight.	4. Attitudes have been found to be relatively enduring attributes that cannot be changed overnight (O'Connell, 1999; Valentine, 2000).
5. Responsibility is an intrinsic stressor.	5. According to Doctor A. Cassard, an authority on stress, responsibility is an intrinsic stressor (Cassard, 1998, 1999).

*All references are fictitious.

tences to conform to a more acceptable form for a research literature review. Many alternative wordings are possible.

Length of a Research Review

There are no easy formulas for how long a review should be. The length depends on several factors, including the complexity of the research question, the extent of prior research, and the purpose for which the review is being prepared. Literature reviews prepared for proposals (*e.g.*, proposals to undertake a study, to test a clinical innovation, or to make a change in practice) tend to be comprehensive. Reviews in theses and dissertations are also lengthy. In these cases, the literature review serves both to summarize knowledge and to document the reviewer's thoroughness.

Because of space limitations in journal articles, literature reviews that appear within research reports are brief. Literature reviews in the introduction to research reports demonstrate the need for the new study and provide a context for the research questions. The literature review sections of qualitative reports tend to be especially brief.

READING AND USING EXISTING RESEARCH REVIEWS

Most of this chapter provided guidance on how to conduct a literature review—how to locate and screen references, what type of information to seek, and how to organize and write a review. In some instances, however, a consumer may not need to conduct a full-fledged review if a recent literature review on the topic of interest has been published. For example, clinical nurses who want to develop a research-based intervention may be fortunate enough to find a relevant review that can offer them adequate direction—although they would probably also want to read the primary sources for the most pertinent studies.

Several different types of review that can be used to support evidence-based nursing practice are briefly described in this section.

Traditional Narrative Reviews

A traditional narrative literature review is a review that synthesizes and summarizes, in narrative terms, a body of research literature. The information offered in this chapter has been designed to help you prepare such a review.

Narrative literature reviews are frequently published in nursing journals, especially in nursing specialty journals. These reviews may have a number of different purposes, including providing practitioners with state-of-the-art research-based information; providing a foundation for the development of innovations for clinical practice; and developing an agenda for further research.

⊞⊞ *Example of a narrative research review:*

Askren and Bloom (1999) did a review of studies that examined the postadoptive reactions of relinquishing mothers. Using CINAHL and other databases, they identified 12 studies meeting specified criteria. Their review indicated that four themes relating to the relinquishment experience emerged: grief reactions, long-term effects, efforts to resolve, and influencing factors. Their review concluded with a discussion of both research and practice implications.

Meta-analysis

Meta-analysis is a method of integrating quantitative research findings statistically. In essence, meta-analysis treats the findings from a study as one piece of data. The findings from multiple studies on the same topic are then combined to create a data set that can be analyzed in a manner similar to that obtained from individuals. Thus, instead of study participants being the **unit of analysis** (the most basic entity on which the analysis focuses), individual studies are the unit of analysis in a meta-analysis. Typically, the meta-analyst takes information about the strength of the relationship between the independent and dependent variables from each study, quantifies that information, and then essentially takes an average across all studies.

Traditional narrative research reviews can be handicapped by some factors that are uncharacteristic of meta-analysis. For example, if there are a large number of studies and the results are inconsistent, it may be difficult in a narrative review to draw conclusions. Furthermore, narrative reviews can be subject to reviewer biases; for example, the reviewer might ignore or minimize the validity of studies with certain findings. Another advantage of meta-analysis is that it can take into account the quality of the studies that are being combined. For example, studies with larger samples can be given more weight than studies with smaller samples. Meta-analysis provides a convenient and objective method of integrating a large body of findings and of observing patterns and relationships that might otherwise have gone undetected. Meta-analysis can thus serve as an important tool in research utilization.

⊞⊞ *Example of a meta-analysis:*

Kleiber and Harper (1999) conducted a meta-analysis to analyze research findings on the effects of distraction on children's pain and distress during a medical procedure. The researchers integrated results from 16 studies on children's distress behavior and 10 studies on children's pain. The aggregated evidence indicated that distraction has a positive effect on children's distress behavior, but that the effect of distraction on pain is moderated by other factors.

Qualitative Metasynthesis

There is an increasing awareness of the need for integrative reviews of qualitative studies so that there can be an accumulation of the understandings gained from such studies. Efforts are underway to develop techniques for qualitative metasynthesis, and several strategies have evolved. An interpretive metasynthesis is more than just a narrative integration and summary of qualitative findings (*i.e.,* a traditional literature review). **Metasynthesis** has been defined as "the theories, grand narratives, generalizations, or interpretive translations produced from the integration or comparison of findings from qualitative studies" (Sandelowski, Docherty, & Emden, 1997, p. 366). Although there are certain thorny issues that pose challenges to the conduct of a metasynthesis, there is little doubt that this is an important avenue for furthering nursing knowledge.

⊞ **Example of a qualitative metasynthesis:**

Beck (in press) conducted a metasynthesis of 14 qualitative studies on the meaning of caring within nursing education. The metasynthesis revealed five themes that permeated caring in nursing education, whether it was faculty caring for each other or their nursing students or nursing students caring for each other or their clients. These themes centered on reciprocal connecting, which consisted of presencing, sharing, supporting, competence, and the uplifting effects of caring.

Critiquing Research Reviews

Some nurses never prepare a written research review, and perhaps you will never be required to do one. Most nurses, however, do read research reviews (including the literature review sections of research reports) and they should be prepared to evaluate them critically. It may be difficult for you to critique a research review because you are likely to be less familiar with the topic than the writer. Therefore, you may not be able to judge whether the author has included all relevant literature and has adequately summarized knowledge on that topic. Many aspects of a research review, however, are amenable to evaluation by readers who are not experts on the topic. Some suggestions for evaluating written research reviews are presented in Box 6-1. Additionally, when a literature review—whether it be a traditional review, a meta-analysis, or a metasynthesis—is published as a stand-alone article, it should include information that will help you understand its scope and evaluate its thoroughness, such as the following:

- What were the criteria for selecting studies to be included in the review? For example, were studies published before a certain date excluded? Were studies involving subjects in a certain age group excluded? Were articles in a language other than English excluded?

BOX 6-1   **GUIDELINES FOR CRITIQUING RESEARCH LITERATURE REVIEWS**

1. Does the coverage of the literature seem thorough? Does it appear that the review includes all or most of the major studies that have been conducted on the topic of interest? Are recent research reports cited?

2. Does the review rely on appropriate materials (*e.g.,* mainly on research reports, using primary sources)?

3. Is the review organized in such a way that the development of ideas is clear?

4. If the review is part of a research report for a new study, does the review support the need for the new research? If the review is designed to guide clinical practice, does the review of the evidence support the need for (or lack of need for) changes in practice?

5. Does the review conclude with a synopsis of the state-of-the-art knowledge on the topic?

6. Is the style of the review appropriate? Does the reviewer paraphrase, or is there an overreliance on quotes? Does the review appear unbiased? Does the reviewer use appropriately tentative language?

- How were the studies identified? Was a computerized search performed, and if so, of what databases?
- What were the key words or terms used in the search?

In assessing a written literature review, the overarching question is whether the review summarizes the current state of research evidence. If the review is written as part of an original research report, an equally important question is whether the review lays a solid foundation for the new study.

EXAMPLES OF RESEARCH LITERATURE REVIEWS

The best way to learn about the style, content, and organization of research literature reviews is to read them. We present two excerpts from reviews here and urge you to read other reviews on a topic of interest to you.

LITERATURE REVIEW OF A QUANTITATIVE RESEARCH REPORT

Lauver, Baggot, and Kruse (1999) conducted a study to delineate the primary concerns of women with abnormal Papanicolaou's (Pap) smear results and colposcopy and to identify women's strategies for coping with these potential stressors. The following excerpt represents a major portion of the literature review section of their research report, which appeared in the *Journal of Obstetric, Gynecologic, and Neonatal Nursing.*

Excerpt From a Review

Learning of an abnormal Pap result can be stressful (Beresford & Gervaize, 1986; Lerman et al., 1991; McDonald, Neutens, Fischer, & Jessee, 1989; Miller, Roussi, Altman, Helm, & Steinberg, 1994; Nugent, Tamlyn-Leaman, Isa, Reardon, & Crumley, 1993). Initial reactions after receiving an abnormal Pap result have included wondering about the seriousness of the findings and feelings of worry (Lauver & Rubin, 1991). Women needing colposcopic follow-up for an abnormal Pap result have reported concerns about cancer, sexual functioning, medical procedures, and sexually transmitted diseases (Beresford & Gervaize, 1986; McDonald et al., 1989). In past research, the stressful dimensions of abnormal Pap results and colposcopy were inferred from questions and comments women expressed. However, researchers have not asked women directly to identify the type of stressors they experience with abnormal Pap results and follow-up colposcopy.

Limited data exist on the coping strategies that women use to deal with the stress of having abnormal Pap results. In Nugent et al. (1993), women who were coping with abnormal Pap results and who sought initial colposcopies were interviewed with open-ended questions. These women spontaneously reported that information, reassurance, and use of escape or avoidance helped to decrease their anxiety (Nugent et al., 1993). In another study, the number of questions women asked about colposcopy was associated with greater confidence regarding their experience, but not with negative moods (Barsevick & Johnson, 1990). In a third study, the coping styles of low-income women with abnormal Pap results were examined. A highly vigilant coping style (*i.e.*, a trait-like quality of attending to threatening cues versus not) was associated with more concerns about the seriousness of the condition and diagnostic follow-up, more self-blame for the condition, and more intrusive thoughts (Miller et al., 1994). However, no data have been published on women's use and reported helpfulness of coping strategies for dealing with abnormal Pap results and follow-up colposcopy.

Clinical Relevance

Lauver and her colleagues found that women's primary concerns involved not understanding the Pap results, and uncertainty about cancer and fertility. Coping strategies they used the most, and rated as helpful throughout their experience, were seeking social support and distraction.

Based on their findings, specific nursing interventions could be designed to help women with the stresses associated with abnormal Pap results. Because the women's most frequently voiced concern was not understanding the Pap test results, providing information is a key intervention that can be provided to women who require colposcopic follow-up. Nurses could assess women's level of knowledge about these abnormal Pap results through phone calls and office contacts. Nurses could also address specific concerns of each woman, such as fear of cancer or infertility. In addition to individualized teaching, nurses can also play a supportive role and can encourage women to seek social support from family and friends. Also, the use of distractions such as working can be suggested and encouraged by nurses.

LITERATURE REVIEW OF A QUALITATIVE RESEARCH REPORT

Boydell, Georing, and Morrell-Bellai (2000) conducted a study of the experiences of 29 homeless people. A portion of the literature review for their research report is presented below.

Excerpt From a Review

Studies show that homelessness involves much more than not having a place to live. Individuals often lose their sense of identity, self-worth, and self-efficacy (Buckner, Bassuk, & Zima, 1993). Hallebone (1997) studied 38 homeless men ethnographically and found that psychosocial identities tend to be fragmented.

Taylor's (1993) study involving qualitative interviews with 10 homeless women indicates that participants shared experiences of depersonalization and stigmatization and the subsequent effects on their personhood. It was found that being or appearing unclean and having an identity without certification (paper proof) greatly affected the women's sense of self-esteem and personhood.

Snow and Anderson (1993) report that those recently dislocated expressed a strong aversion to other homeless individuals. In contrast, those who had been homeless for extended periods of time were more likely than those recently dislocated to embrace self-concepts such as tramp and bum. These unconventional self-concepts may be acquired and reinforced, at least in part, through social comparisons and identification with other homeless people (Grigsby et al., 1990). Montgomery (1994) found that homeless women felt that their hard times contributed to the creation of a new and more positive self. The literature also suggests that there is a spiritual dimension to the experience of homelessness that is often ignored. Matousek (1991) describes how the profound loss of self, which is associated with homelessness, presents a spiritual challenge to define one's very existence.

Clinical Relevance

The researchers undertook an in-depth study of the experiences of 29 homeless men and women. The analysis of the data revealed that the "self" was a process that was continuously developing among the study participants. The process was gradual and entailed considerable loss, including threats to their identity. The researchers also noted that the interview situation in and of itself provided an opportunity for self-reflection.

Boydell and her colleagues noted than one important implication of their research was that health care professionals should focus on the strengths of marginalized people such as the homeless. Their findings led them to conclude that the study participants' sense of hope and positive outlook suggest the need for early interventions to capture and use their motivation to escape homelessness.

• • • • • SUMMARY POINTS

- A research **literature review** is a written summary of the state of existing knowledge on a research problem.
- Researchers prepare literature reviews to determine knowledge on a topic of interest, to provide a context for a study, and to justify the need for a study; consumers review and synthesize evidence-based information to gain knowledge and improve nursing practice.
- An important bibliographic development for locating references is the various **electronic databases**, many of which can be accessed through an **online search** or by way of CD-ROM. For nurses, the **CINAHL database** is especially useful.
- Although electronic information retrieval is widespread, print resources such as **print indexes** and **abstract journals** are also available.
- In writing a research review, the reviewer should carefully organize the relevant materials, which should consist primarily of **primary source** research reports.
- The role of the reviewer is to point out what has been studied to date, how adequate and dependable those studies are, and what gaps exist in the body of research.
- Nurses also need to have skills in critiquing and using research reviews prepared by others, including traditional narrative reviews; **meta-analyses** (the integration of study findings using statistical procedures); and qualitative **metasyntheses** (interpretive translations produced from the integration of findings from qualitative studies).

➤ ➤ ➤ ➤ CRITICAL THINKING ACTIVITIES

Chapter 6 of the accompanying *Study Guide to Accompany Essentials of Nursing Research,* 5th edition offers various exercises and study suggestions for reinforcing the concepts presented in this chapter. In addition, you can address the following:

1. Read the literature review sections from one or both of the actual research studies in the Appendix of this book, and then answer the questions in Box 6-1.

2. Refer to the research report by Lauver, Baggot, & Kruse (1999), an excerpt of which was presented in this chapter. To what extent does the literature review lay the foundation for their study?

For additional review, see questions 62–72 on the study CD provided with Polit: Study Guide to Accompany Essentials of Nursing Research.

▦ WORLD WIDE WEB SITES

The web sites for the literature retrieval service providers are as follows:

Aries Knowledge Finder:
http://www.ariessys.com

Ovid:
http://www.ovid.com

PaperChase:
http://www.paperchase.com

SilverPlatter:
http://www.silverplatter.com

Sigma Theta Tau International Registry:
http://www.stti.iupui.edu

Online Journal of Issues in Nursing:
http://ana.org/ojin

Information about direct online access to CINAHL can be obtained at the CINAHL web site:
http://www.cinahl.com

SUGGESTED READINGS

Methodologic References

Holmes, S. (1996). Systematic search offers a sound evidence base. *Nursing Times, 92,* 37–39.

Martin, P. S. (1997). Writing a useful literature review for a quantitative research project. *Applied Nursing Research, 10,* 159–162.

Sandelowski, M., Docherty, S., & Emden, C. (1997). Qualitative metasynthesis: Issues and techniques. *Research in Nursing & Health, 20,* 365–371.

Sparks, S. M. (1999). Electronic publishing and nursing research. *Nursing Research, 48,* 50–54.

Substantive References

Askren, H. A., & Bloom, K. C. (1999). Postadoptive reactions of the relinquishing mother: A review. *Journal of Obstetric, Gynecologic, and Neonatal Nursing, 28,* 395–400.

Beck, C. T. (in press). Caring within nursing education. *Journal of Nursing Education,* forthcoming.

Boydell, K. M., Goering, P., & Morrell-Bellai, T. L. (2000). Narratives of identity: Representation of self in people who are homeless. *Qualitative Health Research, 10,* 26–38.

Frazier, S. K. (1999). Neurohormonal responses during positive pressure mechanical ventilation. *Heart & Lung, 28,* 149–165.

Kleiber, C., & Harper, D. C. (1999). Effects of distraction on children's pain and distress during medical procedures: A meta-analysis. *Nursing Research, 48,* 44–49.

Lauver, D. R., Baggot, A., & Kruse, K. (1999). Women's experiences in coping with abnormal Papanicolaou results and follow-up colposcopy. *Journal of Obstetric, Gynecologic, and Neonatal Nursing, 28,* 283–290.

Smyer, T., & Chang, B. L. (1999). A typology of consumers of institutional respite care. *Clinical Nursing Research, 8,* 26–50.

Examining Theoretical Frameworks

Student Objectives

On completion of this chapter, the student will be able to:

○ identify the major characteristics of theories, conceptual models, and frameworks
○ describe how theory and research are linked in quantitative and qualitative studies
○ identify several conceptual models of nursing and other conceptual models frequently used by nurse researchers
○ discuss the limitations of a study that does not have a theoretical basis or a study whose link to a theory or conceptual framework is contrived
○ define new terms in the chapter

New Terms

Borrowed theory
Conceptual definition
Conceptual framework
Conceptual map
Conceptual model
Descriptive theory
Framework
Grand theory

Grounded theory
Macro-theory
Middle-range theory
Model
Schematic model
Statistical model
Theoretical framework
Theory

THEORIES, MODELS, AND FRAMEWORKS

Theories and conceptual models are the primary mechanisms by which researchers organize findings into a broader conceptual context. Different terms are used in connection with conceptual contexts for research, including *theories, models, frameworks, schemes,* and *maps.* There is overlap in how these terms are used, partly because they are used differently by different writers. We offer guidance in distinguishing them but note that there is a blurring of these terms in the literature and that our definitions are not universal.

Theories

The term *theory* is used in many ways. For example, nursing instructors and students frequently use the term to refer to the content covered in classrooms, as opposed to the actual practice of nursing. In both lay and scientific language, the term *theory* connotes an abstraction.

Classically, scientists have used **theory** to refer to an abstract generalization that presents a systematic explanation about how phenomena are interrelated. Thus, the traditional definition requires a theory to embody at least two concepts that are related in a manner that the theory purports to explain.

Other researchers use the term *theory* less restrictively to refer to a broad characterization of a phenomenon. Some authors specifically refer to this type of theory as **descriptive theory**—a theory that accounts for (*i.e.*, thoroughly describes) a single phenomenon. Fawcett and Downs (1992) define descriptive theories as empirically driven theories that "describe or classify specific dimensions or characteristics of individuals, groups, situations, or events by summarizing commonalities found in discrete observations" (p. 7). Descriptive theory plays an especially important role in qualitative studies.

Both classical and descriptive theory serve to make research findings meaningful and interpretable. Theories allow researchers to knit together observations into an orderly system. Theories also serve to explain research findings: theory guides the researcher's understanding not only of the "what" of natural phenomena but also of the "why" of their occurrence. Finally, theories help to stimulate research and the extension of knowledge by providing both direction and impetus.

As classically defined, theories consist of concepts and a set of propositions that form a logically interrelated deductive system. This means that the theory provides a mechanism for logically arriving at new statements from the original propositions. To illustrate, consider the theory of reinforcement, which posits that behavior that is reinforced (*i.e.*, rewarded) tends to be repeated and learned. This theory consists of concepts (reinforcement and learning) and a proposition stating the relationship between them. The proposition readily lends itself to deductive hypothesis generation. For example, if the theory of reinforcement is valid, we could deduce that hyperactive children who are praised or rewarded when they are engaged in quiet play will exhibit less acting-out behaviors than similar children who are not praised. This prediction, as well as many others based on the theory of reinforcement, could then be tested in a study.

Theories are abstractions that are created and invented by humans. The building of a theory depends not only on observable facts but also on the theorist's ingenuity in pulling those facts together and making sense of them. Because theories are not just "out there" waiting to be discovered, it follows that theories are tentative. A theory can never be proved—a theory simply represents a theorist's best efforts to describe and explain phenomena. Through research, theories evolve and are sometimes discarded.

Theories are sometimes classified in terms of their level of generality. **Grand theories** (also known as **macro-theories**) purport to explain large segments of the human experience. Some learning theorists, such as Clark Hull, or sociologists, such as Talcott Parsons, developed general theoretical systems to account for broad classes of behavior and social functioning. Within nursing, theories are more restricted in scope, focusing on a narrow range of phenomena. Theories that explain a portion of the human experience are sometimes referred to as **middle-range theories.** For example, there are middle-range theories that attempt to explain such phenomena as decision-making behavior, infant attachment, and stress. This limited scope is consistent with the state of scientific developments in many fields concerned with human behavior.

Models

A **conceptual model** deals with abstractions (concepts) that are assembled because of their relevance to a common theme. Conceptual models provide a conceptual perspective regarding interrelated phenomena, but they are more loosely structured than theories and do not link concepts in a logically derived deductive system. A conceptual model broadly presents an understanding of the phenomenon of interest and reflects the assumptions and philosophical views of the model's designer. There are many conceptual models of nursing that offer broad explanations of the nursing process. Conceptual models are not directly testable by researchers in the same way that theories are. However, conceptual models, like theories, can serve as important springboards for the generation of hypotheses to be tested.

Some writers use the term **model** to designate a mechanism for representing phenomena with a minimal use of words. Words that define a concept can convey different meanings to different people; thus, a visual or symbolic representation of a phenomenon can sometimes help to express abstract ideas in a more understandable or precise form. Two types of models referred to in the research literature are schematic models and statistical models.

Statistical models, not elaborated on here, are mathematic equations that express the nature and magnitude of relationships among a set of variables. These models are tested using sophisticated statistical methods. A **schematic model** (also referred to as a **conceptual map**) represents a phenomenon of interest in a diagram. Concepts and the linkages between them are represented through boxes, arrows, or other symbols. An example of a schematic model is presented in Figure 7-1. This model, known as *Pender's Health Promotion Model* (HPM), is described by its designer as "a multivariate paradigm for explaining and predicting the health-promotion component of lifestyle" (Pender, Walker, Sechrist, & Frank-Stromborg, 1990, p. 326). Schematic models of this type can be useful in clarifying concepts and their associations.

Frameworks

A **framework** is the conceptual underpinnings of a study. Not every study is based on a theory or conceptual model, but every study has a framework. In a study based on a theory, the framework is referred to as the **theoretical framework;** in a study that has its roots in a specified conceptual model, the

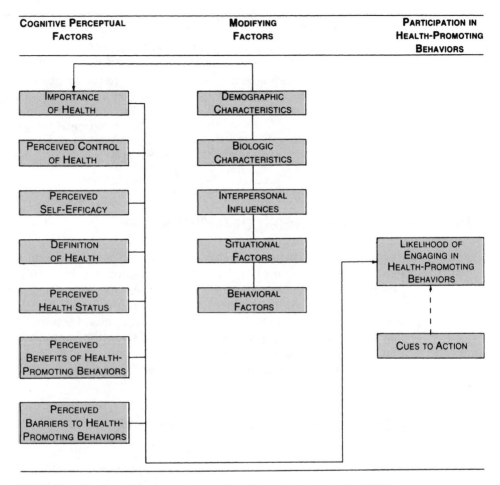

| COGNITIVE PERCEPTUAL FACTORS | MODIFYING FACTORS | PARTICIPATION IN HEALTH-PROMOTING BEHAVIORS |

FIGURE 7-1. The health promotion model. (From Pender et al., 1990.)

framework is often called the **conceptual framework.** (However, the terms *conceptual framework, conceptual model,* and *theoretical framework* are often used interchangeably).

The framework for a study is often implicit (*i.e.,* not formally acknowledged or described by the researcher). World views (and views on nursing) shape how concepts are defined and operationalized; researchers frequently fail to clarify the conceptual underpinnings of their variables. Consider, for example, the concept of caring. Caring can be conceptualized as a human trait, a moral ideal, an affect, an interaction, or an intervention (Morse, Solberg, Neander, Bottorff, & Johnson, 1990). A researcher undertaking a study concerned with caring should make clear what **conceptual definition** of caring he or she has adopted (*i.e.,* what the framework for the study is), just as the researcher must describe the operational definition.

> **⊟⊟**   *Example of a conceptual definition:*
>
> In their study of maternal control style, Sullivan and McGrath (1999) offered the following definitions of maternal involvement:
>
> *Conceptual definition:* Maternal involvement refers to the quality and appropriateness of maternal engagement behavior that a mother displays in interaction with her child. (p. 317)
>
> *Operational definition:* Maternal involvement was rated from a videotaped free play session using the Parent/Caregiver Involvement Scale. Eleven items representing maternal behaviors in interaction were rated on a 5-point scale and summed for a total score. (p. 320)

DEVELOPING AND TESTING THEORY THROUGH RESEARCH

The relationship between theory and research is a reciprocal and mutually beneficial one. Theories and conceptual models are built inductively from observations, and one source of those observations is disciplined research. Concepts and relations that are validated empirically become the foundation for theory development. The theory, in turn, must be tested by subjecting deductions from it (hypotheses) to further scientific inquiry. Thus, research plays a dual and continuing role in theory building and testing. Theory can guide and generate ideas for research; research can assess the worth of the theory and provides a foundation for new ones.

Developing Theory Through Qualitative Research

Qualitative researchers often strive to develop a conceptualization of the phenomena under study that is grounded in actual observations. These researchers seek to develop a **grounded theory**—an empirically based conceptualization for integrating and making sense of a process or phenomenon.

Theory development in a qualitative study is an inductive process. The qualitative researcher seeks to identify patterns, commonalities, and relationships through the scrutiny of specific instances and events. During the ongoing analysis of data, the qualitative researcher moves from specific pieces of data to abstractions that synthesize and give structure to the observed phenomenon. The goal is to use the data, grounded in reality, to provide an explanation of events as they occur in reality—not as they have been conceptualized in preexisting theories.

Not all qualitative studies have theory development as a goal. Moreover, some qualitative researchers acknowledge an existing conceptual model as a framework for their study. For example, a number of qualitative nurse researchers acknowledge that the philosophical roots of their studies lie in such conceptual models of nursing as those developed by Rosemarie Parse (1992) or Martha Rogers (1994).

⊞   *Example of theory in a qualitative study:*

Brown and Olshansky (1997) conducted a qualitative study of the transition to the primary care nurse practitioner role, based on interviews with 35 new nurse practitioners during their first year of practice. The researchers developed a theoretical model of the transition, consisting of a process they called "from limbo to legitimacy."

Testing Theory Through Quantitative Research

There are several ways in which quantitative researchers link research to a theory, but the most common approach is to test hypotheses deduced from an existing theory. Usually, the theory (or conceptual model) was developed on the basis of cumulated research evidence, but sometimes the theory is the product of a theory-generating qualitative inquiry.

The process of theory testing begins when a researcher extrapolates the implications of the theory or conceptual framework for a problem of interest. The researcher asks: If this theory or model is correct, what kinds of behavior would I expect to find in specified situations? and What evidence could be found to support this theory? Through such questioning, the researcher deduces implications of the theory in the form of research hypotheses. These hypotheses are predictions about how the variables would be related, if the theory were correct. For example, a researcher might deduce from reinforcement theory that verbal support and encouragement during primipara's attempts at breastfeeding would result in higher rates of successful continuation with breastfeeding. Theories are never tested directly; it is the hypotheses deduced from theories that are subjected to testing. Comparisons between the observed outcomes of research and the relationship predicted by the hypotheses are the major focus of the testing process.

⊞   *Example of theory in a quantitative study:*

Chang (1999) used Lazarus and Folkman's (1984) Theory of Stress and Coping to develop and test an intervention for homebound caregivers of persons with dementia (PWD). According to the theory, the relationship between stress and a person's coping ability is mediated by primary appraisal—the perception of an experience as stressful or nonstressful. Chang reasoned that an intervention that affects primary appraisal could positively affect caregiver anxiety and depression. She developed a cognitive–behavioral intervention designed to provide caregivers with knowledge and skills to improve the PWD's eating and dressing abilities and to increase caregiver knowledge of coping strategies. In a careful study that compared caregivers who received the intervention with those who did not, Chang found that depression decreased more in the intervention group.

Researchers sometimes base a new study on a theory or model in an effort to explain findings from previous research. For example, suppose that several researchers discovered that nursing home patients demonstrate greater levels of depression, anxiety, and noncompliance with nursing staff around bedtime than at other times. These descriptive findings are interesting, but they shed no light on the underlying cause of the problem and consequently suggest no way to ameliorate it. Several explanations, rooted in such theories as social learning theory, Lazarus and Folkman's stress and coping model, or one or more of the models of nursing, may be relevant in explaining the behavior and moods of the nursing home patients. By directly testing the theory in a new study (*i.e.*, deducing hypotheses derived from the theory), a researcher could gain some understanding of why bedtime is a vulnerable period for the elderly in nursing homes.

CONSUMER TIP:

When a quantitative study is based on a theory or conceptual model, the research report generally states this fact fairly early—often in the first paragraph, or even in the title. Many studies also have a subsection of the introduction called "Conceptual Framework" or "Theoretical Framework." The report usually includes a brief overview of the theory so that even readers with no theoretical background can understand, in a general way, the conceptual context of the study. ■

A few nurse researchers have begun to adopt a useful strategy for furthering knowledge through the direct testing of two competing theories in a single study. Almost all phenomena can be explained in alternative ways. The researcher who directly tests alternative explanations, using a single sample of subjects, is in a position to make powerful comparisons about the utility of the competing theories.

Example of testing competing theories:

Yarcheski, Mahon, and Yarcheski (1999) tested three alternative models of anger in early adolescents: a theory relating anger to stress; a theory attributing anger to differential emotions; and a theory of anger in relation to personality traits. The findings suggested that all three theories are sound and relevant explanations, but the trait theory provided the most powerful explanation.

CONCEPTUAL MODELS AND THEORIES USED BY NURSE RESEARCHERS

Nurse researchers have used both nursing and nonnursing frameworks to provide a conceptual context for their studies. This section discusses some of the more prominent frameworks that have appeared in the nursing research literature.

Conceptual Models of Nursing

Nurses have formulated a number of conceptual models of nursing that constitute formal explanations of what nursing is. As Fawcett (1994) has noted, four concepts are central to models of nursing: person, environment, health, and nursing. The various nursing models define these concepts differently, link them in diverse ways, and give different emphasis to the relationships among them. Moreover, different models emphasize different processes as being central to nursing. For example, Sister Callista Roy's Adaptation Model identifies adaptation of patients as a critical phenomenon (Roy & Andrews, 1998). Martha Rogers (1994), by contrast, emphasizes the centrality of the individual as a unified whole, and her model views nursing as a process in which individuals are aided in achieving maximum well-being within their potential. Nurse researchers increasingly are turning toward these conceptual models for their inspiration in formulating research questions and hypotheses. Other conceptual models of nursing that have been used in nursing studies include King's (1981) Open System Model; Neuman's (1989) Health Care Systems Model; Orem's (1995) Model of Self-Care; and Parse's (1992) Theory of Human Becoming. Table 7-1 lists eight conceptual models of nursing, together with a study for each that claimed the model as its framework.

Let us consider one conceptual model of nursing that has received particular attention among nurse researchers—Roy's Adaptation Model. In this model, human beings are biopsychosocial adaptive systems who cope with environmental change through the process of adaptation. Within the human system, there are four subsystems or response modes: physiologic needs, self-concept, role function, and interdependence. These subsystems constitute adaptive modes that provide mechanisms for coping with environmental stimuli and change. The goal of nursing, according to this model, is to promote patient adaptation during health and illness. Roy's Adaptation Model has been cited as the conceptual framework by many researchers.

Example of a study using Roy's Adaptation Model:

Nuamah, Cooley, Fawcett, and McCorkle (1999) used the Roy Adaptation Model as the conceptual framework for their study of the health-related quality of life among patients with newly diagnosed cancer. Health-related quality of life was viewed as a construct represented by indicators of the four biopsychosocial response modes. The findings of the study supported several, but not all, of the propositions derived from Roy's model.

In addition to conceptual models that describe and characterize the entire nursing process, nurses have developed other models and theories that focus on specific phenomena of interest to nurses. An important example is Nola Pender's Health Promotion Model (1996), a conceptual map for which was presented in Figure 7-1. Another example is Mishel's Uncertainty in Illness

TABLE 7-1.   **Examples of Studies Linked to Conceptual Models of Nursing**

CONCEPTUAL MODEL	RESEARCH QUESTION
King's Open System Model	What is the effect of a nurse–client transactional intervention on female adolescents' oral contraceptive adherence? (Hanna, 1993)
Levine's Conservation Model	What are the dimensions of fatigue as experienced by patients with congestive heart failure? (Schaefer & Potylycki, 1993)
Neuman's Health Care Systems Model	What is the relationship between mood symptoms and daytime ambulatory blood pressure during a 12-hour period in black female caregivers and noncaregivers? (Picot, Zauszniewski, Debanne, & Holston, 1999)
Orem's Model of Self-Care	What is the relationship between self-care agency and abuse on the one hand and physical and emotional health on the other among women in intimate relationships? (Campbell & Soeken, 1999)
Parse's Theory of Human Becoming	What are the factors that influence young women's perceptions of risk for sexually transmitted diseases? (Hutchinson, 1999)
Peplau's Interpersonal Relations Model	What are the factors influencing movement of nurse–patient dyads from Peplau's orientation phase to the working phase of the nurse–client relationship in a psychiatric setting? (Forchuk, Westwell, Martin, Azzapardi, Kosterewa-Tolman, & Hux, 1998)
Rogers' Science of Unitary Human Beings	What is the efficacy of a Rogerian-based intervention of therapeutic touch on anxiety, pain, and plasma T-lymphocyte concentration in burn patients? (Turner, Clark, Gauthier, & Williams, 1998)
Roy's Adaptation Model	Do formal cancer support groups help women to adapt to the physiological and psychosocial sequelae of breast cancer? (Samarel, Fawcett, Krippendorf, Piacentino, Eliasof, Hughes, Kowitski, & Siegler, 1998)

Theory (1988), which focuses on the concept of uncertainty—the inability of a person to determine the meaning of illness-related events. According to this theory, a situation appraised as uncertain will mobilize individuals to use their resources to adapt to the situation. Mishel's conceptualization of uncertainty has been used as a framework for both qualitative and quantitative studies.

Examples of studies based on uncertainty theory:

Leith (1999) studied patients' and family members' perceptions of transfer from an intensive care unit within the context of anxieties stemming from uncertainty. Baier (1995) conducted an in-depth qualitative study focusing on uncertainty in illness of people with schizophrenia.

Other Models Used by Nurse Researchers

Some phenomena of interest to nurse researchers are not unique to nurses, and therefore nursing studies can be linked to frameworks that are not models of nursing. Three conceptual models that have been used frequently in nursing studies are as follows:

- *Becker's Health Belief Model* (HBM). The HBM is a framework for explaining people's health-related behavior, such as health care use and compliance with a medical regimen. According to the model, health-related behavior is influenced by a person's perception of a threat posed by a health problem as well as by the value associated with actions aimed at reducing the threat (Becker, 1978). Nurse researchers have used the HBM extensively—for example, Poss (2000) used the HBM in her study of factors associated with migrant farmworkers' participation in a tuberculosis screening program.
- *Lazarus and Folkman's Theory of Stress and Coping.* This model, which explains people's methods of dealing with stress, posits that coping strategies are learned, deliberate responses to stressors that are used to adapt to or change the stressors. According to this model, people's perception of mental and physical health is related to the ways they evaluate and cope with the stresses of living (Lazarus & Folkman, 1984). An example of a nursing study based on this theory is Delunas and Potempa's (1999) study of the intrapersonal and psychosocial factors that affect adaptation after treatment for heart disease.
- *Azjen and Fishbein's Theory of Reasoned Action* (TRA). The TRA provides a framework for understanding the relationships among a person's attitudes, intentions, and behaviors. According to the TRA, behavioral intentions are the best predictor of a person's behavior, and behavioral intentions are a function of attitude toward performing the behavior and subjective norms—the person's perception of whether others think the behavior should be performed (Azjen & Fishbein, 1980). The TRA has been used in many nursing studies, including a study of the experience of relapse to unsafe sexual behavior among HIV-positive heterosexual men (Sherman & Kirton, 1999).

The use of theories and conceptual models from other disciplines such as psychology (**borrowed theories**) has not been without controversy—some commentators advocate the development of unique nursing theories. However, nursing research is likely to continue on its current path of conducting studies within a multidisciplinary and multitheoretical perspective.

CONSUMER TIP:

Among nursing studies that are linked to a conceptual model or theory, about half are based on borrowed theories. Among the models of nursing, those of Orem, Rogers, and Roy are especially likely to be used as the basis for research. ∎

CRITIQUING CONCEPTUAL AND THEORETICAL FRAMEWORKS

You are likely to find references to theories and conceptual frameworks in some of the studies you read. It is often challenging to critique the theoretical context of a published research report.

In a qualitative study in which a grounded theory is presented, you will not be given enough information to refute the proposed descriptive theory; only evidence supporting the theory is presented. However, you can determine whether the theory seems logical, whether the conceptualization is truly insightful, and whether the evidence is solid and convincing.

Critiquing a theoretical framework in a quantitative report is also difficult. Most of you are not likely to be familiar with the range of relevant models in nursing and other related disciplines. Furthermore, the whole notion of theoretical frameworks, precisely because they are abstract, may be anxiety provoking. Some suggestions for evaluating the conceptual basis of a quantitative study are offered in the following discussion and in Box 7-1 in the hope of lessening some of that anxiety.

The first task is to determine whether the study does, in fact, have a theoretical or conceptual framework. If there is no mention of a theory or conceptual model, you should consider whether the contribution that the study

BOX 7-1

GUIDELINES FOR CRITIQUING THEORETICAL OR CONCEPTUAL FRAMEWORKS

1. Does the research report describe an explicit theoretical or conceptual framework for the study? If not, does the absence of an explicit framework detract from the usefulness or significance of the research?

2. Does the report adequately describe the major features of the framework so that readers can understand the conceptual basis of the study?

3. Is the framework consistent with the research paradigm?

4. Do the research problem and hypotheses naturally flow from the framework, or does the purported link between the problem and the framework seem contrived?

5. Are conceptual definitions of the concepts in the study provided? Are the conceptual definitions consistent with the framework? Are the definitions clear and sufficiently detailed?

6. Did the framework guide the study methods? For example, do the operational definitions correspond to the conceptual definitions? Were hypotheses tested statistically?

7. Does the researcher tie the findings of the study back to the framework at the end of the report? How do the findings support or undermine the framework? Are the findings interpreted within the context of the framework?

is likely to make to knowledge is diminished by the absence of such a framework. Nursing has been criticized for producing many pieces of isolated research that are difficult to integrate because of the absence of a theoretical foundation, but in many cases, the research may be so pragmatic that it does not really need a theory to enhance its usefulness. For example, research designed to determine the optimal frequency of turning patients has a utilitarian goal; it is difficult to see how a theory would enhance the value of the findings.

 CONSUMER TIP:

In most quantitative nursing studies, the research problem is *not* linked to a specific theory or conceptual model. Thus, students may read many studies before finding a study with an explicit theoretical underpinning. ■

If the study does involve an explicit framework, you must then ask whether this particular framework is appropriate. You may not be able to challenge the researcher's use of a particular theory or model or to recommend an alternative because that would require a solid theoretical grounding. However, you can evaluate the logic of using a particular framework and assess whether the link between the problem and the theory is genuine. Does the researcher present a convincing rationale for the framework used? Do the hypotheses flow from the theory? Will the findings contribute to the validation of the theory? Does the researcher interpret the findings within the context of the framework? If the answer to such questions is no, students may have grounds for criticizing the study's framework, even though they may not be in a position to articulate how the conceptual basis of the study could be improved.

 CONSUMER TIP:

Some studies (in nursing as in any other discipline) claim theoretical linkages that are not justified. This is most likely to occur when researchers first formulate the research problem and then find a theoretical context to fit it. An after-the-fact linkage of theory to a research question *may* prove useful, but it is usually problematic because the researcher will not have taken the nuances of the theory into consideration in designing the study. If a research problem is truly linked to a conceptual framework, then the design of the study, the measurement of key constructs, and the analysis and interpretation of data will flow from that conceptualization. ■

RESEARCH EXAMPLES OF THEORETICAL CONTEXTS

This section presents two examples of the linkages between theory and research from the nursing research literature—one from a quantitative study and the other from a qualitative study.

RESEARCH EXAMPLE OF A QUANTITATIVE STUDY: TESTING OREM'S MODEL OF SELF-CARE

Orem's Model of Self-Care (1995) has been used as the conceptual framework in numerous studies. For example, Campbell and Soeken (1999) based their study of women's responses to battering on Orem's Model. Craddock, Adams, Usui, and Mitchell (1999) developed an Orem-based intervention to increase the use and effectiveness of self-care measures among breast cancer chemotherapy patients. Here we describe in some detail another study based on Orem's model.

Research Summary

Orem's (1995) model focuses on a person's ability to perform self-care, defined as "the practice of activities that individuals initiate and perform on their own behalf in maintaining life, health, and well-being" (p. 35). Ability to care for oneself is referred to as *self-care agency,* and the ability to care for others is referred to as *dependent-care agency.* In Orem's model, the goal of nursing is to help people meet their own therapeutic self-care demands.

Renker (1999) used Orem's self-care theory of nursing to study the relationships between self-care, social support, physical abuse, and pregnancy outcomes of older adolescent mothers and their infants. The research variables examined in this study focused on Orem's basic conditioning factors, self-care agency, and self-care. Included in Orem's basic conditioning factors are social/environmental factors and resource availability/adequacy factors. Renker chose physical abuse to represent the social/environmental factor and social support as the resource availability/adequacy factors. The Denyes Self-Care Agency Instrument was used to measure pregnancy self-care agency, and the Denyes Self-Care Practice Instrument measured pregnancy self-care.

Renker hypothesized that the absence of physical abuse and the presence of social support increased self-care agency. Increased levels of self-care agency were expected to enhance self-care practices, which were in turn expected to result in increased infant birth weight and decreased pregnancy complications. The results indicated that abuse, self-care agency, and self-care practice (prenatal care) affected infant birth weight.

Clinical Relevance

A particular strength of Renker's study is that Orem's Self-Care Deficit Theory of Nursing was interwoven throughout its design. For example, the instruments used to collect the data were questionnaires specifically developed to assess components of Orem's theory. Some of these instruments included the Denyes Self-Care Agency Instrument, the Denyes Self-Care Practice Instrument, and Substance Avoidance Self-Care Practice Scores.

In Renker's study, 22% of the adolescents reported they had been physically abused during their pregnancy, which suggests the desirability of routine assessment of adolescents for physical abuse during each trimester of pregnancy. The adolescent's current level of danger—and the possible need for immediate placement in a shelter—need to be assessed. Pregnant teens who are in danger of abuse should be given information that can be of use to them in an emergency.

Renker's study indicated that physical abuse during pregnancy was associated with previous miscarriages, substance abuse, and inadequate prenatal care. Infants whose mothers had been abused in pregnancy had significantly lower birth weights than infants of women who had not been abused. Thus, one implication is that nurses could initiate interventions designed to promote adequate weight gain during pregnancy among high-risk adolescents and provide them with nutritional supplements.

RESEARCH EXAMPLE OF A QUALITATIVE STUDY: DEVELOPMENT OF A THEORY OF CARING

As noted earlier in this chapter, many qualitative studies have theory development as an explicit goal. Here we describe the efforts of a qualitative researcher who developed a middle-range theory of caring on the basis of three separate qualitative inquiries.

Research Summary

Swanson (1991) developed an empirically driven descriptive theory of caring. Using data from three separate qualitative investigations, Swanson inductively derived and then refined a theory of the caring process.

Swanson studied caring in three separate perinatal contexts: as experienced by women who miscarried, as provided by parents and professionals in the newborn intensive care unit, and as recalled by at-risk mothers who had received a long-term public health nursing intervention. Data were gathered through in-depth interviews with study participants and also through observations of care provision. Data from the first study led to the identification and preliminary definition of five caring processes. The outcome of the second study was confirmation of the five processes and refinement of their definitions. In the third study, Swanson confirmed the five processes, redefined one of them, developed subdimensions of each process, and derived a definition of the overall concept of caring: "Caring is a nurturing way of relating to a valued other toward whom one feels a personal sense of commitment and responsibility" (p. 165).

According to Swanson's theory, the five caring processes are as follows:

- *Knowing:* striving to understand an event as it has meaning in the life of the other
- *Being With:* being emotionally present to the other
- *Doing For:* Doing for the other as he or she would do for the self if it were at all possible

- *Enabling:* Facilitating the other's passage through life transitions and unfamiliar events
- *Maintaining Belief:* Sustaining faith in the other's capacity to get through an event or transition and face a future with meaning

In presenting her theory, Swanson described the five processes, supporting each with rich excerpts from her in-depth interviews. Here is an example of the excerpt illustrating the process of knowing:

> When things weren't right, I could say that things were fine and it was only a matter of time. I mean the nurse would ask certain questions and there would be no way that I could be consistent without telling the truth. And then we would talk, and pretty soon instead of saying it was fine, I would start out with what was really wrong. (p. 163)

Swanson noted that her theory of caring was being used in the development and testing of a caring-based nurse counseling program for women who miscarry. Her theory has also been used by other researchers, including a qualitative study of the interactions of acquired immunodeficiency syndrome (AIDS) family caregivers and professional health care providers (Powell-Cope, 1994) and a study of the involvement of relatives in the care of the dying (Andershed & Ternestedt, 1999).

Clinical Relevance

Because caring is a central and unifying focus of nursing, Swanson's middle-range theory of caring is clearly relevant to the profession. This qualitatively based theory has immediate clinical implications for many situations. Incorporating the five caring processes of knowing, being with, doing for, enabling, and maintaining belief into interventions can help to provide a meaningful base for these nursing actions to be perceived as nurturing or helpful by patients. Nurses could profit from examining Swanson's theory of caring for its applicability to other areas of nursing beyond the prenatal context, such as in the specialties of gerontologic and oncologic nursing.

• • • • • SUMMARY POINTS

- A **theory** is a broad and abstract characterization of phenomena. As classically defined, a theory is an abstract generalization that systematically explains the relationships among phenomena. **Descriptive theory** thoroughly describes a phenomenon.
- The overall objective of theory is to make scientific findings meaningful, summarize existing knowledge into coherent systems, stimulate new research by providing direction and impetus, and explain the nature of relationships among variables.

- The basic components of a theory are concepts; classically defined theories consist of a set of propositions about the interrelationships among concepts, arranged in a logically interrelated system that permits new statements to be derived from them.
- Concepts are also the basic elements of **conceptual models**, but the concepts are not linked to one another in a logically ordered, deductive system.
- **Schematic models** (sometimes referred to as **conceptual maps**) are symbolic representations of phenomena that depict a conceptual model through the use of symbols or diagrams.
- A **framework** is the conceptual underpinnings of a study. In many studies, the framework is implicit and not fully explicated.
- Qualitative studies are often used to develop inductively derived theories. Some qualitative researchers specifically seek to develop **grounded theories**—data-driven explanations to account for phenomena under study.
- Quantitative studies test hypotheses developed on the basis of an existing theory or conceptual model.
- Several conceptual models of nursing have been developed and have been used in nursing research (*e.g.,* Orem's Self-Care Model). The concepts central to models of nursing are person, environment, health, and nursing.
- Nonnursing models used by nurse researchers (*e.g.,* Lazarus and Folkman's Theory of Stress and Coping) are referred to as **borrowed theories**.
- Researchers sometimes develop a problem, design a study, and then look for a conceptual framework; such an after-the-fact selection of a framework is less compelling than the systematic testing of a particular theory.

➤ ➤ ➤ ➤ *CRITICAL THINKING ACTIVITIES*

Chapter 7 of the accompanying *Study Guide to Accompany Essentials of Nursing Research,* 5th edition offers various exercises and study suggestions for reinforcing the concepts presented in this chapter. In addition, you can address the following:

1. Read the introduction to one or both of the actual research studies in the Appendix of this book, and then answer the questions in Box 7-1.

2. Select one of the conceptual models of nursing cited in Table 7-1 and read a primary or secondary source description of the model. Prepare a one-page summary of the model.

3. Read a study linked to the model selected for exercise 2. Answer the questions in Box 7-1 regarding this study.

For additional review, see questions 73–80 on the study CD provided with Polit: Study Guide to Accompany Essentials of Nursing Research.

SUGGESTED READINGS

Methodologic References

Azjen, I., & Fishbein, M. (1980). *Understanding attitudes and predicting social behavior.* Englewood Cliffs, NJ: Prentice-Hall.

Becker, M. (1978). The Health Belief Model and sick role behavior. *Nursing Digest, 6,* 35–40.

Fawcett, J. (1994). *Analysis and evaluation of conceptual models of nursing* (3rd ed.). Philadelphia: F. A. Davis.

Fawcett, J., & Downs, F. (1992). *The relationship between theory and research* (2nd ed.). Philadelphia: F. A. Davis.

King, I. M. (1981). *A Theory for nursing: Systems, concept, and process.* NY.: John Wiley & Sons

Lazarus, R. S., & Folkman, S. (1984). *Stress, appraisal, and coping.* New York: Springer.

Levine, M. E. (1973). *Introduction to clinical nursing* (2nd ed.). Philadelphia: F. A. Davis.

Mishel, M. H. (1988). Uncertainty in illness. *Image—The Journal of Nursing Scholarship, 20,* 225–232.

Morse, J. M., Solberg, S. M., Neander, W. L., Bottorff, J. L., & Johnson, J. L. (1990). Concepts of caring and caring as a concept. *Advances in Nursing Science, 13,* 1–14.

Neuman, B. (1989). *The Neuman systems model* (2nd ed.). Norwalk, CT: Appleton & Lange.

Nicoll, L. H. (1997). *Perspectives on nursing theory* (3rd ed.). Philadelphia: Lippincott-Raven.

Orem, D. E. (1995). *Concepts of practice* (5th ed.). New York: McGraw-Hill.

Parse, R. R. (1992). Human becoming: Parse's theory. *Nursing Science Quarterly, 5,* 35–42.

Pender, N., & Pender, A. R. (1996). *Health promotion in nursing practice* (3rd ed.). Norwalk, CT: Appleton & Lange.

Rogers, M. E., Malinski, V. M., & Barrett, E. A. (1994). *Martha E. Rogers: Her life and her work.* Philadelphia: F. A. Davis.

Roy, C. Sr., & Andrews, H. A. (1998). *The Roy Adaptation Model.* Norwalk, CT: Appleton & Lange.

Substantive References

Ailinger, R. L., & Dear, M. R. (1997). An examination of the self-care needs of clients with rheumatoid arthritis. *Rehabilitation Nursing, 22,* 135–140.

Andershed, B., & Ternestedt, B. (1999). Involvement of relatives in care of the dying in different care cultures. *Nursing Science Quarterly, 12,* 45–51.

Baier, M. (1995). Uncertainty in illness for persons with schizophrenia. *Issues in Mental Health Nursing, 16,* 201–212.

Brooks, E. M., & Thomas, S. (1997). The perception and judgment of senior baccalaureate nurses in clinical decision making. *Advances in Nursing Science, 19,* 50–69.

Brown, M., & Olshansky, E. F. (1997). From limbo to legitimacy: A theoretical model of the transition to the primary care nurse practitioner role. *Nursing Research, 46,* 46–51.

Campbell, J. C., & Soeken, K. L. (1999). Women's responses to battering: A test of the model. *Research in Nursing & Health, 22,* 49–58.

Chang, B. L. (1999). Cognitive-behavioral intervention for homebound caregivers of persons with dementia. *Nursing Research, 48,* 173–182.

Craddock, R. B., Adams, P. F., Usui, W. M., & Mitchell, L. (1999). An intervention to increase use and effectiveness of self-care measures for breast cancer chemotherapy patients. *Cancer Nursing, 22,* 312–319.

Delunas, L. R., & Potempa, K. (1999). Adaptation after treatment for heart disease: Preliminary examination within a stress appraisal context. *Heart & Lung, 28,* 186–194.

Forchuk, C., Westwell, J., Martin, M. L., Azzapardi, W. B., Kosterewa-Tolman, D., & Hux, M. (1998). Factors influencing movement of chronic psychiatric patients from the orientation to the working phase of the nurse–client relationship on an inpatient unit. *Perspectives in Psychiatric Care, 34,* 36-44.

Hanna, K. M. (1993). Effect of nurse–client transaction on female adolescents' oral contraceptive adherence. *Image—The Journal of Nursing Scholarship, 25,* 285–290.

Hutchinson, M. K. (1999). Individual, family, and relationship predictors of young women's sexual risk perceptions. *Journal of Obstetric, Gynecologic, and Neonatal Nursing, 28,* 60–67.

Leith, B. A. (1999). Patients' and family members' perceptions of transfer from intensive care. *Heart & Lung, 28,* 210–218.

Nuamah, I. F., Cooley, M. E., Fawcett, J., & McCorkle, R. (1999). Testing a theory for health-related quality of life in cancer patients: A structural equation approach. *Research in Nursing and Health, 22,* 231–242.

Page, C., & Ricard, M. (1996). Conceptual and theoretical foundations for an instrument designed to identify self-care requirements in women treated for depression. *Nursing Research, 28,* 94–112.

Pender, N. J., Walker, S. N., Sechrist, K. R., & Frank-Stromborg, M. (1990). Predicting health-promoting lifestyles in the workplace. *Nursing Research, 39,* 326–332.

Picot, S. J. F., Zauszniewski, J. A., Debanne, S. M., & Holston, E. C. (1999). Mood and blood pressure responses in black female caregivers and noncaregivers. *Nursing Research, 48,* 150–161.

Poss, J. E. (2000). Factors associated with participation by Mexican migrant farmworkers in a tuberculosis program. *Nursing Research, 49,* 20–28.

Powell-Cope, G. M. (1994). Family caregivers of people with AIDS. *Nursing Research, 43,* 324–330.

Renker, P. R. (1999). Physical abuse, social support, self-care, and pregnancy outcomes of older adolescents. *Journal of Obstetric, Gynecologic, and Neonatal Nursing, 28,* 377–388.

Samarel, N., Fawcett, J., Krippendorf, K., Piacentino, J. C., Eliasof, B., Hughes, P., Kowitski, C., & Siegler, E. (1998). Women's perceptions of group support and adaptation to breast cancer. *Journal of Advanced Nursing, 28,* 1259–1268.

Schaefer, K. M., & Potylycki, M. J. S. (1993). Fatigue associated with congestive heart failure: Use of Levine's Conservation Model. *Journal of Advanced Nursing, 18,* 260–268.

Sherman, D. W., & Kirton, C. A. (1999). The experience of relapse to unsafe sexual behavior among HIV-positive, heterosexual, minority men. *Research in Nursing & Health, 12,* 91–100.

Sullivan, M. C., & McGrath, M. M. (1999). Proximal and distal correlates of maternal control style. *Western Journal of Nursing Research, 21,* 313–334.

Swanson, K. M. (1991). Empirical development of middle-range theory of caring. *Nursing Research, 40,* 161–166.

Turner, J. G., Clark, A. J., Gauthier, D. K., & Williams, M. (1998). The effect of therapeutic touch on pain and anxiety in burn patients. *Journal of Advanced Nursing, 28,* 10–20.

Yarcheski, A., Mahon, N. E., & Yarcheski, T. J. (1999). An empirical test of alternate theories of anger in early adolescents. *Nursing Research, 48,* 317–323.

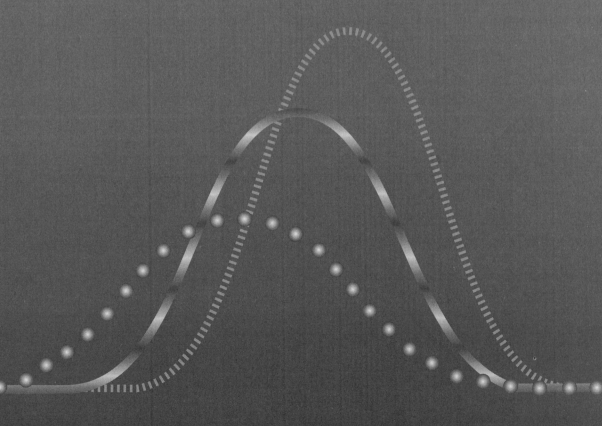

PART III

DESIGNS FOR NURSING RESEARCH

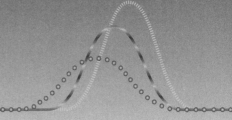

Understanding Quantitative Research Design

● ●

Student Objectives

On completion of this chapter, the student will be able to:

○ describe the decisions that are specified in a research design for a quantitative study

○ describe the characteristics of experimental, quasi-experimental, preexperimental, and nonexperimental designs and discuss their strengths and weaknesses

○ identify several specific designs (*e.g.*, repeated-measures design, nonequivalent control-group design, retrospective design) and describe some of their advantages and disadvantages

○ distinguish between and evaluate cross-sectional and longitudinal designs

○ identify the purposes and some of the distinguishing features of surveys, evaluations, and outcomes research

○ identify and evaluate alternative methods of controlling external and intrinsic extraneous variables

○ describe various threats to the internal and external validity of quantitative studies

○ evaluate a quantitative study in terms of its overall research design and methods of controlling extraneous variables, including the resulting internal and external validity of the design

○ define new terms in the chapter

● ●

New Terms

After-only design	*Ex post facto* research
Analysis of covariance	Experimental research
Attrition	Experimental group
Baseline data	External validity
Before–after design	Extraneous variable
Between-subjects design	Factor
Case-control design	Factorial design
Cell	Follow-up study
Clinical trial	Hawthorne effect
Comparison group	History threat
Constancy of conditions	Homogeneity
Control group	Impact analysis
Correlational research	Implementation analysis
Cost–benefit analysis	Interaction effects
Crossover design	Internal validity
Cross-sectional study	Intervention
Descriptive correlational study	Level
Descriptive research	Longitudinal study
Double-blind experiment	Main effects
Evaluations	Manipulation

Matching
Maturation threat
Mediating variable
Mortality threat
Net effects
Nonequivalent control-group after-only
  design
Nonequivalent control-group
  before–after design
Nonexperimental research
One-group before–after design
Outcome analysis
Outcomes research
Panel study
Posttest data
Posttest-only design
Preexperimental design
Pretest data
Pretest–posttest design
Process analysis
Prospective study

Quasi-experimental research
Random assignment
Randomization
Repeated-measures design
Research control
Research design
Research protocol
Retrospective study
Rival hypothesis
Selection threat
Self-report
Self-selection
Survey
Systematic bias
Table of random numbers
Threats to internal validity
Time-series design
Treatment
Trend study
Within-subjects design

PURPOSES AND DIMENSIONS OF RESEARCH DESIGN IN QUANTITATIVE STUDIES

Research design refers to the researcher's overall plan for answering the research questions or testing the research hypotheses. In a quantitative study, the research design spells out the strategies the researcher plans to adopt to develop information that is accurate and interpretable. Typically, a quantitative research design involves decisions with regard to the following aspects of the study:

- *Will there be an intervention?* In some situations, nurse researchers study the effects of a specific intervention (*e.g.,* an innovative program to promote breast self-examination); in others, researchers gather information about phenomena as they currently exist. This is a distinction between experimental and nonexperimental research. When there is an intervention, the research design specifies its nature and how it is to be implemented.
- *What types of comparison will be made?* Researchers usually plan comparisons within their studies so that their results will be more clearly interpretable. Consider the example presented in Chapter 3, in which the researchers studied the emotional consequences of having an abortion by comparing women who had an abortion with women who delivered a baby. Without a comparison group, the researchers would

not have known whether the abortion group members' emotional status was of special concern. Sometimes, researchers use a before–after comparison (*e.g.*, preoperative and postoperative), and sometimes several comparisons are used.

• *What procedures will be used to control extraneous variables?* The complexity of relationships among variables makes it difficult to test hypotheses unambiguously unless efforts are made to control factors extraneous to the research question (*i.e.*, to control **extraneous variables**). This chapter discusses techniques for achieving control.

• *When and how many times will data be collected from study participants?* In many studies, data are collected from participants at a single point in time, but some studies include multiple contacts with participants, for example, to determine how things have changed over time. The research design designates how often and also when, relative to other events, the data will be collected (*e.g.*, 1 day after surgery).

• *In what setting will the study take place?* Sometimes, data for quantitative studies are collected in real-world settings, such as in clinics or people's homes. Other studies are conducted in laboratory settings (*i.e.*, in highly controlled environments established for research purposes).

The research design incorporates key methodologic decisions. Other aspects of the study—the data collection plan, the sampling plan, and the analysis plan—also involve important decisions, but the research design stipulates the fundamental form the research will take. For this reason, it is crucial for you to understand the implications of researchers' design decisions.

There is no single, easy-to-describe typology of research designs because they vary along a number of dimensions. As shown in Table 8-1, the dimensions involve whether the researcher has control over the independent variable, what type of comparison is made, how many times data are collected, whether the researcher looks forward or backward in time for the occurrence of the independent and dependent variables, and what setting is used for data collection. Each dimension is, with a few exceptions, independent of the others. For example, an experimental design can be a between-subjects or within-subjects design; experiments can also be cross-sectional or longitudinal, and so on (these terms are discussed later). Moreover, within any one category, there are a number of variants; for example, there are several alternative experimental designs. The sections that follow elaborate on different designs for quantitative nursing research. Qualitative research design is discussed in Chapter 9.

◪ CONSUMER TIP:

Research reports typically present information about the research design early in the method section. Complete information about the design is not always provided, however, and some researchers use terminology that is different from that used in this book. (Occasionally, researchers even misidentify the study design.) ■

TABLE 8-1.　Dimensions of Quantitative Research Designs

DIMENSION	DESIGN	MAJOR FEATURES
Control over independent variable	Experimental	Manipulation of independent variable, control group, randomization
	Quasi-experimental	Manipulation of independent variable but no randomization or no control group
	Nonexperimental	No manipulation of independent variable
Type of group comparisons	Between-subjects	Participants in groups being compared are different people.
	Within-subjects	Participants in groups being compared are the same people.
Number of data collection points	Cross-sectional	Data collected at one point in time
	Longitudinal	Data collected at multiple points in time over extended period
Occurrence of independent and dependent variable	Retrospective	Study begins with dependent variable and looks backward for cause or influence.
	Prospective	Study begins with independent variable and looks forward for the effect.
Setting	Naturalistic	Data collected in a real-world setting
	Laboratory	Data collected in artificial, contrived setting

EXPERIMENTAL, QUASI-EXPERIMENTAL, AND NONEXPERIMENTAL DESIGNS

This section reviews designs that differ with regard to the amount of control the researcher has over the independent variable. We begin with research designs that offer the greatest amount of control: experimental designs.

Experimental Research

Experimental research differs from nonexperimental research in one important respect: The researcher using an experimental design is an active agent rather than a passive observer. Early physical scientists found that, although observation of natural phenomena is valuable, the complexity of naturally occurring events often obscures relationships. This problem was addressed by isolating phenomena in a laboratory setting and controlling the conditions under which they occurred. The procedures developed by physical scientists were adopted by biologists during the 19th century, resulting in many achievements in physiology and medicine. Researchers interested in human behavior and psychological states began using experimental methods in the 20th century.

Characteristics of Experiments

Experiments are not necessarily performed in laboratories; they can be conducted in any setting. To qualify as an experiment, a research design need only possess the following three properties:

1. *Manipulation.* The experimenter does something to participants in the study.
2. *Control.* The experimenter introduces controls over the experimental situation, including the use of a control group.
3. *Randomization.* The experimenter assigns participants to control experimental groups randomly.

Using **manipulation**, the experimenter controls and consciously varies the independent variable and then observes its effect on the dependent variable. The investigator manipulates the independent variable by administering an experimental **treatment** (or **intervention**) to some subjects while withholding it from others (or administering an alternative treatment, such as a placebo). As an illustration, suppose we were investigating the effect of physical restraint with a Posey belt on heart rate, using rats as subjects. One experimental design for this research problem is a **before–after design** (also known as a **pretest–posttest design**). This design involves the observation of the dependent variable (heart rate) at two points in time: before and after the treatment. Each of the rats in the experimental group is restrained with a Posey belt, whereas those in the control group are not. This design permits us to examine what changes in heart rate were *caused* by the restraint because only some rats were restrained, providing an important comparison. In this example, we met the first criterion of a true experiment by manipulating physical restraint of the rats, the independent variable.

This example also meets the second requirement for experiments, the use of a control group. Campbell and Stanley (1963), in a classic monograph on research design, noted that scientific evidence requires at least one comparison. But not all comparisons provide equally persuasive evidence. Let us look at an example. If we were to supplement the diet of a sample of premature neonates with special nutrients for 2 weeks, the infants' weight at the end of the 2-week period would give us no information about the treatment's effectiveness. At a bare minimum, we would need to compare their posttreatment weight with their pretreatment weight to determine whether, at least, their weights had increased. But suppose we find an average weight gain of half a pound. Does this finding indicate that there is a causal relationship between the nutritional supplements (the independent variable) and weight gain (the dependent variable)? No, it does not. Infants normally gain weight as they mature. Without a control group—a group that does not receive the supplements—it is impossible to separate the effects of maturation from those of the treatment. The term **control group** refers to a group of participants whose performance on a dependent variable is used as a basis for evaluating the performance of the **experimental group** (the group that receives the treatment of interest to the researcher) on the same dependent variable.

To qualify as an experiment, the design must also involve the assignment of subjects to groups randomly. Through **randomization** (or **random assignment**), every participant has an equal chance of being included in any group. If people are randomly assigned, there is no **systematic bias** in the groups with respect to attributes that may affect the dependent variable. *Randomly assigned groups are expected to be comparable, on average, with respect to an infinite number of biologic, psychological, and social traits at the outset of the study.* Any group differences that emerge after random assignment can therefore be attributed to the treatment.

Random assignment can be accomplished by flipping a coin or pulling names from a hat. Researchers typically either use computers to perform the randomization or rely on a **table of random numbers**, a table displaying hundreds of digits arranged in a random order.

Experimental Designs

Basic Designs. The most basic experimental design involves the random assignment of subjects to two groups and the subsequent collection of data after the intervention. This design is sometimes called an **after-only** (or **posttest-only**) **design.** A more refined design, discussed previously, is the pretest–posttest or before–after design, which involves the collection of **pretest data** (also known as **baseline data**) before the experimental manipulation and **posttest data** after it.

⊞⊞ **Example of an after-only design:**

Leitch (1999) studied the effect of a videotaped intervention to promote positive mother–infant interactions. First-time mothers were randomly assigned to either an intervention or control group, and the intervention group received the special instruction. Mother–infant interaction was then observed, and group differences were assessed.

Factorial Design. Researchers sometimes manipulate two or more variables simultaneously. Suppose, for example, that we were interested in comparing the effects of tactile stimulation versus auditory stimulation on cardiac responsiveness in premature infants, and that we were also interested in learning whether the daily *amount* of stimulation had any effects. Figure 8-1 illustrates the structure of this experiment.

This type of study, which involves a **factorial design**, permits the testing of three hypotheses. Here, the three research questions are (1) Does auditory stimulation have a different effect on cardiac responsiveness in premature infants than tactile stimulation? (2) Is the amount of stimulation (independent of modality) related to cardiac responsiveness? and (3) Is auditory stimulation most effective when linked to a certain dose and tactile stimulation most effective when coupled with a different dose?

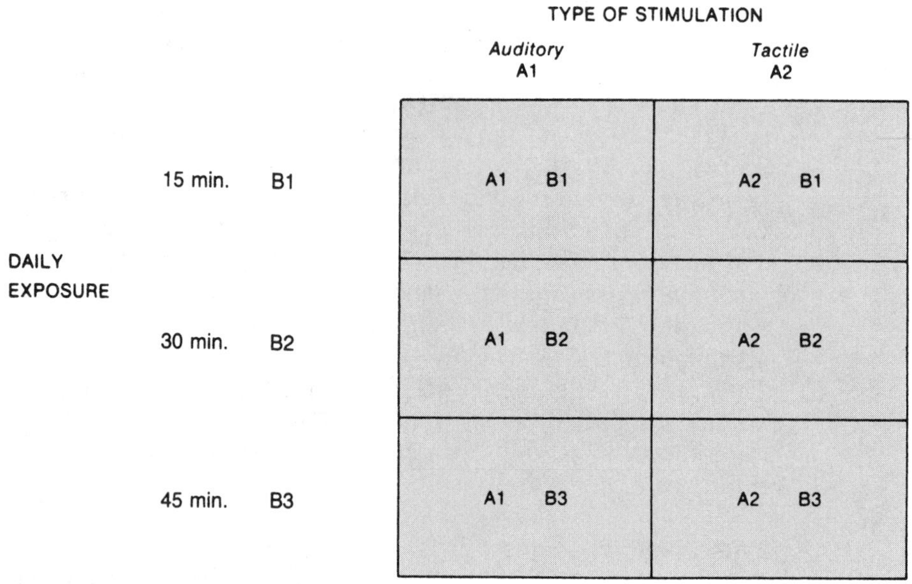

FIGURE 8-1. Schematic diagram of a factorial experiment.

The third question demonstrates a major strength of factorial designs: they permit us to evaluate not only **main effects** (effects resulting from the manipulated variables, as exemplified in questions 1 and 2) but also **interaction effects** (effects resulting from combining the treatment methods). Our results may indicate, for example, that 15 minutes of tactile stimulation and 45 minutes of auditory stimulation are the most beneficial treatments. We could not have learned this by conducting two separate experiments that manipulated one independent variable at a time.

In factorial experiments, subjects are assigned at random to a combination of treatments. In our example, premature infants would be assigned randomly to one of the six cells. The term **cell** is used in experimental research to refer to a treatment condition and is represented in a schematic diagram as a box. In a factorial design, the independent variables are referred to as **factors**. Type of stimulation is factor A and amount of exposure is factor B. Each factor must have two or more **levels**. Level one of factor A is *auditory,* and level two of factor A is *tactile.* The research design in Figure 8-1 would be described as a 2 × 3 design: two levels of factor A times three levels of factor B.

🔳 *Example of a factorial design:*

Pridham and her colleagues (1999) used a 2 × 2 design to study the effects of two factors—prescribed versus *ad libitum* infant feedings, and two caloric densities of the formula—on weight gain in premature infants. The 78 infant subjects were randomly assigned to one of four treatment conditions, and weight change was then assessed over a 5-day period.

Repeated-Measures Design.　Thus far, we have described experimental studies in which the subjects who are randomly assigned to groups are different people. For instance, the infants given 15 minutes of auditory stimulation in the factorial experiment are not the same infants as those exposed to the other treatment conditions. This broad class of designs is referred to as **between-subjects designs** because the comparisons made are between different people. When the same subjects are compared, the general class of designs is known as **within-subjects designs.**

A **repeated-measures design** (sometimes called a **crossover design**) involves the exposure of the same study participants to more than one treatment. Such studies are true experiments only if the participants are randomly assigned to different orderings of treatment. For example, if a repeated-measures design were used to compare the effects of auditory and tactile stimulation on infants, some subjects would be randomly assigned to receive auditory stimulation first, and others would receive tactile stimulation first. In such a study, the three conditions for an experiment have been met: there is manipulation, randomization, and control—with *subjects serving as their own control group.*

A repeated-measures design has the advantage of ensuring the highest possible equivalence among subjects exposed to different conditions. Repeated-measures designs are inappropriate for certain research questions, however, because of possible carryover effects. When subjects are exposed to two different treatments, they may be influenced in the second condition by their experience in the first. Drug studies rarely use a repeated-measures design because drug B administered after drug A is not the same treatment as drug B before drug A.

Some nonexperimental studies use a *statistical* repeated-measures feature for dealing with multiple points of data collection. A design is an experimental repeated-measures design only when the researcher introduces two or more treatments and randomizes the order of presentation of the treatments.

⊞　***Example of a repeated-measures or crossover design:***

Foster-Fitzpatrick and her co-researchers (1999) studied the effects of leg position on blood pressure measurements. Fifty subjects had their blood pressure measured with their feet flat on the floor and then again with their legs crossed at the knee. The ordering was reversed for the other 50 subjects in the sample.

Clinical Trials.　Medical researchers and epidemiologists often evaluate an innovative treatment through the use of a randomized clinical trial. **Clinical trials** involve the testing of a clinical treatment; random assignment of subjects to experimental and control conditions; collection of outcome information, sometimes after a long period has elapsed; and, generally, the use of a large, heterogeneous sample of subjects, frequently from multiple, geographically dispersed sites to ensure that the findings are not unique to a single setting. Clinical trials typically use a before–after or after-only design and are thus not so much a specific design type as a distinctive application of experimental design.

> **Example of a clinical trial:**
>
> Using a sample of more than 1,800 newborns from two hospitals, Dore and her colleagues (1998) assessed the effects of two different methods of umbilical cord care on umbilical infection and cord-separation time. The infants were randomly assigned to either umbilical cleansing with alcohol at each diaper change or natural drying of the umbilical site without special treatment.

Advantages and Disadvantages of Experiments

Experiments are the most powerful designs for testing hypotheses of cause-and-effect relationships. Because of its special controlling properties, an experiment offers greater corroboration than any other research approach that the independent variable (*e.g.,* diet, drug dosage, teaching approach) affects the dependent variable (*e.g.,* weight loss, recovery of health, learning).

Lazarsfeld (1955) identified three criteria for causality. First, a cause must precede an effect in time. To test the hypothesis that saccharin causes bladder cancer, it would be necessary to demonstrate that the subjects had not developed cancer before exposure to saccharin. Second, there must be an empirical relationship between the presumed cause and the presumed effect. In the saccharin and cancer example, the researcher would have to demonstrate an association between the ingestion of saccharin and the presence of a carcinoma (*i.e.,* that people who used saccharin experienced a higher incidence of cancer than those who did not). The final criterion for causality is that the relationship cannot be due to the influence of a third variable. Suppose, for instance, that people who use saccharin tend also to drink more coffee than nonusers. Thus, a relationship between saccharin use and bladder cancer may reflect an underlying causal relationship between a substance in coffee and bladder cancer. It is particularly because of this third criterion that the experimental approach is so strong. Through the controlling properties of manipulation, control groups, and randomization, alternative explanations to a causal interpretation can often be ruled out or discredited.

Despite the advantages of experiments, they have some limitations. First, a number of interesting variables simply are not amenable to manipulation. A large number of human characteristics, such as disease or health habits, cannot be randomly conferred on people.

Second, there are many variables that could technically—but not ethically—be manipulated. For example, to date there have been no experiments to study the effect of cigarette smoking on lung cancer. Such an experiment would require us to assign people randomly to a smoking group (people forced to smoke) or a nonsmoking group (people prohibited from smoking). Experimentation with humans, therefore, is subject to a number of ethical constraints.

In many health care settings, experimentation may not be feasible because it is impractical. It may, for instance, be impossible to secure the necessary cooperation from administrators or other key people to conduct an experiment.

Another potential problem is the **Hawthorne effect,** a term derived from a series of experiments conducted at the Hawthorne plant of the Western Electric Corporation in which various environmental conditions (*e.g.,* light, working hours) were varied to determine their effect on worker productivity. Regardless of what change was introduced (*i.e.,* whether the light was made better or worse), productivity increased. Thus, knowledge of being in a study may cause people to change their behavior, thereby obscuring the effect of the research variables.

In a hospital situation, the researcher might have to contend with a double Hawthorne effect. For example, if an experiment investigating the effect of a new postoperative patient routine were conducted, nurses as well as patients might be aware of participating in a study, and both groups could alter their actions accordingly. It is for this reason that **double-blind experiments**, in which neither the subjects nor those administering the treatment know who is in the experimental or control group, are so powerful. Unfortunately, the double-blind approach is not feasible in most nursing research because nursing interventions are harder to disguise than medications.

In summary, experimental designs have some limitations that make them difficult to apply to real-world problems; nevertheless, experiments have a clear-cut superiority for testing causal hypotheses.

 CONSUMER TIP:

Researchers using an experimental design generally note this in their reports, but they may also refer to the designs as randomized designs or as clinical trials. After-only, before–after, and repeated-measures designs are the most commonly used experimental designs. The research report does not always identify which specific experimental design was used; this may have to be inferred from information about the data collection plan (in the case of after-only and before–after designs) or from such statements as: The subjects were used as their own controls (in the case of a repeated-measures design). ■

Quasi-Experimental Research

Quasi-experimental research looks much like experiments because quasi-experiments also involve the manipulation of an independent variable (*i.e.,* the institution of a treatment). Quasi-experiments, however, lack either the randomization or control-group features that characterize true experiments, or both—features that strengthen the ability to make causal inferences.

Quasi-Experimental Designs
There are several quasi-experimental designs, but only the two most commonly used by nurse researchers are discussed here.

Nonequivalent Control Group Design.   The most frequently used quasi-experimental design is the **nonequivalent control-group before–after design**, which involves a treatment and two or more groups of subjects observed before and after its implementation. As an example, suppose we wanted to study the effect of primary nursing on nursing staff morale in a large metropolitan hospital. Because the new system of nursing care delivery is being implemented throughout the hospital, randomization is not possible. Therefore, we decide to collect comparison data from nurses in another similar hospital that is not instituting primary nursing. We decide to gather data on staff morale in both hospitals before implementing primary nursing delivery system (the pretest) and again after its implementation in the first hospital (the posttest).

This quasi-experimental research design is identical to the before–after experimental design discussed in the previous section, *except* subjects were not randomly assigned to the groups. The quasi-experimental design is weaker because, without randomization, *it cannot be assumed that the experimental and comparison groups are equivalent at the outset.* The design is, nevertheless, a strong one because the collection of pretest data allows us to determine whether the groups had similar morale initially. If the comparison and experimental groups responded similarly, on the average, at the pretest, we could be relatively confident that any posttest difference in self-reported morale was the result of the experimental treatment. (Note that in quasi-experiments, the term **comparison group** is generally used in lieu of *control group* to refer to the group against which outcomes in the treatment group are evaluated.)

Now suppose we had been unable to collect pretest data before primary nursing care was introduced (*i.e.,* only posttest data were collected). This design has a serious flaw because we have no basis for judging the initial equivalence of the two nursing staffs. If we found higher morale in the experimental group, could we conclude that primary nursing caused an improvement in staff morale? There could be several alternative explanations for posttest differences. Campbell and Stanley (1963), in fact, would call this **nonequivalent control group after-only design** a **preexperimental design** rather than a quasi-experimental design because the researcher is severely constrained from making the desired inferences. Thus, even though quasi-experiments lack some of the controlling properties of experiments, the hallmark of quasi-experiments is the effort to introduce some controls.

Example of a nonequivalent control group before–after design:

Johnson and her colleagues (1999) evaluated the effect of a nurse-delivered smoking cessation intervention on smoking status and smoking self-efficacy among patients hospitalized with cardiac disease. Experimental subjects were admitted to one cardiac unit, and comparison subjects were admitted to another. The researchers preferred this approach to randomization within units because information sharing among patients in the same unit would have contaminated the treatment conditions. By collecting pretest data, the researchers learned that the two groups were comparable with regard to demographic characteristics and preintervention smoking histories.

Time-Series Design.   In the designs just described, a control group was used, but randomization was not. The next design has neither a control group nor randomization. Let us suppose that a hospital is adopting a requirement that all its nurses accrue a certain number of continuing education units before being eligible for a promotion or raise. The nurse administrators want to assess the consequences of this mandate on turnover rate, absentee rate, and number of raises and promotions awarded. For the purposes of this example, assume there is no other hospital that can serve as a reasonable comparison for this study. In such a case, the only kind of comparison that can be made is a before–after contrast. If the requirement were inaugurated in January, one could compare the turnover rate, for example, for the 3-month period before the new rule with the turnover rate for the subsequent 3-month period.

This **one-group before–after design** seems logical, but it has a number of problems. What if one of the 3-month periods is atypical, apart from the mandate? What about the effect of any other rules instituted during the same period? What about the effects of external factors, such as changes in the local economy? The design in question, which is also preexperimental, offers no way of controlling any of these factors.

The inability to obtain a meaningful control group, however, does not eliminate the possibility of conducting research with integrity. The previous design could be modified so that at least some of the alternative explanations for change in nurses' turnover rate could be ruled out. One such design is the **time-series design**, which involves the collection of data over an extended time period and the introduction of the treatment during that period. The present study could be designed with four observations before the new continuing education rule and four observations after it. For example, the first observation might be the number of resignations between January and March in the year before the new rule, the second observation might be the number of resignations between April and June, and so forth. After the rule is implemented, data on turnover similarly would be collected for four consecutive 3-month periods, giving us observations 5 through 8.

Although the time-series design does not eliminate all the problems of interpreting changes in turnover rate, the extended time perspective strengthens a researcher's ability to attribute change to the intervention. This is because the time-series design rules out the possibility that changes in resignations represent a random fluctuation of turnover measured at only two points.

⊞⊞ *Example of a time-series design:*

Neuberger and her colleagues (1997) used a time-series design to study the effect of a low-impact aerobic exercise program on fatigue and aerobic fitness among people with rheumatoid arthritis. The researchers obtained measures of their outcome variables before the intervention, at midtreatment (after 6 weeks of exercise), at the end of treatment (12 weeks of exercise), and at a 15-week follow-up.

Advantages and Disadvantages of Quasi-Experiments

A strength of quasi-experiments is that they are practical. It is sometimes not feasible to conduct true experiments. Nursing research often occurs in natural settings, where it is difficult to deliver an innovative treatment randomly to some people but not to others. Quasi-experimental designs introduce some research control when full experimental rigor is not possible.

The major disadvantage of quasi-experiments is that cause-and-effect inferences that researchers often seek cannot be made as easily as with experiments. With quasi-experiments, there are alternative explanations for observed results. Suppose we wanted to evaluate the effect of a nursing intervention for infants of heroin-addicted mothers on infants' weight gain. If we use no comparison group or if we use a nonequivalent control group and then observe a weight gain, we must ask the following questions: Is it plausible that some external factor influenced the gain? Is it plausible that pretreatment group differences resulted in differential weight gains? Is it plausible that the changes would have occurred without an intervention? If the answer to any of these **rival hypotheses** is yes, inferences about treatment effectiveness are weakened. With quasi-experiments, there is almost always at least one plausible rival explanation.

CONSUMER TIP:

Researchers often do not identify their studies as quasi-experimental or preexperimental. If a study involves a treatment or intervention (*i.e.*, if the researcher has control over the independent variable) and if the report does not explicitly mention random assignment or the use of an experimental design, it is probably safe to conclude that the design is quasi-experimental or preexperimental. ■

Nonexperimental Research

Many research problems cannot be addressed with an experimental or quasi-experimental design. For example, suppose we are interested in studying the effect of widowhood on physical and psychological functioning. Our independent variable here is widowhood versus nonwidowhood. Clearly, we cannot manipulate widowhood; people lose their spouses by a process that is neither random nor subject to research control. Thus, we would have to proceed by taking the two groups (widows and nonwidows) as they naturally occur and comparing their psychological and physical well-being. There are various reasons for doing **nonexperimental research**, including situations in which the independent variable is inherently nonmanipulable or in which it would be unethical to manipulate the independent variable. There are also research questions for which an experimental design is not appropriate, such as studies whose purpose is description.

Types of Nonexperimental Research

One class of nonexperimental research is known as *ex post facto* (or **correlational**) **research.** The literal translation of the Latin term *ex post facto* is "from after the fact," indicating that the research has been conducted after variation in the independent variable has occurred.

The basic purpose of *ex post facto* or correlational research is essentially the same as that of experimental research: to study relationships among variables. However, it is difficult to infer causal relationships in *ex post facto* studies. In experiments, the investigator makes a prediction that a deliberate variation in *X,* the independent variable, will result in changes to *Y,* the dependent variable. In *ex post facto* research, on the other hand, the investigator does not control the independent variable—the presumed causative factor—because it has already occurred. It is risky to draw cause-and-effect conclusions in such a situation. A famous research dictum is relevant: *correlation does not prove causation.* That is, the mere existence of a relationship between variables is not enough to warrant the conclusion that one variable caused the other, even if the relationship is strong.

Ex post facto research that is designed to shed light on causal relationships is sometimes described as either retrospective or prospective. **Retrospective studies** are *ex post facto* investigations in which a phenomenon observed in the present is linked to phenomena occurring in the past. In a retrospective study, the investigator focuses on a presently occurring outcome and then tries to ascertain the antecedent factors that have caused it. For example, in retrospective lung cancer research, the investigator begins with a sample of those who have lung cancer and a sample of those who do not. The researcher then looks for differences between the groups in antecedent behaviors or conditions, such as smoking habits.

Prospective studies, by contrast, start with an examination of a presumed cause and then go forward to the presumed effect. For example, in prospective lung cancer studies, researchers start with samples of smokers and nonsmokers and later compare the two groups in terms of lung cancer incidence. Prospective studies are more costly than retrospective studies but are considerably stronger. For one thing, any ambiguity concerning the temporal sequence of phenomena is resolved in prospective research (*i.e.,* the smoking is known to precede the lung cancer). In addition, samples are more likely to be representative of smokers and nonsmokers, and investigators may be in a position to impose controls to rule out competing explanations for observed effects.

Example of a prospective study:

McGrath & Sullivan (1999) studied the motor outcomes of children aged 4 years who had been born with varying degrees of medical risk. Five groups of children born at a tertiary medical center (full-term infants; healthy preterm infants; small-for-gestational-age preterm infants; sick preterm infants; and neurological preterm infants) were followed over a 4-year period to study the relationship between degree of medical risk and subsequent motor deficits.

Researchers can sometimes strengthen a retrospective study, using a **case-control design.** This design involves comparing "cases" with a certain condition (*e.g.,* women with breast cancer) with controls (women without breast cancer) who are selected to be similar to the cases with regard to key background factors (*e.g.,* age, family history of breast cancer). If the researcher can demonstrate similarity between cases and controls with regard to extraneous traits, the inferences regarding the presumed cause of the disease are enhanced.

Example of a retrospective case-control study:

Pressler and her co-researchers (1999) compared the behavioral responses of newborns of insulin-dependent diabetic mothers with newborns of nondiabetic mothers. The two groups were matched to be comparable in terms of type of delivery, parity, labor and delivery medications, race, and maternal education, so that any group differences in the newborns' responses could not be attributed to these factors.

A second broad class of nonexperimental research is **descriptive research.** The purpose of descriptive studies is to observe, describe, and document aspects of a situation. For example, an investigator may wish to determine the percentage of teenaged mothers who receive inadequate prenatal care. Sometimes, a report refers to the study design as a **descriptive correlational study,** meaning that the researcher was interested primarily in describing relationships among variables, without necessarily seeking to establish a causal connection. For example, a researcher might be interested in documenting the relationship between fatigue and psychological distress. Because the intent in these situations is not to explain or to understand the underlying causes of the variables of interest, a nonexperimental design is appropriate.

Example of a descriptive study:

Berg (1999) conducted a study to describe the biologic, psychological, social, and cultural dimensions of the perimenopausal transition of Filipino American women in midlife. For example, Berg described the Filipino women's level of depression, menstrual cyclicity, and good health and risk behaviors.

Advantages and Disadvantages of Nonexperimental Research

The major disadvantage of nonexperimental research is its inability to reveal causal relationships conclusively. *Ex post facto* studies are susceptible to faulty interpretation because the researcher works with preexisting groups that have formed through self-selection. Kerlinger (1986), a noted research methodologist, indicates that "**self-selection** occurs when the members of the groups being studied are in the groups, in part, because they differentially possess traits or characteristics extraneous to the research problem, characteristics that possibly influence or are otherwise related to the variables of the research problem" (p. 349). In other words, preexisting differences may be a plausible alternative explanation for any observed group differences on the dependent variable.

As an example of the interpretive problems in *ex post facto* studies, suppose we were interested in studying differences in the level of depression of cancer patients who do or do not have adequate social support (*i.e.,* assistance and emotional sustenance through a social network). The independent variable is social support, and the dependent variable is depression. Suppose we found that patients without social support are more depressed than the patients with adequate social support. We could interpret this finding to mean that people's emotional state is influenced by the adequacy of their social supports. This relationship is diagrammed in Figure 8-2*A*. There are, however, alternative explanations for the findings. Perhaps there is a third variable that influences *both* social support and depression, such as the patients' family structure (*e.g.,* whether they are married). It may be that the availability of a significant other is a powerful influence on how depressed cancer patients feel *and* on the quality of their social support. These relationships are diagrammed in Figure 8-2*B*. A third possibility may be reversed causality, as shown in Figure 8-2*C*. Depressed cancer patients may find it more difficult to elicit needed social support from others than patients who are more cheerful. In this interpretation, it is the person's emotional state that causes the amount of received social support, and not the other way around. The point here is that *ex post facto* results should be interpreted cautiously, especially if the research has no theoretical basis.

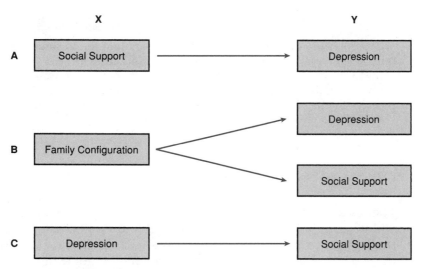

FIGURE 8-2. Alternative explanations for relationship between depression and social support in cancer patients.

CONSUMER TIP:

Be prepared to think critically when a researcher claims to be studying the "effects" or "impacts" of an independent variable on a dependent variable in a nonexperimental study. For example, if the title of a report were "The Effects of Dieting on Depression," the study would likely be nonexperimental (*i.e.,* subjects were not randomly assigned to dieting or not dieting). In such a situation, you might ask, Did dieting have an effect on depression? or, Did depression have an affect on dieting? or, Did a third variable (*e.g.,* being overweight) have an effect on both? ■

Despite the interpretive problems associated with *ex post facto* studies, they continue to play a crucial role in nursing because many interesting problems are not amenable to experimentation. Correlational research is often an efficient and effective means of collecting a large amount of data about a problem area. For example, it would be possible to collect extensive information about the health histories and eating habits of a large number of people. Researchers could then examine which health problems correlate with which diets. By doing this, a large number of interrelationships could be discovered in a relatively short time. By contrast, an experimenter looks at only a few variables at a time. For example, one experiment might manipulate foods with different cholesterol levels to observe the effects on physical symptoms, whereas another experiment might manipulate protein consumption, and so forth.

One final advantage is that nonexperimental research tends to be high in realism. Correlational and descriptive research can seldom be criticized for their artificiality.

 CONSUMER TIP:

Retrospective *ex post facto* studies are more common in nursing than prospective studies. Research reports, however, rarely point out that the design is retrospective. You will have to determine whether the researcher measured the dependent variable in the present and then attempted to identify its antecedent causes or determinants. By contrast, researchers almost always make explicit reference to the use of a prospective design. ■

RESEARCH DESIGN AND THE TIME DIMENSION

The research design incorporates decisions about when and how often data will be collected in a study. In many nursing studies, data are collected at a single point in time; other studies involve data collection on more than one occasion. Indeed, several designs involving multiple measurements have already been discussed, such as the pretest–posttest experimental design, the time-series design, and the prospective design.

There are four situations in which it is appropriate to design a study with multiple points of data collection:

1. *Time-related processes.* Certain research problems involve phenomena that evolve over time. Examples include healing, learning, growth, recidivism, and physical development.
2. *Time-sequenced phenomena.* It is sometimes important to ascertain the sequencing of phenomena. For example, if it is hypothesized that infertility contributes to depression, it would be important to determine that depression did not precede the fertility problem.
3. *Comparative purposes.* Sometimes, multiple data points are used to compare phenomena over time. For example, a study might document trends in the incidence of child abuse over a 10-year period. Another example is a time-series study, in which the intent is to determine whether changes over time can be attributed to an intervention.
4. *Enhancement of research control.* Some research designs collect data at multiple points to enhance the interpretability of the results. For example, in nonequivalent control-group designs, the collection of preintervention data allows the researcher to detect and control for initial group differences.

Because of the importance of the time dimension in designing research, studies are often categorized in terms of how they deal with time. The major distinction is between cross-sectional and longitudinal designs.

Cross-Sectional Designs

Cross-sectional studies involve the collection of data at one point in time. The phenomena under study are captured during one data collection period. Cross-sectional designs are especially appropriate for describing the status of phenomena or relationships among phenomena at a fixed point. For example, a researcher might study whether psychological symptoms in menopausal women are correlated contemporaneously with physiologic symptoms. Retrospective studies are almost always cross-sectional. Data with regard to the independent and dependent variables are collected concurrently (*e.g.,* the lung cancer status of respondents and their smoking habits), but the independent variable usually captures events or behaviors occurring in the past.

When cross-sectional designs are used to study time-related phenomena, the designs are weaker than longitudinal ones. Suppose, for example, we were studying changes in nursing students' attitudes toward nursing research as they progress through a 4-year baccalaureate program. One way to investigate this would be to survey students when they are freshmen and resurvey them again as seniors. On the other hand, we could use a cross-sectional design by surveying members of these two classes at one point in time and then comparing their responses. If seniors had more positive attitudes toward research than freshmen, it might be inferred that nursing students become socialized professionally by their educational experiences. To make this kind of inference, the researcher must assume that the seniors would have responded as the freshmen responded had they been questioned 3 years earlier, or, conversely, that freshmen would be more favorable toward research if they were surveyed again 3 years later.

The main advantage of cross-sectional designs is that they are economical and easy to manage. There are, however, problems in inferring changes and trends over time using a cross-sectional design. The amount of social and technological change that characterizes our society makes it questionable to assume that differences in the behaviors, attitudes, or characteristics of different age groups are the result of the passage through time rather than cohort or generational differences. In the previous example, seniors and freshmen may have different attitudes toward nursing research independent of any experiences they had during their 4 years of education. In cross-sectional studies, there are frequently alternative explanations for any observed differences.

Example of a cross-sectional study:

Morse and Fife (1998) used a cross-sectional design to study the development of coping and adjustment patterns among the spouses and partners of cancer patients. Their sample included patients at four stages of the illness trajectory: diagnosis, first remission, first recurrence, and metastatic disease.

Longitudinal Designs

Research projects designed to collect data over an extended time period are referred to as **longitudinal studies.** The main value of longitudinal designs is their ability to demonstrate changes over time and the temporal sequencing of phenomena, which is an essential criterion for establishing causality.

Three types of longitudinal studies deserve special mention: trend, panel, and follow-up studies. **Trend studies** are investigations in which samples from a general population are studied over time with respect to some phenomenon. Different samples are selected at repeated intervals, but the samples are always drawn from the same population. Trend studies permit researchers to examine patterns and rates of change and to make predictions about future directions. For example, trend studies have been conducted to analyze the number of students entering nursing programs and to forecast future supplies of nursing personnel.

In **panel studies,** the same participants supply the data at two or more points in time. The term *panel* refers to the sample of people involved in the study. Panel studies typically yield more information than trend studies because the investigator can examine patterns of change and reasons for the changes. The same people are contacted at two or more points in time; therefore, the researcher can identify those who did and did not change and then isolate the characteristics of the subgroups in which change occurred. Panel studies are appealing as an approach to studying change but are difficult and expensive to manage. The most serious problem is the loss of participants at different points in the study. Subject **attrition** causes problems for the researcher because those who drop out of the study may differ in important respects from those who continue to participate; hence, the generalizability of the findings may be impaired.

EE | *Example of a panel study:*

Wilson and co-researchers (2000) explored relationships among family dynamics, paternal–fetal and maternal–fetal attachment, and infant temperament. They first gathered data from pregnant women and their partners during the third trimester of pregnancy. Parental data from the first round of data collection were then linked to the infant's temperament about 1 year later when they were 8 to 9 months old.

Follow-up studies are undertaken to determine the subsequent status of subjects with a specified condition or those who have received a specified intervention. For example, patients who have received a particular nursing intervention or clinical treatment may be followed up to ascertain the long-term effects of the treatment. To take a nonexperimental example, samples of premature infants may be followed up to assess their later perceptual and motor development. Prospective studies generally fall in this category.

EE | *Example of a follow-up study:*

Miles, Holditch-Davis, Burchinal, and Nelson (1999) conducted a follow-up study of 67 mothers whose infants had a serious life-threatening illness. Data on the mothers' level of depression and their personal growth and development were collected at hospital discharge and then 6, 12, and 16 months after birth.

In longitudinal studies, the number of data collection periods and the time intervals between data collection points depend on the nature of the study. When change or development is rapid, numerous time points at relatively short intervals may be required to document the pattern and to make accurate forecasts. By convention, however, the term *longitudinal* implies multiple data collection points over an extended period of time. Our earlier example of a time-series study, which involved the collection of data on nurse turnover rates over a 2-year period, would be considered longitudinal. However, a time-series design involving the collection of patient data on vital signs preoperatively and postoperatively at hourly intervals over a 2-day period would not be described as longitudinal.

SPECIFIC TYPES OF QUANTITATIVE RESEARCH

This section describes some specific types of quantitative nursing research that vary according to the study's purpose rather than the dimensions outlined in Table 8-1.

Surveys

A **survey** obtains information regarding the prevalence, distribution, and interrelationships of variables within a population. Political opinion polls, such as those conducted by Gallup, are examples of surveys. Surveys collect information on people's actions, knowledge, intentions, opinions, and attitudes. Survey data are based on **self-reports**; that is, the respondents answer questions posed by the researcher. The three most common methods of collecting survey data are personal, face-to-face interviews; interviews by telephone; and self-administered questionnaires distributed through the mail. Survey research is highly flexible: it can be applied to many populations, it can focus on a wide range of topics, and its information can be used for many purposes. Survey information tends, however, to be relatively superficial. Survey research is better suited to extensive rather than intensive analysis. Although surveys can be performed within the context of large-scale experiments, surveys are usually done as part of a nonexperimental study.

> *Example of a survey:*
>
> Paul-Allen and Ostrow (2000) were interested in learning about critical care nurses' use of closed-system versus open-system suctioning, and the use of hyperoxygenation and hyperinflation among those using closed-system suctioning. Using mailed questionnaires, the researchers surveyed 241 critical care nurses in a tristate area.

Evaluations

Evaluations are used to find out how well a program, treatment, practice, or policy works. Clinical nurses, nurse administrators, and nursing educators often need to pose such questions as the following: How are current practices working? Is there a more effective way to do things? Should a new practice be adopted? Which approach is most effective? In this era of accountability, evaluations of the effectiveness of nursing actions are common. Evaluations can employ experimental, quasi-experimental, or nonexperimental designs and can be either cross-sectional or longitudinal.

There are various types of evaluations. A **process analysis** (or an **implementation analysis**) is undertaken to obtain descriptive information about the process of implementing a new program or procedure and about its functioning in actual operation. An **outcome analysis** documents the extent to which the goals of a program are attained (*i.e.*, the extent to which positive outcomes occur). An **impact analysis** attempts to identify (usually using an experimental design) the impacts or **net effects** of an intervention (*i.e.,* the effects over and above what would have occurred in the absence of the intervention). Finally, evaluations sometimes include a **cost–benefit analysis** to determine whether the monetary benefits of the program outweigh the costs.

> **Example of an evaluation:**
>
> Parker and her colleagues (1999) evaluated a nursing intervention designed to prevent further abuse of pregnant women who had been abused by their partners. Using a nonequivalent control-group design, the researchers compared women who received the three-session intervention with those who did not and found less violence reported by women in the intervention group both 6 months and 12 months after delivery.

Outcomes Research

Outcomes research, designed to document the effectiveness of health care services, is gaining momentum in nursing and health care fields. Outcomes research overlaps with evaluation research, but evaluations typically appraise a specific new intervention, whereas outcomes research is a more global assessment of health care services. The impetus for outcomes research comes from the quality assessment and quality assurance functions that grew out of the professional standards review organizations (PSROs) in the 1970s. Outcomes research represents a response to the increasing demand from policy makers, insurers, and the public to justify care practices and systems in terms of both improved patient outcomes and costs. Specific efforts to appraise and document the quality of nursing care—as distinct from the care provided by the overall health care system—are not numerous. A major obstacle is attribution, that is, linking the outcomes of interest to specific nursing actions or interventions, distinct from the actions or interventions of other members of the health care team.

> **Example of outcomes research:**
>
> Alexy and Elnitsky (1998) conducted an outcomes study to document the experiences of a Mobile Health Unit that was designed to increase access to nursing services among rural elderly residents. The research project found, for example, that the Mobile Health Unit resulted in reduced use of the emergency room and increased breast and cervical cancer screenings.

TECHNIQUES OF RESEARCH CONTROL

A major purpose of research design in quantitative studies is to maximize the researcher's control over the research situation. This section describes what is meant by research control and then discusses methods of achieving it.

Research Control

Research control is concerned with eliminating possible extraneous influences on the dependent variable so that the true relationship between the independent and dependent variables can be understood. Research control attempts to exclude contaminating factors that might obscure the relationship between the variables that are of central interest. A detailed example should clarify this point.

Suppose we wanted to study whether teenaged women are at higher risk than older mothers of having low-birth-weight infants because of their age. In other words, we want to test whether something about the maturational development of women causes differences in the birth weights of their infants. Existing studies have shown that, in fact, teenagers have a higher rate of low-birth-weight infants than women in their 20s. The question, however, is whether age itself causes this difference or whether there are other **mediating variables** that intervene in the relationship between maternal age and infant birth weight.

We would want a study design that controls other influences on the dependent variable. But which variables should be controlled? To answer this, we must ask the following crucial question: What variables affect the dependent variable and at the same time are related to the independent variable?

In the present study, the dependent variable is infant birth weight and the independent variable is maternal age. Two variables that are candidates for concern (there are other possibilities) are the nutritional habits of the mother and the amount of prenatal care received. Teenagers have been found to have less-adequate diets during pregnancy and are also less likely to obtain adequate prenatal care than older women. Both nutrition and the amount of care could, in turn, affect the baby's birth weight. Thus, if these two mediating factors are not controlled, any observed relationship between the mother's age and her baby's weight at birth could be caused by the mother's age, by her diet, or by her prenatal care.

These three possible explanations are shown schematically.

1. Mother's age → infant birth weight
2. Mother's age → adequacy of prenatal care → infant birth weight
3. Mother's age → nutritional adequacy → infant birth weight

The arrows symbolize a causal mechanism or an influence. The researcher's task is to design a study in which the true explanation is made clear. If the researcher is testing the first explanation, then both nutrition and prenatal care must be controlled.

How can the researcher impose this control? The general principle underlying various control methods is this: the competing influences—the extraneous variables—must be held constant. The extraneous variables must somehow be handled in such a way that, *in the context of the study,* they are not related to the independent variable or dependent variable.

Research control is a fundamental feature of quantitative studies. The world is complex, and variables are interrelated in complicated ways. In quantitative studies, it is difficult to examine this complexity directly. Researchers analyze a few relationships at one time and put the pieces together like a jigsaw puzzle. That is why even modest quantitative studies can make contributions to knowledge. The extent of the contribution, however, is often related to how well a researcher controls contaminating influences. In reading reports, you will need to consider whether the researcher has, in fact, appropriately controlled extraneous variables.

Controlling External Factors

Various external factors, such as the research environment, can affect study variables. In carefully controlled quantitative research, steps are taken to minimize situational contaminants (*i.e.*, to achieve **constancy of conditions** for the collection of data) so that the researcher can be confident that the conditions are not influencing the data.

The environment has been found to influence people's emotions and behavior, and therefore investigators strive to control the environmental context of the study. Control over the environment is most easily achieved in laboratory experiments, in which all subjects are brought into an environment structured by the researcher. Researchers have less freedom to control studies that occur in natural settings, but some opportunities exist. For example, in interview studies, researchers can restrict data collection to one type of setting (*e.g.*, the respondents' homes).

A second external factor that may need to be controlled is time. Depending on the research topic, the dependent variable may be influenced by the time of day or the time of year in which the data are collected. In these cases, the researcher should ensure that constancy of time is maintained. If an investigator were studying fatigue or perceptions of well-being, it would matter whether the data were gathered in the morning, afternoon, or evening or in the summer as opposed to the winter.

Another aspect of maintaining constancy of conditions concerns the communications to the subjects. To ensure constancy of communication, formal scripts are often prepared. In research involving the implementation of a treatment, formal **research protocols**, or specifications for the interventions, are developed. For example, in an experiment to test the effectiveness of a new medication, care would be needed to ensure that the subjects in the experimental group received the same chemical substance and the same dosage, that the substance was administered in the same way, and so forth.

Controlling Intrinsic Factors

Control of study participants' characteristics is especially important. For example, suppose we were investigating the effects of an innovative physical training program on the cardiovascular functioning of nursing home residents. In this study, variables such as the subjects' age, gender, and smoking history would be extraneous variables; each is likely to be related to the outcome variable (cardiovascular functioning), independent of the physical training program. In other words, the effects that these variables have on the dependent variable are extraneous to the research topic. In this section, we review methods of controlling extraneous subject characteristics.

Methods of Controlling Subject Characteristics

Randomization. We have already discussed the most effective method of controlling subject characteristics: randomization. The primary function of randomization is to secure comparable groups, that is, to equalize the groups with respect to the extraneous variables. A distinct advantage of random assignment, compared with other methods of controlling extraneous variables, is that randomization controls all possible sources of extraneous variation, without any conscious decision on the researcher's part about which variables need to be controlled. In our example of the physical training intervention, random assignment of subjects to an experimental (intervention) group and control (no intervention) group would be the ideal control mechanism. Presumably, these two groups would be comparable in terms of age, gender, smoking history, and thousands of other preintervention characteristics. Randomization within a repeated-measures context is especially powerful. In a repeated-measures design, participants serve as their own controls, thereby totally controlling all extraneous variables.

Example of randomization:

Roberts and her colleagues (1999) tested the effects of problem-solving counseling for the caregivers of the cognitively impaired using an experimental before–after design. The researchers found that the randomly assigned experimental group was similar to the control group in terms of pretreatment income, employment status, marital status, depression levels, health status, age, and gender.

Homogeneity. When randomization is not feasible, other methods of controlling extraneous subject characteristics can be used. The first alternative is **homogeneity**, in which only subjects who are homogeneous with respect to the extraneous variables are included in the study. The extraneous variables, in this case, are not allowed to vary. In the example of the physical training program, if gender were considered a confounding variable, the researcher could recruit only men (or only women) as participants. If the researcher were concerned about the confounding effect of the participants' ages on physical fitness, participation could be limited to those within a specified age range. This strategy of using a homogeneous subject pool is easy, but its limitation is that the findings can be generalized only to the type of subjects who participated. If the physical training program was found to have beneficial effects on the cardiovascular functioning of men aged 65 to 75 years, its usefulness for improving the cardiovascular status of women in their 80s would need to be tested in a separate study.

> **Example of homogeneity:**
>
> Lee, Portillo, and Miramontes (1999) studied the fatigue experience of women with human immunodeficiency virus (HIV) in relation to physiologic variables such as age, sleep, and CD4 cell count. Women with certain characteristics were excluded from the study to avoid confounding effects; for example, women with grade II neuropathy were excluded because they are "often taking medications that confound the validity of the findings" (p. 195).

Matching. A third method of dealing with extraneous variables is matching. **Matching** involves using information about subject characteristics to form comparison groups. For example, suppose the researcher began with a sample of nursing home residents already participating in the physical training program. A comparison group of nonparticipating residents could be created by matching subjects, one by one, on the basis of important extraneous variables (*e.g.,* age and gender). This procedure results in groups known to be comparable in terms of the extraneous variables of concern. Matching is the technique used to form comparable groups in case-control designs.

Matching has some drawbacks as a control technique. To match effectively, the researcher must know in advance what the relevant extraneous variables are. Second, after two or three variables, it becomes difficult to match. Suppose we wanted to control the age, gender, race, and length of nursing home stays of the participants. Thus, if participant 1 in the physical training program is an African American woman, aged 80 years, whose length of stay is 5 years, the researcher must seek another woman with these same or similar characteristics as a comparison group counterpart. With more than three variables, the matching procedure becomes extremely cumbersome. Thus, matching as a control technique is generally used only when more powerful procedures are not feasible.

> **Example of matching:**
>
> Walker and O'Brien (1999) studied the relationship between method of pain management (epidural and nonepidural) during labor on the one hand and birth outcomes such as cesarean delivery, length of second stage labor, and infant Apgar scores on the other. To keep the groups similar, the nonepidural women were matched with the epidural women in terms of cervical dilation on admission and birthing day.

Statistical Control. Yet another method of controlling extraneous variables is through statistical analysis. Many readers are unfamiliar with basic statistical procedures, let alone sophisticated techniques such as those referred to here. Therefore, a detailed description of powerful statistical control mechanisms, such as **analysis of covariance**, will not be attempted. You should recognize, however, that nurse researchers are increasingly using powerful statistical techniques to control extraneous variables. A brief description of analysis of covariance is presented in Chapter 13.

Example of statistical control:

Kim, Bramlett, Wright, and Poon (1998) studied racial differences in the health status and health behaviors of older adults. The researchers knew that race is related to socioeconomic variables, which in turn are related to health outcomes. The researchers therefore statistically controlled income and education. Through statistical control, the two racial groups (African Americans and whites) were made comparable in terms of education and income, so that observed racial differences in health could not be attributed to these socioeconomic indicators.

Evaluation of Control Methods

Overall, random assignment is the most effective approach to controlling extraneous variables because randomization tends to cancel out individual variation on all possible extraneous variables. Repeated-measures designs are especially powerful, but they cannot be applied to all nursing research problems because of the possibility of carryover effects. The three remaining alternatives described here have two disadvantages in common. First, the researcher must know the relevant extraneous variables in advance. To select homogeneous samples, match, or perform an analysis of covariance, researchers must decide which variables to control. Second, these three methods control only for pre-identified characteristics, possibly leaving others uncontrolled.

Although randomization is the best mechanism for controlling extraneous subject characteristics, randomization is not always possible. If the independent variable cannot be manipulated, other techniques must be used. It is far better to use matching or analysis of covariance than simply to ignore the problem of extraneous variables.

 CONSUMER TIP:

In nursing studies that are not experimental, statistical procedures such as analysis of covariance are the most frequently used methods of controlling extraneous variables. Matching, which was a commonly used control technique a few decades ago, has become much less prevalent since computers have become widely available for statistical analysis. ■

INTERNAL AND EXTERNAL VALIDITY

In evaluating the merits of a quantitative study, you will need to pay careful attention to its research design. One useful framework for evaluating the adequacy of a research design in a quantitative study is an assessment of its internal and external validity.

Internal Validity

Campbell and Stanley (1963), in a classic monograph, use the term **internal validity** to refer to the extent to which it is possible to make an inference that the independent variable is truly influencing the dependent variable. Experiments possess a high degree of internal validity because randomization to different groups enables the researcher to rule out competing explanations. With quasi-experiments and correlational studies, the investigator must always contend with rival hypotheses. Competing explanations, or **threats to internal validity**, have been grouped into several classes.

Threats to Internal Validity

History.   The **history threat** is the occurrence of events concurrent with the independent variable that can affect the dependent variable. For example, suppose we were studying the effectiveness of an outreach program to encourage flu shots among the community-dwelling elderly using a time-series design. Now let us further suppose that, at about the same time the outreach program was initiated, there was a national public media campaign focusing on the flu. Our dependent variable in this case, number of flu shots administered, is now subject to the influence of at least two forces, and it becomes impossible for us to disentangle the two effects. In an experiment, history is not typically an issue because external events are as likely to affect one group as another; however, history can be a threat in quasi-experimental and nonexperimental studies.

Selection.   The **selection threat** encompasses biases resulting from preexisting differences between groups. When people are not assigned randomly to groups, the possibility always exists that groups being compared are not equivalent. In such a situation, the researcher contends with the possibility that any difference in the dependent variable is due to extraneous factors rather than to the independent variable. Selection biases are the most problematic threats to the internal validity of studies not using an experimental design but can be partially addressed using the control mechanisms described in the previous section.

Maturation.   In a research context, the **maturation threat** arises from processes occurring within the subjects as a result of time (*e.g.,* growth, fatigue) rather than the independent variable. For example, if we wanted to evaluate the effect of a special sensorimotor-development program for developmentally retarded children, we would have to contend with the fact that progress would occur even without the intervention. Maturation is a relevant consideration in many areas of nursing research. Remember that the term here does not refer to developmental changes exclusively but rather to any kind of change that occurs as a function of time. Thus, phenomena such as wound healing, postoperative recovery, and other bodily changes can occur with little nursing intervention, and thus maturation may be a rival explanation for posttreatment results. The one-group before–after design is particularly vulnerable to the maturation threat.

Mortality. The **mortality threat** arises from differential attrition from groups. The loss of subjects during the study may differ among groups because of initial differences in interest, motivation, and the like. For example, suppose we used a nonequivalent control-group design to assess nurses' morale in two different hospitals, one of which initiated primary nursing. The dependent variable, nursing staff satisfaction, is measured before and after the intervention. The comparison group, which may have no particular commitment to the study, may be reluctant to complete a posttest questionnaire. Those who do fill it out may be totally unrepresentative of the group as a whole; they may be highly critical of their work environment, for example. Thus, on the average, it may appear that the morale of nurses in the comparison hospital declined, but this might only be an artifact of the mortality of a select segment of this group.

Internal Validity and Research Design

Quasi-experimental, preexperimental, and correlational studies are especially susceptible to threats to internal validity. The four threats described previously represent alternative explanations that compete with the independent variable as an influence on the dependent variable. *The aim of a good quantitative research design is to rule out these competing explanations.* The control mechanisms previously reviewed are strategies for improving the internal validity of studies.

Experimental designs normally eliminate competing explanations, but this is not always the case. For example, if constancy of conditions is not maintained for experimental and control groups, history might be a rival explanation for obtained results. Experimental mortality is, in particular, a salient threat in experiments. Because the experimenter does different things with the experimental and control groups, participants may drop out of the study differentially among these groups. This is particularly likely to happen if the experimental treatment is stressful, inconvenient, or time-consuming or if the control condition is boring or aggravating. When this happens, the participants remaining in the study may differ from those who left, thereby nullifying the initial equivalence of the groups.

You should pay careful attention to the possibility of competing explanations for reported results, especially in studies that do not use an experimental design. When the investigator does not have control over critical extraneous variables, caution in interpreting the results and drawing conclusions from them is appropriate.

External Validity

The term **external validity** refers to the generalizability of the research findings to other settings or samples. Quantitative studies are rarely conducted with the intention of discovering relationships among variables for a single group of people. If a nursing intervention is found to be successful, others would want to adopt the procedure. Therefore, an important question is whether the intervention would work in another setting or with different patients.

One aspect of a study's external validity concerns the adequacy of the sampling design. If the characteristics of the sample are representative of those of the population, the generalizability of the results is enhanced. Sampling designs are described in Chapter 10.

Various characteristics of the environment or research situation also affect the study's external validity. For example, when a treatment is new (*e.g.*, a new curriculum for nursing students), subjects and researchers alike might alter their behavior. People may be either enthusiastic or skeptical about new methods of doing things. Thus, the results may reflect reactions to the novelty rather than to the intrinsic qualities of the treatment.

Sometimes, the demands for internal and external validity conflict. If a researcher exercises tight control over a study to maximize internal validity, the setting may become too artificial to generalize to a more naturalistic environment. Therefore, a compromise must sometimes be reached. The importance of replicating studies in different settings with new subjects cannot be overemphasized.

CRITIQUING QUANTITATIVE RESEARCH DESIGNS

The overriding consideration in evaluating a research design is whether the design enables the researcher to answer the research question. This must be determined in terms of both substantive and methodologic issues.

Substantively, the issue is whether the researcher selected a design that matches the aims of the research. If the research purpose is descriptive or exploratory, an experimental design is inappropriate. If the researcher is searching to understand the full nature of a phenomenon about which little is known, a highly structured design that allows little flexibility might block insights (flexible designs are discussed in Chapter 9). We have discussed research control as a mechanism for reducing bias, but in certain situations, too much control can introduce bias, for example, when the researcher tightly controls the ways in which the phenomena under study can be manifested and thereby obscures their true nature.

Methodologically, the main design issues in quantitative studies are whether the research design provides the most accurate, unbiased, interpretable answers possible to the research question and whether it yields replicable results. Box 8-1 provides questions to assist you in evaluating the methodologic aspects of quantitative research designs.

RESEARCH EXAMPLES

Following are descriptions of the research designs used in three actual nursing studies. Use the guidelines in Box 8-1 to evaluate the research designs, referring to the full reports (cited at the end of the chapter), if necessary.

| BOX 8-1 | **GUIDELINES FOR CRITIQUING RESEARCH DESIGNS IN QUANTITATIVE STUDIES** |

1. Given the nature of the research question, what type of design is most appropriate? How does this correspond to the type of design used?

2. Does the design used in the study involve an intervention? If yes, was an experimental, quasi-experimental, or preexperimental design used—and was this the most appropriate design?

3. If the design is nonexperimental, why didn't the researcher manipulate the independent variable? Was the decision regarding manipulation appropriate?

4. Was the study longitudinal or cross-sectional? Was the number of points of data collection appropriate, given the research question?

5. What type of comparisons were called for in the research design (*e.g.*, was the study design within-subjects or between-subjects)? Are these comparisons the most appropriate for illuminating the relationship between the independent and dependent variables?

6. Can the study be described as a survey, an evaluation, or outcomes research?

7. What procedures, if any, did the researcher use to control external (situational) factors and intrinsic (subject characteristic) factors? Were these procedures appropriate and adequate?

8. To what extent is the study internally valid? What types of alternative explanations must be considered (*i.e.*, what are the threats to the study's internal validity)? Does the research design enable the researcher to draw causal inferences about the relationship among study variables?

9. To what extent is the study externally valid?

10. What are the major limitations of the design used? Are these limitations acknowledged by the researcher and taken into account in interpreting the results?

RESEARCH EXAMPLE OF AN EXPERIMENTAL EVALUATION

York and her colleagues (1997) conducted a clinical trial to evaluate an intervention for high-risk childbearing women—pregnant women diagnosed with diabetes or hypertension. The evaluation included both an impact analysis and a cost–benefit analysis.

Research Summary

In York's study, women meeting the study criteria and agreeing to participate were randomly assigned to either a control or an experimental intervention group after signing informed consent forms. The sample consisted of

52 women in the control group and 42 women in the intervention group. Women in the control group were discharged normally from the hospital. Those in the experimental group had an early hospital discharge, combined with in-hospital education and follow-up care in the form of home visits and telephone contacts from a clinical nurse specialist.

The research team was interested in evaluating the effect of the intervention in terms of three broad areas: (1) maternal outcomes, such as acute care visits, rehospitalizations, return to normal activities, and satisfaction with care; (2) infant outcomes, such as birth weight, acute care visits, and rehospitalizations; and (3) costs of care.

The results indicated that the intervention group had fewer rehospitalizations than the control group during pregnancy and that diabetic women in the control group were three times as likely to have a low-birth-weight infant (less than 2500 g) than those in the intervention group. The two groups were similar in terms of postpartum hospitalizations, acute care visits, postpartum functional status, and satisfaction with care. The cost–benefit analysis, however, revealed that a net savings of $13,327 was realized for each mother–infant dyad in the intervention group.

Clinical Relevance

Women with high-risk pregnancies are at risk of numerous antepartum and postpartum complications and may thus experience prolonged hospitalizations or rehospitalizations after childbirth for treatment of those complications. Hospital care for these women is costly and also poses certain health risks. Thus, York and her colleagues addressed a problem of considerable significance to health care providers.

Their findings are persuasive because they used a rigorous research design. By randomly assigning the high-risk women to either the standard care control group or the special intervention group, the researchers could be reasonably confident that the intervention, rather than any preexisting group differences, resulted in fewer rehospitalizations. In fact, the researchers documented that the experimental and control groups were comparable in terms of such factors as maternal age, parity, education, marital status, ethnicity, type of health insurance, income, method of delivery, and type of health risk—attesting to the success of the randomization.

The effectiveness of advanced nursing practice was given high visibility by the study's findings. Not only did substantial savings result from this model of clinical nurse specialist transitional care, but also patient outcomes were improved (*i.e.,* prevention of low-birth-weight infants). The clinical implications of this study are directed at hospital administrators. As health care costs continue to spiral upward, it may be financially beneficial for hospitals to consider programs similar to that of York and her colleagues, in which in-hospital education is combined with home visits and telephone contacts by clinical nurse specialists. The value of this quality/cost model lies in the improved and extended care it can provide to high-risk pregnant women and their families.

RESEARCH EXAMPLE OF A QUASI-EXPERIMENTAL STUDY

Pickler, Higgins, and Crummette (1993) used a strong quasi-experimental design to study the effects of nonnutritive sucking on the physiologic and behavioral stress reactions of preterm infants at early bottle feedings.

Research Summary

The sample in this study consisted of 20 preterm infants. Ten of the infants were provided nonnutritive sucking for 5 minutes before and 5 minutes after an early bottle feeding. The other 10 infants, who served as the comparison group, received no nonnutritive sucking. The experimental and comparison group infants were matched on the basis of gender, race, birth weight, and gestational age.

Physiologic stress was measured in terms of heart rate and oxygen saturation rate. For each, mean rates were computed for three periods: the 5 minutes before feeding, the first 5 minutes of bottle feeding, and the 5 minutes after feeding. Behavioral stress was measured by observation of the infants' behavioral state at four points: before the 5-minute prefeeding period, after the initiation of bottle feeding, after the conclusion of bottle feeding, and after the conclusion of the 5-minute postfeeding period.

The results indicated that infants who received nonnutritive sucking before and after bottle feedings were more likely to be in a quiescent behavior state 5 minutes after feeding. However, there were no treatment, time, or time $\times$ treatment interaction effects for heart rate. Oxygen saturation was unaffected by the treatment but did change between different measurements in time.

Clinical Significance

The immature feeding ability of preterm infants puts them at risk for behavioral stress, such as fatigue and agitation, and physiologic stress, such as lowered heart rate and changes in their breathing patterns. Thus, it is important to identify strategies that may help prevent or decrease some of these stress reactions in these fragile infants.

Although Pickler and her colleagues did not randomly assign the infants to groups, this nonequivalent control group design was strengthened by matching the infants in the experimental and comparison groups on a number of important extraneous variables. Despite the small sample size and lack of randomization, the findings do suggest that nurses can help preterm infants in mastering the stress associated with bottle feeding by using the simple and inexpensive intervention of nonnutritive sucking. The evidence from this study suggests that nonnutritive sucking may help preterm infants return to restful states sooner after feeding. This nursing strategy could also help these infants conserve much needed energy for the next feeding.

RESEARCH EXAMPLE OF A NONEXPERIMENTAL SURVEY

Heikkilä, Paunonen, Virtanen, and Laippala (1999) conducted a longitudinal survey of patients undergoing a coronary arteriography (CA). The purpose of the survey was to document the type and intensity of fears experienced by these patients in relation to CA. The researchers sought to compare the fears of men and women and to describe how the fears evolved over time.

Research Summary

The survey sample for this study consisted of 54 women and 166 men scheduled for CA at a 1360-bed university hospital. Study participants were surveyed before and after the procedure and then again 6 months later. The survey instrument, which was self-administered in questionnaire format, included measures of CA-specific fears as well as general anxiety and depression. Because patients' age had been found in prior research to be related to their fears, and because the women in their study were significantly older than the men, the researchers statistically controlled age in their comparison of men's and women's fears.

Heikkilä and her colleagues found that women had higher average fear scores at all points in time, even after controlling for age, but that changes in fear over time were similar for men and women. For both genders, the most intense fear during the hospitalization was uncertainty about the illness and the fear of needing coronary artery bypass grafting. Six months later, fear of myocardial infarction was the most intense fear. There were relatively few gender differences in specific fears, although men were more likely than women to experience intense fears of problems in their sex life. The researchers surmised that the few existing gender differences could be explained by the specific treatment chosen for the patients.

Clinical Relevance

Previous studies had demonstrated that many patients are anxious about the possibility of coronary artery bypass grafting and fear serious illness and death. By conducting a longitudinal study, the researchers were able to describe the evolution of patients' concerns over time and to document gender-specific issues. The study was also strengthened by the use of statistical procedures that controlled for the patients' age, which allowed the researchers to rule out the possibility that gender differences were a function of the age differences of the men and women in their sample.

This study took place in Finland; therefore, the study should be replicated to determine its applicability in other countries. However, the major implication for practice centers on providing much-needed information regarding aspects of coronary artery disease to help decrease patients' fears. The findings suggest that nurses have to address different fears in CA patients at different points in time and that men and women may have different concerns.

● ● ● ● ● ● *SUMMARY POINTS*

- The **research design** is the researcher's overall plan for answering the research question. In quantitative studies, the design indicates whether there is an intervention, the type of intervention, the nature of any comparisons, the methods used to control extraneous variables, and the timing and location of data collection.
- **Experimental Research** involve **manipulation** (the researcher manipulates the independent variable by introducing a **treatment**), control (including the use of a **control group** that is compared to the experimental group), and **randomization** (wherein subjects are allocated to experimental and control groups at random to make the groups comparable at the outset).
- The **after-only design** involves collecting data only once—after random assignment and the introduction of the treatment.
- In the **before–after** (or **pretest–posttest**) design, data are collected both before and after the experimental manipulation.
- **Factorial designs**, in which two or more variables are manipulated simultaneously, allow researchers to test both **main effects** (effects from the experimentally manipulated variables) and **interaction effects** (effects resulting from combining the treatments).
- **Between-subjects designs**, in which different groups of people are compared, contrast with **within-subjects designs**, which involve comparisons of the same subjects.
- In a **repeated-measures design** (or **crossover design**), research subjects are exposed to more than one experimental condition and serve as their own controls.
- When an experiment is used to test the efficacy of a clinical treatment in a large, heterogeneous population, the study is referred to as a **clinical trial.**
- **Quasi-experimental research** involves manipulation but lacks a comparison group or randomization. Quasi-experiments are designs in which controls are introduced to compensate for these missing components. By contrast, **preexperimental designs** have no such safeguards.
- **The nonequivalent control-group before–after design** involves the use of a **comparison group** that was not created through random assignment and the collection of pretreatment data that permits an assessment of initial group equivalence.
- In a **time-series design**, there is no comparison group; information on the dependent variable is collected over a period of time before and after the treatment.
- **Nonexperimental research** includes **descriptive research**—studies that summarize the status of phenomena—and *ex post facto* (or **correlational**) studies that examine relationships among variables but involve no manipulation of the independent variable.
- Researchers use **retrospective** and **prospective** *ex post facto* designs to infer causality, but the findings from such studies are generally open to several interpretations.

- **Cross-sectional designs** involve the collection of data at one point in time, whereas longitudinal designs involve data collection at two or more points over an extended time period. Three types of **longitudinal studies**, which are used to study changes or development over time, are **trend studies, panel studies,** and **follow-up studies.**
- **Survey research** examines the characteristics, attitudes, behaviors, and intentions of a group of people by asking individuals to answer questions either through interviews or self-administered questionnaires.
- **Evaluations** involve the collection and analysis of information relating to the effects and functioning of a program or procedure.
- **Outcomes research** is undertaken to document the effectiveness and quality of health care services and the end results of patient care.
- **Research control** is used to control external factors that could affect the study outcomes (*e.g.,* the environment) and to control intrinsic subject characteristics that are extraneous to the research question.
- Techniques for controlling subject characteristics include **homogeneity** (restricting the selection of subjects to eliminate variability on the extraneous variable); **matching** (matching subjects on a one-to-one basis to make groups comparable on the extraneous variables); statistical procedures, such as **analysis of covariance**; and randomization—the most effective control procedure because it controls all possible extraneous variables without the researcher having to identify or measure them.
- **Internal validity** concerns the degree to which the results of a study can be attributed to the independent variable. **Threats to internal validity** include **history, selection, maturation,** and **mortality** (caused by subject attrition).
- **External validity** refers to the generalizability of study findings to other samples and settings.

> > > > ➤ *CRITICAL THINKING ACTIVITIES*

Chapter 8 of the accompanying *Study Guide to Accompany Essentials of Nursing Research,* 5th edition offers various exercises and study suggestions for reinforcing the concepts presented in this chapter. In addition, you can address the following:

1. Read the first of the actual research studies in the Appendix of this book and then answer the questions in Box 8-1.

2. Read the full study by York and colleagues (1997) that was briefly described as a research example of an experimental study. What were the independent and dependent variables in this study? What, in your opinion, were the key extraneous variables? To what extent did the research design control these variables?

3. In the study by Heikkilä, Paunonen, Virtanen, and Laippala (1999) that was used as an example of a nonexperimental survey, men were signifi-

cantly more likely than women to have had a prior coronary arteriography. What does this suggest about how the study was designed?

For additional review, see questions 81–105 on the study CD provided with Polit: Study Guide to Accompany Essentials of Nursing Research.

SUGGESTED READINGS

Methodologic References

Campbell, D. T., & Stanley, J. C. (1963). *Experimental and quasi-experimental designs for research.* Chicago: Rand McNally.

Cook, T. D., & Campbell, D. T. (1979). *Quasi-experimental design and analysis issues for field settings.* Chicago: Rand McNally.

Kerlinger, F. N. (1986). *Foundations of behavioral research* (3rd ed.). New York: Holt, Rinehart and Winston.

Lazarsfeld, P. (1955). Foreword. In H. Hyman (Ed.), *Survey design and analysis.* New York: The Free Press.

Polit, D. F., & Hungler, B. P. (1999). *Nursing Research: Principles and Methods.* Philadelphia: Lippincott Williams & Wilkins.

Substantive References

Alexy, B. B., & Elnitsky, C. (1998). Rural mobile health unit: Outcomes. *Public Health Nursing, 15,* 3–11.

Berg, J. A. (1999). The perimenopausal transition of Filipino American midlife women: Biopsychosociocultural dimensions. *Nursing Research, 48,* 71–77.

Dore, S., Buchan, D., Coulas, S., Hamber, L., Stewart, M., Cowan, D., & Jamieson, L. (1998). Alcohol versus natural drying for newborn cord care. *Journal of Obstetric, Gynecologic, and Neonatal Nursing, 27,* 621–627.

Foster-Fitzpatrick, L., Ortiz, A., Sibilano, H., Marcantonio, R., & Braun, L. T. (1999). The effects of crossed leg on blood pressure measurement. *Nursing Research, 48,* 105–108.

Heikkilä, J., Paunonen, M., Virtanen, V., & Laippala, P. (1999). Gender differences in fears related to coronary arteriography. *Heart & Lung, 28,* 20–30.

Johnson, J. L., Budz, B., Mackay, M., & Miller, C. (1999). Evaluation of a nurse-delivered smoking cessation intervention for hospitalized patients with cardiac disease. *Heart & Lung, 28,* 55–64.

Kim, J., Bramlett, M. H., Wright, L. K., & Poon, L. W. (1998). Racial differences in health status and health behaviors of older adults. *Nursing Research, 47,* 243–250.

Lee, K. A., Portillo, C. J., & Miramontes, H. (1999). The fatigue experience for women with human immunodeficiency virus. *Journal of Obstetric, Gynecologic, and Neonatal Nursing, 28,* 193–200.

Leitch, D. B. (1999). Mother-infant interaction: Achieving synchrony. *Nursing Research, 48,* 55–58.

McGrath, M. M., & Sullivan, M. C. (1999). Medical and ecological factors in estimating motor outcomes of preschool children. *Research in Nursing & Health, 22,* 155–167.

Miles, M. S., Holditch-Davis, D., Burchinal, P., & Nelson, D. (1999). Distress and growth outcomes in mothers of medically fragile infants. *Nursing Research, 48,* 129–140.

Morse, S. R., & Fife, B. (1998). Coping with a partner's cancer: Adjustment at four stages of the illness trajectory. *Oncology Nursing Forum, 25,* 751–760.

activity measures in persons with rheumatoid arthritis. *Research in Nursing & Health, 20,* 195–204.

Parker, B., McFarlane, J., Soeken, K., Silva, C., & Reel, S. (1999). Testing an intervention to prevent further abuse to pregnant women. *Research in Nursing & Health, 22,* 59–66.

Paul-Allen, J., & Ostrow, C. L. (2000). Survey of nursing practices with closed-system suctioning. *American Journal of Critical Care, 9,* 9–19.

Pickler, R. H., Higgins, K. E., & Crummette, B. D. (1993). The effect of nonnutritive sucking on bottle-feeding stress in preterm infants. *Journal of Obstetric, Gynecologic, and Neonatal Nursing, 22,* 230–234.

Pressler, J., Hepworth, J., LaMontagne, L., Sevcik, & Hesselink, L. (1999). Behavioral responses of newborns of insulin-dependent and nondiabetic, healthy mothers. *Clinical Nursing Research, 8,* 103–118.

Pridham, K., Kosorok, M. R., Greer, F., Carey, P., Kayata, S., & Sondel, S. (1999). The effects of ad libitum feelings and formula caloric density on premature infant dietary intake and weight gain. *Nursing Research, 48,* 86–93.

Roberts, J., Browne, G., Milne, C., Spooner, L., Gafni, A., Drummond-Young, M., LeGris, J., Watt, S., LeClair, K., Beaumont, L., & Roberts, J. (1999). Problem-solving counseling for caregivers of the cognitively impaired. *Nursing Research, 48,* 162–172.

Walker, N. C., & O'Brien, B. (1999). The relationship between method of pain management during labor and birth outcomes. *Clinical Nursing Research, 8,* 119–134.

Wilson, M. E., White, M. A., Cobb, B., Curry, R., Greene, D., & Popovich, D. (2000). Family dynamics, parental-fetal attachment, and infant temperament. *Journal of Advanced Nursing, 31,* 204–210.

York, R., Brown, L. P., Samuels, P., Finkler, S. A., Jacobsen, B., Persely, C. A., Swank, A., & Robbins, D. (1997). A randomized trial of early discharge and nurse specialist transitional follow-up care of high-risk childbearing women. *Nursing Research, 46,* 254–261.

Understanding Qualitative Research Design

Student Objectives

On completion of this chapter, the student will be able to:

○ describe the characteristics of and rationale for an emergent design in qualitative research

○ describe the three major phases typical in the design of a qualitative study

○ identify the major research traditions for qualitative research and describe the domain of inquiry of each

○ describe the characteristics of ethnographic, phenomenologic, and grounded theory studies

○ identify several advantages of an integrated qualitative and quantitative design and describe specific applications

○ define new terms in the chapter

New Terms

Being-in-the-world	Ethology
Black box	Etic perspective
Bracketing	Grounded theory
Bricolage	Hermeneutics
Cognitive anthropology	Historical research
Constant comparison	Integrated design
Corporeality	Intuiting
Discourse analysis	Macroethnography
Ecological psychology	Microethnography
Embodiment	Multimethod research
Emergent design	Phenomenology
Emic perspective	Relationality
Essence	Researcher as instrument
Ethnography	Spatiality
Ethnomethodology	Symbolic interaction
Ethnonursing research	Tacit knowledge
Ethnoscience	Temporality

THE DESIGN OF QUALITATIVE STUDIES

As we have seen, quantitative researchers specify a research design before collecting any data and adhere to that design after the study is underway. In qualitative research, by contrast, study design elements typically evolve over the course of the project. Decisions about how best to obtain data, from whom to obtain data, how to schedule data collection, and how long each data collection session should last are made in the field, as the study unfolds.

The design for a qualitative study is an **emergent design**—a design that emerges as the researcher makes ongoing decisions reflecting what has already been learned. As noted by Lincoln and Guba (1985), an emergent design in qualitative studies is not the result of researchers' sloppiness or laziness, but rather of their desire to base the inquiry on the realities and viewpoints of those under study—realities and viewpoints that are not known or understood at the outset.

 CONSUMER TIP:

Design decisions for a qualitative study are usually summarized in the method section of a report (e.g., a decision to interview a subset of study participants a second time), but the decision-making process for design decisions is rarely described. ∎

Characteristics of Qualitative Research Design

Qualitative inquiry has been guided by a number of different disciplines, and each has developed methods best suited to address questions of particular interest. However, some general characteristics of qualitative research design tend to apply across disciplines. Qualitative design:

- is flexible and elastic, capable of adjusting to what is being learned during the course of data collection;
- typically involves a merging together of various data collection strategies;
- tends to be holistic, striving for an understanding of the whole;
- requires the researcher to become intensely involved, usually remaining in the field for lengthy periods of time;
- requires the researcher to become the research instrument; and
- requires ongoing analysis of the data to formulate subsequent strategies and to determine when field work is done.

With regard to the second characteristic, qualitative researchers tend to put together a complex array of data, derived from various sources. This tendency has been described as **bricolage**, and the qualitative researcher has been referred to as a *bricoleur,* a person who "is adept at performing a large number of diverse tasks, ranging from interviewing to observing, to interpreting personal and historical documents, to intensive reflection and introspection" (Denzin & Lincoln, 1994, p. 2).

Qualitative Design and Planning

Although design decisions are not specified in advance, the qualitative researcher typically does advance planning that can support an emergent design. In the absence of planning, flexibility in the design might actually be constrained. For example, a researcher might project a 6-month period for data collection but might also plan (financially and emotionally) for the possibility of spending longer in the field to pursue emerging data collection opportunities. In other words, the qualitative researcher plans for broad contingencies that may be expected to pose decision opportunities after the study has begun. Advance planning is especially important with regard to the following:

- Selection of a broad research tradition (described in the next section) that will guide certain design and analytic decisions
- Selection of the study site and identification of settings within the site that are likely to be especially fruitful for data collection
- Identification of the key "gatekeepers" who can provide (or deny) access to important sources of data and can make arrangements for gaining entrée
- Determination of the maximal time available for the study, given costs and other constraints
- Identification of all needed equipment for the collection and analysis of data in the field (*e.g.,* audio and video recording equipment, laptop computers, and so forth)

Thus, a qualitative researcher plans for various circumstances, but decisions about how he or she will deal with them must be resolved when the social context of time, place, and human interactions is better understood.

Phases in a Qualitative Study

Although the exact form of a qualitative study is not specified in advance, Lincoln and Guba (1985) noted that a naturalistic inquiry typically progresses through three broad phases while the researcher is in the field:

1. *Orientation and overview.* Quantitative researchers generally believe they know what they do not know (*i.e.,* they know the type of knowledge they expect to obtain by doing a study and then strive to obtain it). A qualitative researcher, by contrast, enters the study "not knowing what is not known" (*i.e.,* not knowing what it is about the phenomenon that will drive the inquiry forward). Therefore, the first phase of many qualitative studies is to get a handle on what is salient about the phenomenon of interest.
2. *Focused exploration.* The second phase is a more focused scrutiny and in-depth exploration of aspects of the phenomenon judged to be salient. The questions asked and the types of people invited to participate in the study are shaped by the understandings developed in the first phase.
3. *Confirmation and closure.* In the final phase, qualitative researchers undertake efforts to establish that their findings are trustworthy, often by going back and discussing their understanding with study participants. Phase 3 activities are described in Chapter 12.

The three phases are not discrete but rather overlap to a greater or lesser degree in different projects. For example, even the first few interviews or observations are typically used as a basis for selecting subsequent informants, even though the researcher is still striving to understand the scope of the phenomenon and to identify its major dimensions. The various phases might take only a few weeks to complete—or they may take many months.

Qualitative Design Features

Some of the design features of quantitative studies (see Chap. 8) also apply to qualitative studies. However, qualitative design features are often *post hoc* characterizations of what happened in the field rather than features specifically planned in advance. To further contrast qualitative and quantitative research design, we refer to the design elements identified in Table 8-1 in Chapter 8.

Control Over the Independent Variable

Qualitative researchers do not conceptualize their studies as having independent and dependent variables, and they rarely control or manipulate any aspect of the setting under study. Qualitative research is almost always nonexperimental—although, as we discuss later in this chapter, a qualitative study sometimes can be embedded within an experimental project.

Type of Group Comparisons

Qualitative researchers typically do not plan in advance to make group comparisons because the intent of most qualitative studies is to describe thoroughly and explain a phenomenon. Nevertheless, patterns emerging in the data sometimes suggest that certain comparisons are relevant and illuminating.

Example of qualitative comparisons:

Newshan (1998) studied the experience of pain in hospitalized patients with acquired immunodeficiency syndrome (AIDS). Newshan discovered that, although there were commonalities in the experiences of chemically dependent and non–chemically dependent participants, those who were chemically dependent experienced unique challenges.

Number of Data Collection Points

Qualitative research, like quantitative research, can be either cross-sectional, with one data collection point, or longitudinal, with multiple data collection points over an extended time period, to observe the evolution of some phenomenon. Sometimes, a qualitative researcher plans in advance for multiple sessions, but in other cases, the decision to study a phenomenon longitudinally may be made in the field after preliminary data have been collected and analyzed.

> **Examples of the time dimension in qualitative studies:**
>
> *Cross-sectional:* Dickerson (1998) studied in single sessions the evolving help-seeking experiences of cardiac patients' spouses over the course of the illness, in retrospective accounts of experiences from diagnosis to homecoming from the hospital.
>
> *Longitudinal:* Brown and Stetz (1999) studied the influence that chronic and potentially fatal illness has on the caregiving process over time. They interviewed 26 caregivers of patients with AIDS or cancer three times over a 4-month period to examine how the caregiving process evolved.

Occurrence of the Independent and Dependent Variables

Qualitative researchers typically would not apply the terms *retrospective* or *prospective* to their studies. Nevertheless, in trying to elucidate the full nature of some phenomenon, they may look back retrospectively (with the assistance of study participants) for antecedent events leading to the occurrence of some phenomenon. Qualitative researchers may also study the evolution of some phenomenon prospectively.

> **Examples of exploring influences and causes in qualitative designs:**
>
> *Retrospective exploration:* Paterson, Thorne, Crawford, and Tarko (1999) studied the process of transformation as it had been experienced by patients with type I diabetes that had been diagnosed for at least 15 years.
>
> *Prospective exploration:* Gray and Smith (1999) conducted a prospective study to explore the effects of mentorship on nursing students. A sample of 10 students were interviewed over the course of 3 years; these students also kept a diary of their experiences during practice placements. The researchers found that mentors played a crucial role in the professional socialization of the students.

Research Setting

Qualitative researchers collect their data in real-world, naturalistic settings. And, whereas a quantitative researcher usually strives to collect data in one type of setting to maintain constancy of conditions (*e.g.*, conducting all interviews in study participants' homes), qualitative researchers may deliberately strive to study their phenomena in a variety of natural contexts.

> **Examples of variation in settings:**
>
> Nicholas (1999) studied the lived experience of mothers who were caring for their children with end-stage renal disease. The everyday lives of the mothers were observed in various natural settings—in the participants' homes, in clinics, in the children's schools, in stores, and so on.

QUALITATIVE RESEARCH TRADITIONS

There are many different types of qualitative studies, but there unfortunately is no readily agreed-upon taxonomy for the various approaches. Some authors have categorized qualitative studies in terms of analysis styles; others have classified studies according to their focus. One useful system is to describe qualitative research according to disciplinary traditions. These traditions vary in their conceptualization of what questions are important to ask to understand human experiences. This section provides an overview of qualitative research traditions, and subsequent sections describe three traditions that have been especially useful for nurse researchers.

Overview of Qualitative Research Traditions

The research traditions that have provided an underpinning for qualitative studies come primarily from anthropology, psychology, and sociology. As shown in Table 9-1, each discipline has tended to focus on one or two broad domains of inquiry.

The discipline of anthropology is concerned with human cultures. **Ethnography** is the primary research tradition within anthropology and provides a framework for studying the meanings, patterns, and experiences

TABLE 9-1. Overview of Qualitative Research Traditions

DISCIPLINE	DOMAIN	RESEARCH TRADITION	AREA OF INQUIRY
Anthropology	Culture	Ethnography	Holistic view of a culture
		Ethnoscience (cognitive anthropology)	Mapping of the cognitive world of a culture; a culture's shared meanings, semantic rules
Psychology or philosophy	Lived experience	Phenomenology	Experiences of individuals within their lifeworld
		Hermeneutics	Interpretations and meanings of individuals' experiences
Psychology	Behavior and events	Ethology	Behavior observed over time in natural context
		Ecological psychology	Behavior as influenced by the environment
Sociology	Social settings	Grounded theory	Social structural processes within a social setting
		Ethnomethodology	Manner by which shared agreement is achieved in social settings
Sociolinguistics	Human communication	Discourse analysis	Forms and rules of conversation

of a defined cultural group in a holistic fashion. **Ethnoscience** (or **cognitive anthropology**) focuses on the cognitive world of a culture, with particular emphasis on the semantic rules and the shared meanings that shape behavior. Ethnoscience often relies on quantitative as well as qualitative data.

Phenomenology, which has its disciplinary roots in both philosophy and psychology, is concerned with the lived experiences of humans. A closely related research tradition is **hermeneutics**, which uses the lived experiences of people as a tool for better understanding the social, cultural, political, and historical context in which those experiences occur. Hermeneutic inquiry often focuses on meaning—how socially and historically conditioned individuals interpret the world within their given context.

The discipline of psychology has several qualitative research traditions that focus on human behavior. Human **ethology**, which is sometimes described as the biology of human behavior, studies human behavior as it evolves in its natural context. Human ethologists use observational methods to discover universal behavioral structures. **Ecological psychology** focuses more specifically on the environment's influence on human behavior and attempts to identify principles that explain the interdependence of humans and their environmental context.

Sociologists study the social world and have developed several research traditions of importance to qualitative researchers. The **grounded theory** tradition (described briefly in Chap. 7 and elaborated on in a later section of this chapter) seeks to understand the key social psychological and structural processes that occur in a social setting. **Ethnomethodology** seeks to discover how people make sense of everyday activities and interpret their social world in order to behave in socially acceptable ways. Within this tradition, researchers attempt to understand a social group's norms and assumptions that are so deeply ingrained that members no longer think about the underlying reasons for their behaviors.

The domain of inquiry for sociolinguists is human communication. The tradition often referred to as **discourse analysis** seeks to understand the rules, mechanisms, and structure of conversations. The data for discourse analysis typically are transcripts from naturally occurring conversations, such as those between nurses and their patients.

Finally, **historical research**—the systematic collection and critical evaluation of data relating to past occurrences—is also a tradition that relies primarily on qualitative data. Generally, historical research is undertaken to answer questions concerning causes, effects, or trends relating to past events that may shed light on present behaviors or practices. It is important not to confuse historical research with a review of the literature about historical events. Like other types of research, historical inquiry has as its goal the discovery of new knowledge, not the summary of existing knowledge. Nurses have used historical research methods to examine a wide range of phenomena in both the recent and more distant past.

CONSUMER TIP:

Some qualitative research reports do not identify a research tradition (*e.g.,* ethnography or phenomenology) but simply describe the study as qualitative. A research tradition may need to be inferred from information about the types of questions that were asked and the methods used to collect and analyze data. ■

Researchers in each of the qualitative research traditions have developed methodologic guidelines for the design and conduct of relevant studies. Thus, after a researcher has identified what aspect of the human experience is of greatest interest, there is typically a wealth of advice available with regard to methods likely to be productive.

 CONSUMER TIP:

A research report will sometimes identify more than one tradition as having provided the framework for a qualitative inquiry. For example, Gibson and Kenrick (1998) studied the experience of living with peripheral vascular disease in a sample of nine patients who had had vascular bypass surgery. They described their investigation as a phenomenologic study that used a grounded theory method. However, such "method slurring" (Baker, Wuest, & Stern, 1992) has been criticized because each research tradition has different intellectual assumptions and methodologic prescriptions. ■

Ethnography

Ethnography, as noted previously, focuses on the culture of a group of people. Ethnographic researchers can study both broadly defined cultures (*e.g.,* a Samoan village culture), in what is sometimes referred to as a **macroethnography**, and more narrowly defined ones (*e.g.,* the culture of homeless shelters) in a **microethnography.** An underlying assumption of the ethnographer is that every human group evolves a culture that guides the members' view of the world and the way they structure their experiences.

The aim of the ethnographer is to learn from (rather than to study) members of a cultural group. Ethnographic researchers sometimes refer to emic and etic perspectives. An **emic perspective** is the way the members of the culture envision their world—it is the insiders' view. The **etic perspective**, by contrast, is the outsiders' interpretation of the experiences of that culture. Ethnographers strive to acquire an emic perspective of cultures. Moreover, they strive to reveal **tacit knowledge**, information about the culture that is so deeply embedded in cultural experiences that members do not talk about it or may not even be consciously aware of it.

Ethnographers undertake extensive field work to learn about the cultural group in which they are interested. Ethnographic research typically is a labor-intensive and time-consuming endeavor—months and even years of field work may be required. The study of a culture requires a certain level of intimacy with members of the cultural group, and such intimacy can only be developed over time and by working directly with those members as an active participant. The concept of **researcher as instrument** is frequently used by anthropologists to describe the significant role the ethnographer plays in analyzing and interpreting a culture.

Three types of information are usually sought by ethnographers: cultural behavior (what members of the culture do); cultural artifacts (what members of the culture make and use); and cultural speech (what people say). This implies that the ethnographer relies on various data sources, including observations, in-depth interviews, records, charts, and other types of physical evidence (photographs, diaries, letters, and so forth). Ethnographers typically conduct in-depth interviews with about 25 to 50 informants.

The products of ethnographic research are rich and holistic descriptions of the culture under study. Ethnographers also make interpretations of the culture, describing normative behavioral and social patterns. Among health care researchers, ethnography provides information about the health beliefs and health practices of a culture or subculture. Ethnographic inquiry can thus facilitate understanding of behaviors affecting health and illness. Many nurse researchers have undertaken ethnographic studies. Indeed, Madeleine Leininger has coined the phrase **ethnonursing research**, which she defines as "the study and analysis of the local or indigenous people's viewpoints, beliefs, and practices about nursing care behavior and processes of designated cultures" (1985, p. 38).

⊟⊟   *Example of an ethnographic study:*

Higgins and Learn (1999) conducted an ethnography focused on the health practices of adult Hispanic women. The study involved four to seven interviews each with a sample of adult Hispanic women living in New Mexico. Through these interviews, the researchers learned that the women tended to take better care of their families than of themselves.

Phenomenology

Phenomenology, rooted in a philosophical tradition developed by Husserl and Heidegger, is an approach to thinking about people's life experiences. The phenomenologic researcher asks the question: What is the essence of this phenomenon as experienced by these people and what does it *mean?* The phenomenologist assumes there is an **essence**—an essential invariant structure—that can be understood, in much the same way that the ethnographer assumes that cultures exist. The phenomenologist investigates subjective phenomena in the belief that critical truths about reality are grounded in people's lived experiences.

There are two "schools" of phenomenology: descriptive phenomenology and interpretive phenomenology (hermeneutics). Descriptive phenomenology was developed first by Husserl (1962), who was primarily interested in the question: What do we know as persons? His philosophy emphasized descriptions of the meaning of human experience. Heidegger, a student of Husserl, moved away from his professor's philosophy into interpretive phenomenology. To Heidegger (1962), the critical question is: What is being? He stressed interpreting and understanding—not just describing—human experience. The focus of phenomenologic inquiry, then, is what people experience in regard to a phenomenon (descriptive phenomenology) and how they interpret those experiences (hermeneutics). The phenomenologist believes that lived experience gives meaning to each person's perception of a particular phenomenon. The goal of phenomenologic inquiry is to describe fully lived experience and the perceptions to which it gives rise. Four aspects of lived experience that are of interest to phenomenologists are lived space, or **spatiality**; lived body, or **corporeality**; lived time, or **temporality**; and lived human relation, or **relationality.**

Phenomenologists believe that human existence is meaningful and interesting because of people's consciousness of that existence. The phrase **being-in-the-world** (or **embodiment**) is a concept that acknowledges people's physical ties to their world—they think, see, hear, feel, and are conscious through their bodies' interaction with the world.

In a phenomenologic study, the main data source is in-depth conversations, with the researcher and informant as full co-participants. The researcher helps the informant to describe lived experiences without leading the discussion. Through in-depth conversations, the researcher strives to gain entrance into the informants' world, to have full access to their experiences as lived. Sometimes, two separate interviews or conversations may be needed. Typically, phenomenologic studies involve a small number of study participants—often 10 or fewer. For some phenomenologic researchers, the inquiry includes not only gathering information from informants but also efforts to experience the phenomenon in the same way, typically through participation, observation, and introspective reflection.

Although there are a number of methodologic interpretations of phenomenology, a descriptive phenomenologic study often involves the following four steps: bracketing, intuiting, analyzing, and describing. **Bracketing** refers to the process of identifying and holding in abeyance preconceived beliefs and opinions about the phenomenon under study. The researcher brackets out the world and any presuppositions in an effort to confront the data in pure form. **Intuiting** occurs when the researcher remains open to the meanings attributed to the phenomenon by those who have experienced it. Phenomenologic researchers then proceed to the analysis phase (*i.e.,* extracting significant statements, categorizing, and making sense of the essential meanings of the phenomenon). (Chap. 14 provides further information regarding the analysis of data collected in phenomenologic studies.) Finally, the descriptive phase occurs when the researcher comes to understand and define the phenomenon. An important distinction between descriptive and interpretive phenomenology is that in an interpretive phenomenologic study, bracketing does not occur. For Heidegger, it was not possible to bracket one's being-in-the-world. Hermeneutics presupposes prior understanding on the part of the researcher.

The phenomenologic approach is especially useful when a phenomenon of interest has been poorly defined or conceptualized. The topics appropriate to phenomenology are ones that are fundamental to the life experiences of humans; for health researchers, these include such topics as the meaning of stress, the experience of bereavement, and the quality of life with a chronic illness.

Example of a phenomenologic study:

Beck (1998) conducted a phenomenologic study of the lived experience of panic disorders in mothers during the postpartum period. The study involved in-depth interviews with a sample of six women who had ongoing panic attacks after childbirth.

Grounded Theory

Grounded theory has become a strong research tradition that began more as a systematic method of qualitative research than as a philosophy. Grounded theory was developed in the 1960s by two sociologists, Glaser and Strauss (1967), whose theoretical roots were in **symbolic interaction**, which focuses on the manner in which people make sense of social interactions and the interpretations they attach to social symbols, such as language.

Grounded theory is an approach to the study of social processes and social structures. The focus of most grounded theory studies is the evolution of a social experience—the social and psychological stages and phases that characterize a particular event or process. As noted in Chapter 7, the primary purpose of the grounded theory approach is to generate comprehensive explanations of phenomena that are grounded in reality.

Grounded theory methods constitute an entire approach to the conduct of field research. For example, a study that truly follows Glaser and Strauss' precepts does not begin with a focused research question; the question emerges from the data. A fundamental feature of grounded theory research is that data collection, data analysis, and sampling of participants occur simultaneously. A procedure referred to as **constant comparison** is used to develop and refine theoretically relevant categories and to identify the basic problem. The categories elicited from the data are constantly compared with data obtained earlier so that commonalities and variations can be determined, and categories can be condensed and collapsed. As data collection proceeds, the inquiry becomes increasingly focused on emerging theoretical concerns and on core processes. Data analysis within a grounded theory framework is described more fully in Chapter 14.

In-depth interviews are the most common data source in a grounded theory study, but observational methods and existing documents may also be used. Typically, a grounded theory study involves interviews with a sample of about 25 to 50 informants.

Grounded theory has become an important research method for the study of nursing phenomena and has contributed to the development of many middle-range theories of phenomena relevant to nurses. Most qualitative nursing studies that identify a research tradition claim grounded theory as the tradition to which they are linked.

Example of a grounded theory study:

Ingram and Hutchinson (2000) conducted a grounded theory study that focused on the reproductive and mothering experience of human immunodeficiency virus (HIV)-positive women. The basic social psychological problem these women faced was the double-bind of living in a society where motherhood is valued while at the same time being stigmatized by having children because of their HIV status.

INTEGRATION OF QUALITATIVE AND QUANTITATIVE APPROACHES

An emerging trend, and one that we believe will gain momentum, is the integration of qualitative and quantitative data within single studies or coordinated clusters of studies. This section discusses the rationale for such **integrated designs** and presents a few applications.

Rationale for Integrated Designs

The dichotomy between quantitative and qualitative data represents the key epistemologic and methodologic distinction within the social and behavioral sciences. Some argue that the paradigms that underpin qualitative and quantitative research are fundamentally incompatible. Others, however, believe that many areas of inquiry can be enriched through the judicious blending of qualitative and quantitative data—that is, by undertaking **multimethod research.** The advantages of an integrated design include the following:

- *Complementarity.* Qualitative and quantitative data are complementary, representing words and numbers, the two fundamental languages of human communication. Researchers address their problems with methods that are fallible, but the strengths and weaknesses of quantitative and qualitative data are complementary. By using multiple methods, the researcher can allow each method to do what it does best, possibly avoiding the limitations of a single approach.
- *Incrementality.* It is sometimes argued that qualitative methods are well suited to hypothesis-generating research early in the development of a research problem area, and that quantitative methods are needed as the problem area matures for verification. However, the evolution of

knowledge is rarely linear and unidirectional. The need for in-depth insights is rarely confined to the beginning of an inquiry in an area, and subjective experiences may need to be tested continuously. Thus, progress on a topic tends to be incremental, relying on multiple feedback loops. It can be productive to build a loop into the design of a single study, thereby potentially speeding progress toward understanding.

- *Enhanced validity*. When a researcher's hypothesis or model is supported by multiple and complementary types of data, the researcher can be more confident about the validity of the results. The integration of qualitative and quantitative data can provide opportunities for testing alternative interpretations of the data and for examining the extent to which context helped to shape the results.
- *Creating new frontiers*. Researchers sometimes find that qualitative and quantitative data are inconsistent with each other. This lack of congruity—when it happens in the context of a single investigation—can lead to insights that can push a line of inquiry further. Inconsistencies in separate studies may reflect differences in study participants and circumstances rather than theoretically meaningful distinctions that merit further study. In a single study, discrepancies can be used as a springboard for further exploration.

 CONSUMER TIP:

Integrated studies rarely combine qualitative and quantitative findings in a single report. Typically, the quantitative findings are reported in one journal article, and the qualitative findings appear in a separate article in a different journal. However, the authors often summarize the results of the other component of the study in the introduction or discussion section of the report. ■

Applications of Integrated Designs

Researchers make decisions about study design and procedures based on the specific objectives of their investigations. The integration of qualitative and quantitative data can be used to address various research goals.

1. *Instrumentation*. Qualitative data are sometimes collected for the development and validation of formal, quantitative instruments for research or clinical purposes. The questions for a formal instrument are sometimes derived from clinical experience, theory, or prior research. When a construct is new, however, these mechanisms may be inadequate to capture its full complexity and dimensionality. A researcher's knowledge base, no matter how rich, is personal and limited, and thus nurse researchers sometimes gather qualitative data as the basis for generating questions for quantitative instruments that are subsequently subjected to rigorous testing.

> **Example of instrumentation:**
>
> Beck (2000) developed the Postpartum Depression Screening Scale, an instrument that screens new mothers for the mood disorder that can develop after delivering a baby. The items in the scale were based on in-depth interviews of three different samples of mothers suffering from postpartum depression.

2. *Explicating and validating constructs.* Multimethod research is often used to develop a comprehensive understanding of a construct or to validate the construct's dimensions. Such research may be undertaken when a little-researched phenomenon has been identified as worthy of further scrutiny or when there is a body of existing research in which some serious gaps have been identified or doubts have been raised about the prevailing conceptualization.

> **Example of explication and validation:**
>
> Reece and Harkless (1996) conducted a multimethod study to examine the maternal experiences of women older than 35 years. The researchers administered an existing quantitative measure of maternal experience and also asked their respondents probing questions about their motherhood experience, which they analyzed qualitatively for emerging themes. They found that several new dimensions arose in the qualitative portion of the research not captured by the quantitative scale.

3. *Illustration.* Qualitative data are sometimes used to illustrate the meaning of quantitative descriptions or relationships. Such illustrations help to clarify important concepts and further serve to corroborate the findings from the statistical analysis. The illustrations help to illuminate the analysis and give guidance to the interpretation of results. Qualitative materials can be used to illustrate specific statistical findings and to provide more global and dynamic views of the phenomena under study, often in the form of illustrative case studies.

> **Example of illustrating with qualitative data:**
>
> Polit, London, and Martinez (2000) used data from the ethnographic component of a study of poor urban families to illustrate how food insecurity and hunger—reported by more than half of the sample from the survey component of the study—were experienced and managed.

4. *Understanding relationships and causal processes.* Quantitative methods can demonstrate that variables are systematically related but may fail to provide insights about why they are related. Interpretations are often speculative, representing new hypotheses that could be tested in another study. When a study integrates qualitative and quantitative

data, however, the researcher may be in a stronger position to derive meaning immediately from the statistical findings.

> **Example of illuminating with qualitative data:**
>
> In the previously mentioned multicomponent study of poor urban families, Polit and colleagues (2000) found from the survey data that differences in the food insecurity of poor women were related to differences in their sources of income, and yet the differences in the hunger of their children were more modest. The ethnographic data revealed that differences were small largely because of the lengths to which mothers, regardless of income source, went to protect their children from hunger.

5. *Theory building, testing, and refinement.* The most ambitious application of an integrated approach is in the area of theory development. A theory gains acceptance as it escapes disconfirmation, and the use of multiple methods provides great opportunity for potential disconfirmation of a theory. If the theory can survive these assaults, it can provide a stronger context for the organization of clinical and intellectual work.

> **Example of theory building:**
>
> Salazar and Carter (1993) conducted a study that promoted the development of theory in the area of decision making. These researchers sought to identify the factors that influence the decision of working women to practice breast self-examination (BSE). The first phase of the study involved in-depth interviews with 19 women, selected on the basis of how frequently they practiced BSE. The qualitative analysis led to the development of a hierarchical scheme of factors influencing the BSE decision. The researchers then used the hierarchy as the basis for developing a questionnaire that was administered to 52 women. A complex statistical analysis was used to identify factors in the decision hierarchy that best distinguished BSE performers and nonperformers.

Integration Strategies

The ways in which a researcher can design a study to integrate qualitative and quantitative methods are almost limitless. The three following scenarios are especially common:

1. *Embedding qualitative approaches within a survey.* After the researcher has gained the cooperation of a survey sample, he or she may be in a good position to collect more in-depth data with a subset of the initial respondents. If the collection of in-depth data can be postponed until after the analysis of quantitative data, the researcher can probe into the reasons for any obtained results. The second-stage respondents, in

other words, can be used as informants to help the researcher interpret outcomes.

Example of embedding qualitative approaches into a survey:

Boydell, Goering, and Morrell-Bellai (2000) directed a large-scale multimethod study of homeless people in Toronto. Some 330 homeless adults were surveyed, using a formal interview that yielded quantitative data. Subsequently, some 29 participants were purposively selected from the larger sample for in-depth questioning about their inner view of their lives and experiences.

---

2. *Embedding quantitative measures into field work.* Although qualitative data prevail in field studies, field researchers can sometimes profit from the collection of more structured information, either from the study participants or from a larger or more representative sample. Having already gained entrée into the community and the trust and cooperation of its members, the field researcher may be in an ideal position to pursue a survey or a record-extraction activity. For example, if the researcher's in-depth field work focused on family violence, community-wide police and hospital records could be used to gather systematic data amenable to statistical analysis.

Example of quantitative measures in field work:

Moore (1999) conducted an in-depth study of social interaction in a special care unit for cognitively impaired older people. The rich qualitative data were gathered through observations and in-depth interviews with staff and family members. The researcher contextualized the study and developed a better understanding of the participants by administering several structured, quantitative instruments, such as the Mini-Mental State Examination and the Katz Index of Activities of Daily Living.

---

3. *Qualitative data in experimental and quasi-experimental research.* Qualitative data can often enrich experimental or quasi-experimental studies. Through in-depth, unstructured approaches, the researcher can better understand qualitative differences between groups, including differences in the experiences and processes underlying experimental effects. Qualitative data may be especially useful when the researcher is evaluating complex interventions. When an experimental treatment is straightforward (*e.g.*, a new drug), it might be easy to interpret the results. However, many nursing interventions are more complicated; they may involve new ways of interacting with patients or new approaches to organizing the delivery of care. At the end of the experiment, even when hypothesized results are obtained, people may ask, What was it that really caused the group differences? In-depth qualita-

tive data may help researchers to address the **black box** question—understanding what it is about the intervention that is driving any observed effects. Finally, the use of qualitative methods in nursing intervention studies can play a role in making nursing work more visible and accessible to other nurses, policy makers, and the public (Sandelowski, 1996).

Example qualitative data in an experiment:

Morgan & Stewart (1999) conducted a quasi-experimental (nonequivalent control group design) study of the effect of an environmental intervention (reduced density and increased privacy) for people with dementia in special care units. The qualitative part of the study involved in-depth interviews to obtain a more complete picture of the environment–behavior relationship for the patients.

CRITIQUING QUALITATIVE AND INTEGRATED DESIGNS

Evaluating a qualitative design is often difficult. Qualitative researchers do not always document design decisions and are even less likely to describe the process by which such decisions were made. Researchers often do, however, indicate whether the study was conducted within a specific qualitative tradition. This information can be used to come to some conclusions about the study design. For example, if a report indicated that the researcher conducted 1 month of field work for an ethnographic study, there would be reason to suspect that insufficient time had been spent in the field to obtain a true emic perspective of the culture under study.

Most qualitative studies—quite appropriately—do not collect any quantitative data. However, it might be useful to consider how and in what way the addition of quantitative data might have improved the study design. Conversely, not all integrated studies are well suited to a multimethod approach; hence, integrated studies should be carefully evaluated in terms of the incremental value of having both types of data in a single study.

The guidelines in Box 9-1 are designed to assist you in critiquing the designs of qualitative and integrated studies.

RESEARCH EXAMPLES

Nurse researchers have conducted studies within all of the qualitative research traditions described in this chapter. Table 9-2 provides several examples of research questions addressed within various traditions. In this section, we present more detailed descriptions of three nursing studies, including two multimethod investigations.

BOX 9-1

GUIDELINES FOR CRITIQUING QUALITATIVE AND INTEGRATED DESIGNS

1. Is the research tradition within which the qualitative study was undertaken identified? What was that tradition? If no research tradition is identified, can one be inferred?

2. Does the research question appear to be congruent with the research tradition (*i.e.*, is the domain of inquiry for the study congruent with the domain encompassed by the tradition)? Do the data sources and general methods of the study appear consistent with the tradition?

3. How well is the research design described? Are design decisions explained and justified?

4. Does the design appear thoughtful and appropriate? Does the design lend itself to a thorough, in-depth, intensive examination of the phenomenon of interest? What design elements might have strengthened the study (*e.g.*, would a longitudinal perspective have been preferable, although a cross-sectional design was used)?

5. Is the study exclusively qualitative, or were both qualitative and quantitative data collected? Could the study have been strengthened by the inclusion of some quantitative data?

6. If both qualitative and quantitative data were collected, were they used in a complementary fashion? How (if at all) did the inclusion of both types of data contribute to enhanced theoretical insights, enhanced validity, or movement toward new frontiers?

TABLE 9-2. Examples of Qualitative Studies Within Various Traditions

RESEARCH TRADITION	RESEARCH QUESTION
Ethnography	What is the process by which elders adapt to the dual nature of the nursing home as an institution and as a home? (Kahn, 1999)
Phenomenology	What are the lived experiences of micturition problems, indwelling catheter treatment, and sexual life consequences of men with prostate cancer? (Jakobsson, Hallberg, & Loven, 2000)
Ethology	What are the interaction dynamics between nurses and patients at transitions from one type of nurse attending to another? (Bottorff & Varcoe, 1995)
Grounded theory	How do family members manage disclosure to a child who has perinatally acquired HIV disease? (Ledlie, 1999)
Ethnomethodology	How do nurses define and redefine medication error? (Baker, 1997)
Discourse analysis and history	What historically situated discourse was used at the Hadamar trial in defense of the actions and inactions of nurses in Nazi Germany? (Lagerwey, 1999)

RESEARCH EXAMPLE OF A GROUNDED THEORY STUDY

Sayre (2000) conducted a grounded theory study about adults' perceptions of being a psychiatric patient. Her research report appeared in *Qualitative Health Research*.

Research Summary

Sayre (2000) conducted biweekly interviews, from admission to discharge, with 35 patients diagnosed with schizophrenia who had been hospitalized in psychiatric units of an urban public facility. The central question of the inquiry was: How do individuals explain their admission to a psychiatric facility? Subquestions included (a) What contextual and intervening experiences influenced their explanation? (b) What strategies resulted? and (c) What were the consequences of those strategies?

The constant comparison method of data analysis revealed that managing self-worth was the process inpatients used to cope with the stigma of being a mental patient. Factors that affected individual responses to psychiatric hospitalization included substance abuse, lack of social capital (especially lack of stable housing), and medication noncompliance. Six attribution styles, rated on a continuum from acceptance to rejection of the psychiatric treatment model, emerged from the analysis: problem, disease, crisis, punishment, ordination, and violation. These attribution styles helped the patients to maintain their sense of self-worth during the stigmatizing process of psychiatric hospitalization.

Clinical Relevance

Individuals' negative reactions to psychiatric hospitalization can result in their refusal to cooperate with necessary treatments. Thus, information about how these patients explain their admission to an inpatient psychiatric unit and how these patients cope with their hospitalization can be valuable in their treatment.

Sayre's study has a number of strengths that enhance its clinical relevance. In particular, Sayre strategically combined data from multiple sources to develop a thorough and comprehensive understanding of the patients' perceptions and strategies. Data were collected through in-depth interviews with the patients, observations, review of medical records, and informal conversations with staff. Two hundred hours of interview data were obtained.

The findings suggest that clinicians need to view stigma as an important issue that should be addressed with patients in psychiatric units. Patients may need help to separate their own concept of self from their views of mental patients in general. Another clinical implication focuses on a shift in health care providers' attention on symptoms as indicative of disease to considering that patient behaviors may be their attempts at coping with the stressful experience of psychiatric hospitalization and a psychotic episode. It appears that treatment could be enhanced by paying more attention to the subjective experiences of psychotic patients.

RESEARCH EXAMPLE OF AN ETHNOGRAPHIC STUDY

Dreher and Hayes (1993) studied marijuana use among pregnant Jamaican women and subsequent effects on the offspring. The researchers combined two types of investigations: an ethnographic study of perinatal use of marijuana in rural Jamaican communities, and a quantitative clinical study of a sample of women (including both users and nonusers of marijuana) and their children.

Research Summary

Dreher and Hayes spent 6 years in the field living in a rural Jamaican parish and had regular contact with each of the families in the study. The ethnographic portion of the study involved in-depth observations and interviews related to perinatal use of marijuana (called *ganja* in Jamaica). The researchers found that most female users prepared and consumed ganja for themselves and their families in the form of teas and tonics for medicinal or health-rendering purposes. Ganja smoking was less common among Jamaican women than Jamaican men, although the researchers found that smoking increased among women over the course of the field work. Women who smoked ganja often smoked throughout pregnancy, during labor, and into the breastfeeding period.

In the clinical portion of the study, the researchers compared the offspring of 30 ganja users and 30 nonusers using standardized measures of development (*e.g.,* the Bayley Scales of Infant Development). The ethnographic work proved to be critical in suggesting adaptations that made these instruments appropriate for a different culture.

Clinical Relevance

Increasing numbers of women are smoking ganja (marijuana) in Jamaica. To compound matters, Jamaican women are smoking it during pregnancy, during labor, and while breastfeeding. This research was important in revealing patterns of ganja use and in evaluating the effects of ganja on children whose mothers smoked it during pregnancy and lactation.

Triangulation of the two research methods of ethnography and standardized measurements of development proved to be an essential feature of this cross-cultural research. The findings emphasize the importance of exercising caution when using an instrument developed in the United States with patients in other cultures, such as in the Jamaican culture. The items on U.S.-designed instruments may need to be modified to be sensitive to the inhabitants of differing cultures. In-depth ethnographic field work proved to be essential in making such modifications.

RESEARCH EXAMPLE OF AN INTEGRATED STUDY

Connelly, Bott, Hoffart, and Taunton (1997) conducted a multimethod research project that focused on the retention of staff nurses. Their research is an example of construct explication and theory building through the integration of qualitative and quantitative methods.

Research Summary

The study by Connelly and her colleagues was primarily quantitative and involved the development of a sophisticated statistical model designed to predict nurse retention. The researchers measured four types of factors that they believed could predict retention: characteristics of the managers (*e.g.,* leadership style); characteristics of the organization (*e.g.,* promotional opportunity); work characteristics (*e.g.,* group cohesion); and characteristics of the nurses themselves (*e.g.,* education, marital status). The variables in the model had all been verified in the research literature; nevertheless, their cumulative predictive power was relatively low.

In the final year of the project, the researchers did a qualitative study to examine whether a different research approach might produce an additional construct that belonged in the retention model. A total of 21 staff nurses who had low scores on an Intent to Stay Scale that had been administered to them in the first year of the project—but who had nevertheless remained working in the same hospital—were interviewed in depth about their reasons for staying, their possible reasons for leaving, and the positive and negative aspects of their employment.

The researchers found that there was some correspondence between the information obtained through the in-depth interviews and the variables included in their model, thereby validating aspects of the model. However, new themes also emerged during the qualitative interviews—for example, variables such as location close to home, fringe benefits, ability to provide high-quality care, and ability to transfer among units within the hospital. The advantages of having used a multimethod design were described as follows:

> Triangulation helped us attain three benefits. First, the careful comparison of quantitative and qualitative data added support for the variables in the retention model. Second, the comparison also showed new dimensions about nurse retention, thereby contributing to a more complete understanding of nurse retention. . . . Third, the researchers were able to make suggestions for revision of the quantitative instrument. (Connelly et al., 1997, p. 301)

Clinical Relevance

The study by Connelly and co-researchers has implications for nursing administrators, who are routinely confronted with the disruptive effects of staff turnover. The findings suggest that certain factors should be of particular concern to administrators attempting to achieve nurse retention. These include personal job stress, situational job stress, routinization, instrumental communication, and distributive justice—all of which are amenable to modification through carefully conceived institutional policies. It is noteworthy that these factors, which were significant predictors of nurse retention in the quantitative portion of the study, were validated through the in-depth qualitative interviews, adding credibility to these findings.

Administrators also need to consider the new dimensions discovered in the qualitative data as critical pieces in the puzzle of retaining nurses in their workforce. For example, the issue of nurses' ability to give quality time can be addressed through nurse-to-patient ratios: nurses need time to be caring and to sit with their patients and give their full attention.

● ● ● ● ● *SUMMARY POINTS*

- Qualitative research typically involves an **emergent design**—a design that emerges in the field as the study unfolds.
- As **bricoleurs**, qualitative researchers tend to be creative and intuitive, putting together an array of data drawn from many sources in an effort to arrive at a holistic understanding of a phenomenon.
- Although qualitative design is elastic and flexible, qualitative researchers nevertheless can plan for broad contingencies that can be expected to pose decision opportunities for the design of the study in the field.
- A naturalistic inquiry typically progresses through three broad phases in the field: an orientation and overview phase to determine what it is about the phenomenon under investigation that is salient; a focused exploration phase that closely examines important aspects of the phenomenon; and a confirmation and closure phase to confirm findings.
- Qualitative research traditions have their roots in anthropology (*e.g.,* **ethnography** and **ethnoscience**); philosophy (**phenomenology** and **hermeneutics**); psychology (**ethology, ecological psychology**); sociology (**grounded theory, ethnomethodology, symbolic interaction**); and sociolinguistics (**discourse analysis**).
- Ethnography focuses on the culture of a group of people and relies on extensive field work. The ethnographer strives to acquire an **emic**, or insider's, perspective of the culture under study; the outsider's perspective is known as **etic**.
- Phenomenology seeks to discover the essence and meaning of a phenomenon as it is experienced by people. In descriptive phenomenology, the researcher strives to **bracket** out any preconceived views and to **intuit** the essence of the phenomenon by remaining open to the meanings attributed to it by those who have experienced it. Bracketing is not a feature of interpretive (hermeneutic) phenomenology.
- **Grounded theory**, an approach to studying social psychological processes and social structures, aims to discover theoretical precepts grounded in the

data. This approach uses **constant comparison**: categories elicited from the data are constantly compared with data obtained earlier so that shared themes and variations can be determined.

- In some studies, an **integrated design** that combines qualitative and quantitative data in a single investigation (multimethod research) can be advantageous because qualitative and quantitative approaches have complementary strengths and weaknesses.

- In nursing, one of the most frequent uses of **multimethod research** has been in the area of instrument development. Integrated designs are also used in efforts to illustrate, to interpret relationships and causal processes, and to develop theory.

➤ ➤ ➤ ➤ CRITICAL THINKING ACTIVITIES

Chapter 9 of the accompanying *Study Guide to Accompany Essentials of Nursing Research,* 5th edition offers various exercises and study suggestions for reinforcing the concepts presented in this chapter. In addition, you can address the following:

1. Read the introduction and method section from the qualitative study in the Appendix of this book, and then answer relevant questions in Box 9-1.

2. In Chapter 8, one of the research examples was a quantitative study by York and her colleagues (1997), who evaluated an intervention for high-risk child-bearing women. How might qualitative data have enriched this study? (*Nursing Research,* volume 46, pp. 254–261)

3. In Dreher and Hayes' study, used as an example of an ethnographic study in this chapter, what might the focal research question have been in a phenomenologic study? In a hermeneutic study? In a grounded theory study?

For additional review, see questions 106–124 on the study CD provided with Polit: Study Guide to Accompany Essentials of Nursing Research.

SUGGESTED READINGS

Methodologic References

Baker, C., Wuest, J., & Stern, P. N. (1992). Method slurring: The grounded theory/phenomenology example. *Journal of Advanced Nursing, 17,* 1355–1360.

Carey, J. W. (1993). Linking qualitative and quantitative methods: Integrating cultural factors into public health. *Qualitative Health Research, 3,* 298–318.

Chesla, C. A. (1992). When qualitative and quantitative findings do not converge. *Western Journal of Nursing Research, 14,* 681–685.

Creswell, J. W. (1998). *Qualitative inquiry and research design: Choosing among five traditions.* Thousand Oaks, CA: Sage.

Denzin, N. K. & Lincoln, Y. S. (Eds.). (1994). *Handbook of qualitative research.* Thousand Oaks, CA: Sage.

Glaser, B. G., & Strauss, A. L. (1967). *The discovery of grounded theory: Strategies for qualitative research.* Chicago: Aldine.

Heidegger, M. (1962) *Being and time.* New York: Harper & Row.

Husserl, E. (1962). *Ideas: General introduction to pure phenomenology.* New York: MacMillan.

Leininger, M. M. (Ed.). (1985). *Qualitative research methods in nursing.* New York: Grune & Stratton.

Lincoln, Y. S., & Guba, E. G. (1985). *Naturalistic inquiry.* Newbury Park, CA: Sage.

Morse, J. M. (1991). *Qualitative nursing research: A contemporary dialogue.* Newbury Park, CA: Sage.

Morse, J. M. (1999). Qualitative methods: The state of the art. *Qualitative Health Research, 9,* 393–406.

Morse, J. M., & Field, P. A. (1995). *Qualitative research methods for health professionals* (2nd ed.). Thousand Oaks, CA: Sage.

Sandelowski, M. (1996). Using qualitative methods in intervention studies. *Research in Nursing & Health, 19,* 359–364.

Streubert, H. J., & Carpenter, D. R. (1995). *Qualitative research in nursing: Advancing the humanistic imperative.* Philadelphia: J. B. Lippincott.

Substantive References

Baker, H. M. (1997). Rules outside the rules for administration of medication. *Image— The Journal of Nursing Scholarship, 29,* 155–158.

Beck, C. T. (1998). Postpartum onset of panic disorder. *Image—The Journal of Nursing Scholarship, 30,* 131–135.

Beck, C. T. (2000). Postpartum Depression Screening Scale: Development and psychometric testing. *Nursing Research, 49.*

Bottorff, J. L., & Varcoe, C. (1995). Transitions in nurse-patient interactions: A qualitative ethology. *Qualitative Health Research, 5,* 315–331.

Boydell, K. M., Goering, P., & Morrell-Bellai, T. L. (2000). Narratives of identity: Representation of self in people who are homeless. *Qualitative Health Research, 10,* 26–38.

Brown, M. A., & Stetz, K. (1999). The labor of caregiving: A theoretical model of caregiving during potentially fatal illness. *Qualitative Health Research, 9,* 182–197.

Connelly, L. M., Bott, M., Hoffart, N., & Taunton, R. L. (1997). Methodological triangulation in a study of nurse retention. *Nursing Research, 46,* 299–302.

Dickerson, S. S. (1998). Cardiac spouses' help-seeking experiences. *Clinical Nursing Research, 7,* 6–28.

Dreher, M. C., & Hayes, J. S. (1993). Triangulation in cross-cultural research of child development in Jamaica. *Western Journal of Nursing Research, 15,* 216–229.

Eastland, L. S. (1995). Recovery as an interactive process: Explanation and empowerment in 12-step programs. *Qualitative Health Research, 5,* 292–314.

Gibson, J. M. E., & Kenrick, M. (1998). Pain and powerlessness: The experience of living with peripheral vascular disease. *Journal of Advanced Nursing, 27,* 737–745.

Gray, M., & Smith, L. N. (1999). The professional socialization of diploma of higher education in nursing students. *Journal of Advanced Nursing, 29,* 639–647.

Higgins, P. G., & Learn, C. D. (1999). Health practices of adult Hispanic women. *Journal of Advanced Nursing, 29,* 1105–1112.

Ingram, D., & Hutchinson, S. A. (2000). Double binds and the reproductive and mothering experiences of HIV-positive women. *Qualitative Health Research, 10,* 117–132.

Jakobsson, L., Hallberg, I. R., & Loven, L. (2000). Experiences of micturition problems, indwelling catheter treatment, and sexual life consequences in men with prostate cancer. *Journal of Advanced Nursing, 31,* 59–67.

Kahn, D. L. (1999). Making the best of it: Adapting to the ambivalence of a nursing home environment. *Qualitative Health Research, 9,* 119–132.

Lagerwey, M. D. (1999). Nursing ethics at Hadamar. *Qualitative Health Research, 9,* 759–772.

Ledlie, S. W. (1999). Diagnosis disclosure by family caregivers to children who have perinatally acquired HIV disease. *Nursing Research, 48,* 141–149.

Lowenberg, J. S. (1997). Who's responsible? Clients in a stress management clinic. *Qualitative Health Research, 7,* 448–467.

Mayo, K. (1992). Physical activity practices among American black working women. *Qualitative Health Research, 4,* 51–71.

Moore, K. D. (1999). Dissonance in the dining room: A study of social interaction in a special care unit. *Qualitative Health Research, 9,* 133–155.

Morgan, D. G., & Stewart, N. J. (1999). The physical environment of special care units: Needs of residents with dementia from the perspective of staff and family caregivers. *Qualitative Health Research, 9,* 105–118.

Newshan, G. (1998). Is anybody listening? A phenomenological study of pain in hospitalized persons with AIDS. *Journal of the Association of Nurses in AIDS Care, 9,* 57–67.

Nicholas, D. B. (1999). Meanings of maternal caregiving: Children with end stage renal disease. *Qualitative Health Research, 9,* 468–478.

Paterson, B., Thorne, S., Crawford, J., & Tarko, M. (1999). Living with diabetes as a transformational experience. *Qualitative Health Research, 9,* 786–802.

Polit, D. F., London, A. S., & Martinez, J. M. (2000). *Food security and hunger in poor, mother-headed families in four U. S. cities.* New York: MDRC.

Reece, S. M., & Harkless, G. (1996). Divergent themes in maternal experience in women older than 35 years of age. *Applied Nursing Research, 9,* 148–153.

Salazar, M. K., & Carter, W. B. (1993). Evaluation of breast self-examination beliefs using a decision model. *Western Journal of Nursing Research, 15,* 403–418.

Sayre, J. (2000). The patient's diagnosis: Explanatory models of mental illness, *Qualitative Health Research, 10,* 71–83.

Examining Sampling Plans

• •

Student Objectives

On completion of this chapter, the student will be able to:

○ describe the rationale for sampling in research studies
○ distinguish between nonprobability and probability samples and compare their advantages and disadvantages
○ identify several types of nonprobability and probability samples and describe their main characteristics
○ identify differences in the logic and evaluation criteria used in sampling approaches for quantitative versus qualitative studies
○ identify several approaches to theoretical/purposive sampling in qualitative studies
○ evaluate the sampling method and sample size in a research study
○ define new terms in the chapter

• •

New Terms

Accessible population	Quota sampling
Accidental sampling	Random selection
Cluster sampling	Response rate
Convenience sampling	Sample size
Data saturation	Sampling
Disproportionate sample	Sampling bias
Elements	Sampling error
Eligibility criteria	Sampling frame
Extreme/deviant case sampling	Sampling interval
Judgmental sampling	Simple random sampling
Maximum variation sampling	Snowball sampling
Multistage sampling	Strata
Network sampling	Stratified random sampling
Nonprobability sampling	Systematic sampling
Nonresponse bias	Target population
Population	Theoretical sampling
Power analysis	Typical case sampling
Probability sampling	Volunteer sample
Proportionate sample	Weighting
Purposive (purposeful) sampling	

Sampling is a process familiar to all of us—we gather information, make decisions, and formulate predictions about phenomena based on contact with a limited portion of them. Researchers, too, derive knowledge and draw conclusions from samples. In testing the efficacy of a nursing intervention for cancer patients, a nurse researcher reaches conclusions without testing the intervention with every victim of the disease. However, researchers cannot afford to draw conclusions about the effectiveness of nursing interventions based on faulty samples. The consequences of erroneous inferences are more momentous in nursing research than in private decision making.

Quantitative and qualitative researchers have different approaches to sampling. Quantitative researchers select samples that allow them to generalize their results by developing an appropriate plan before data collection begins. Qualitative researchers are not as concerned with issues of generalizability but rather want to achieve an in-depth, holistic understanding of the phenomenon of interest. They allow sampling decisions to emerge during the course of data collection based on informational and theoretical needs. Because formal sampling designs are more relevant to quantitative than to qualitative research, most of this chapter is devoted to sampling plans for quantitative studies.

BASIC SAMPLING CONCEPTS IN QUANTITATIVE RESEARCH

Sampling is an important step in the research process for quantitative studies. Let us first consider some terms associated with sampling—terms that are used primarily (but not exclusively) in connection with quantitative studies.

Populations

A **population** is the entire aggregation of cases that meets a specified set of criteria. For instance, if a nurse researcher were studying American nurses with doctoral degrees, the population could be defined as all U.S. citizens who are RNs and who have acquired a PhD, DNSc, or other doctoral-level degree. Other possible populations might be: all the cardiac patients hospitalized in Memorial Hospital in 1998; all Canadian women older than 60 years of age who have Alzheimer's disease; or all the children in Atlanta with cystic fibrosis. Thus, a population may be broadly defined, involving millions of people, or narrowly specified to include only several hundred people.

Populations are not restricted to human subjects. A population might consist of all the hospital records on file in the Belleview Hospital, or all the U.S. high schools with a school-based clinic that dispenses contraceptives. Whatever the basic unit, the population comprises the aggregate of entities in which the researcher is interested.

Quantitative researchers specify the characteristics that delimit the population through the **eligibility criteria** for inclusion in their studies. For example, consider the population of American nursing students. Would this population include part-time students? Would RNs returning to school for a bachelor's degree be included? The researcher establishes these criteria to determine whether a person qualifies as a member of the population. A reader of a research report needs to know the eligibility criteria to understand the population to which the findings can be generalized.

 Example of eligibility criteria:

Sinclair and colleagues (1999) studied the effects of a cognitive-behavioral intervention for women with arthritis. The eligibility criteria for the study included the following: (1) female; (2) 24 to 80 years of age; (3) diagnosed with rheumatoid arthritis by a rheumatologist; (4) no history of organic brain syndrome or a major psychotic disorder; (5) no other uncontrolled medical or communicative disorders; and (6) able to read and speak English.

Researchers sample from an accessible population in the hope of generalizing to a target population. The **target population** is the entire population in which the researcher is interested. The **accessible population** comprises cases from the target population that are accessible to the researcher as a pool of subjects. For example, the researcher's target population might consist of all diabetic patients in the United States, but, in reality, the population that is accessible to a researcher might consist of diabetic patients who are members of a particular health plan.

CONSUMER TIP:

In some quantitative research reports, the researchers do not clearly identify the population under study. In others, the population is not clarified until the discussion section, when an effort is made to discuss the group to which the study findings can be generalized. ∎

Samples and Sampling

Sampling is the process of selecting a portion of the population to represent the entire population. A **sample**, then, is a subset of the population. The entities that make up the samples and populations are **elements.** In nursing research, the elements are usually humans.

Samples and sampling plans vary in their adequacy. *The overriding consideration in assessing a sample in a quantitative study is its representativeness*—the extent to which the sample is similar to the population. Unfortunately, there is no method for ensuring that a sample is representative. Certain sampling plans are less likely to result in biased samples than others, but there is never a guarantee of a representative sample. Researchers operate under conditions in which error is possible, but an important role of the researcher is to minimize or control those errors. Consumers must assess the researcher's success in having done so.

There are two broad categories of sampling plans: **probability sampling** and **nonprobability sampling.** With a probability sample, researchers are able to specify the probability that each element of the population will be included in the sample. Probability samples use random selection in choosing the sample units, and therefore some confidence can be placed in their representativeness. In nonprobability samples, elements are selected by nonrandom methods. There is no way to estimate the probability of including each element in a nonprobability sample, and every element usually does not have a chance for inclusion.

Strata

Populations consist of subpopulations, or **strata.** Strata are mutually exclusive segments of a population based on a specified characteristic. For instance, a population consisting of all RNs in the United States could be divided into two strata based on gender. Alternatively, we could specify three strata consisting of nurses younger than 30 years, nurses aged 30 to 45 years, and nurses aged 46 years or older. Strata are used in the sample selection process to enhance the sample's representativeness.

Sampling Rationale

Researchers work with samples rather than with populations because it is more economical and efficient to do so. Researchers have neither the time nor the resources to study all members of a population. Furthermore, it is unnecessary to do so because it is usually possible to obtain reasonably accurate information from a sample. Samples, thus, are practical means of collecting data.

Still, data from samples can lead to erroneous conclusions. Finding 50 subjects to participate in a study is easy, but it is difficult to select 50 subjects who are not a biased subset of the population. **Sampling bias** is the systematic overrepresentation or underrepresentation of some segment of the population in terms of a characteristic relevant to the research question.

Sampling bias is affected by the homogeneity of the population. If the elements in a population were all identical on the critical attribute, any sample would be as good as any other. Indeed, if the population were completely homogeneous (*i.e.,* exhibited no variability at all), a single element would be a sufficient sample for drawing conclusions about the population. For many physical or physiologic attributes, it may be safe to assume a reasonable degree of homogeneity. For example, the blood in a person's veins is relatively homogeneous; hence, a single blood sample chosen haphazardly from a patient is adequate for clinical purposes. Most human attributes, however, are not homogeneous. Variables, after all, derive their name from the fact that traits vary from one person to the next. Age, blood pressure, stress level, and health habits are all attributes that reflect the heterogeneity of humans.

CONSUMER TIP:

The sampling plan is usually discussed in the method section of a research report, sometimes in a separate subsection with the heading "Sample," "Subjects," or "Study Participants." A description of sample characteristics, however, may be reported in the results section. If the researcher has undertaken analyses to detect sample biases in a quantitative study, these may be described in either the method or results section (e.g., the researcher might compare the characteristics of patients who were invited to participate in the study but who declined to do so with those of patients who actually became subjects). ■

NONPROBABILITY SAMPLING

Three primary methods of nonprobability sampling are used in quantitative studies: convenience, quota, and purposive sampling.

Convenience Sampling

Convenience sampling (or **accidental sampling**) entails the use of the most conveniently available people as study participants. A nurse who distributes questionnaires about breastfeeding intentions to the first 100 available pregnant women is using a convenience sample. The problem with convenience sampling is that available subjects might be atypical of the population; therefore, the price of convenience is the risk of bias and erroneous findings. Convenience samples do not necessarily comprise people known to the researchers. Stopping people at a street corner to ask them questions is sampling by convenience. People select themselves as pedestrians on certain streets, and self-selection generally leads to bias.

Another type of convenience sampling is **snowball sampling** (or **network sampling**). With this approach, early sample members are asked to refer others who meet the study's eligibility criteria. This method of sampling is most often used when the population consists of people with specific traits who might be difficult to identify by ordinary means (*e.g.,* women who stopped breastfeeding their infants within 1 month after birth).

Convenience sampling is the weakest form of sampling for quantitative studies. When the phenomena of interest are heterogeneous, there is no other sampling method in which the risk of bias is greater—and there is no way to evaluate the biases. You should exercise caution in interpreting findings and generalizing results from quantitative studies that used convenience samples.

⊞ *Example of convenience sampling:*

Brown, Whittemore, and Knapp (2000) conducted a study to determine whether a person's height could be accurately estimated based on a measure of arm span. Their subjects were a convenience sample of 83 people between the ages of 20 and 61 years.

Quota Sampling

With **quota sampling**, the researcher uses knowledge about the population to build some representativeness into the sampling plan. A quota sample is one in which the researcher identifies strata of the population and specifies the number (the quota) of elements needed from those strata in the sample. By using information about the composition of the population, the investigator can ensure that diverse segments are represented.

Let us use as an example a researcher interested in studying the attitudes of undergraduate nursing students toward working on an AIDS unit. The accessible population for this study is a nursing school with an enrollment of 1000 undergraduates, and a sample size of 200 students is desired. With a convenience sample, the researcher could simply distribute questionnaires to students in classrooms. Suppose, however, that the researcher suspects that male and female students, as well as members of the four classes, have different attitudes toward working with AIDS victims. A convenience sample could easily sample too many or too few students from these subgroups. Table 10-1

TABLE 10-1. **Numbers and Percentages of Students in Strata of a Population, Convenience Sample, and Quota Sample**

	FRESHMEN	SOPHOMORES	JUNIORS	SENIORS	TOTAL
POPULATION					
Males	25 (2.5%)	25 (2.5%)	25 (2.5%)	25 (2.5%)	100 (10%)
Females	225 (22.5%)	225 (22.5%)	225 (22.5%)	225 (22.5%)	900 (90%)
TOTAL	250 (25%)	250 (25%)	250 (25%)	250 (25%)	1000 (100%)
CONVENIENCE SAMPLE					
Males	2 (1%)	4 (2%)	3 (1.5%)	1 (0.5%)	10 (5%)
Females	98 (49%)	36 (18%)	37 (18.5%)	19 (9.5%)	190 (95%)
TOTAL	100 (50%)	40 (20%)	40 (20%)	20 (10%)	200 (100%)
QUOTA SAMPLE					
Males	5 (2.5%)	5 (2.5%)	5 (2.5%)	5 (2.5%)	20 (10%)
Females	45 (22.5%)	45 (22.5%)	45 (22.5%)	45 (22.5%)	180 (90%)
TOTAL	50 (25%)	50 (25%)	50 (25%)	50 (25%)	200 (100%)

presents some fictitious data showing the numbers of students in each strata, both for the population and for a hypothetical convenience sample. As this table shows, the convenience sample seriously overrepresents freshmen and women and underrepresents men and upperclassmen. In a quota sample, the researcher can guide the selection of subjects so that the sample includes an appropriate number of cases from each stratum. The bottom panel of Table 10-1 shows the number of cases that would be required from each stratum in a quota sample.

If we continue with this example, you may better appreciate the problem of inadequate representation of the strata. Suppose a key question in this study was: Would you be willing to work on a unit that cared exclusively for AIDS patients? The percentage of students in the population who would respond "yes" to this question is shown in the first column of Table 10-2. Of course, these values would not be known by the researcher; they are displayed to illustrate a point. Within the population, males and older students are more likely than females and younger students to express willingness to work on a unit with AIDS patients, yet these are the groups underrepresented in the convenience sample. Thus, there is a sizable discrepancy between the population and sample values: nearly twice as many students in the population are favorable toward working with AIDS victims (12.5%) than in the convenience sample (6.5%). The quota sample, on the other hand, does a reasonably good job of reflecting the population's views.

Quota sampling is a relatively easy way to enhance the representativeness of a nonprobability sample. Researchers stratify on the basis of extraneous variables that, in their estimation, would reflect important differences in the

TABLE 10-2. Students Willing to Consider Working with AIDS Patients

	NUMBER IN POPULATION	NUMBER IN CONVENIENCE SAMPLE	NUMBER IN QUOTA SAMPLE
Freshmen males	2	0	0
Sophomore males	6	1	1
Junior males	8	1	2
Senior males	12	0	3
Freshmen females	6	2	1
Sophomore females	16	2	3
Junior females	30	4	7
Senior females	45	3	9
Number of willing students	125	13	26
Total number of students	1000	200	200
Percentage	12.5%	6.5%	13.0%

dependent variable under investigation. Such variables as age, gender, ethnicity, socioeconomic status, and medical diagnosis are most likely to be used.

Except for the identification of the key strata, quota sampling is procedurally similar to convenience sampling. The subjects are a convenience sample from each stratum of the population. Because of this fact, quota sampling shares many of the same weaknesses as convenience sampling. For instance, if the researcher were required by the quota sampling plan to interview 20 male nursing students, a trip to the dormitories might be a convenient method of recruiting those subjects. Yet this approach would fail to give any representation to male students living off campus, who may have distinctive views about working with AIDS patients. Despite its problems, however, quota sampling is an important improvement over convenience sampling for quantitative studies.

Example of quota sampling:

Wilbur, Miller, Montgomery, and Chandler (1998) developed a method of categorizing patterns of women's activities by describing their frequency, intensity, and duration. The study was designed as a 24-cell quota sample of 200 women, stratified by four occupations, two racial groups, and three age groups.

Purposive Sampling

Purposive sampling, (or judgmental sampling), is based on the assumption that a researcher's knowledge about the population can be used to hand pick the cases to be included in the sample. The researcher might decide purposely to select the widest possible variety of respondents or might choose subjects who are judged to be typical of the population in question or particularly knowledgeable about the issues under study. Sampling in this subjective manner, however, provides no external, objective method for assessing the typicalness of the selected subjects. Nevertheless, this method can be used to advantage in certain instances. For example, newly developed instruments can be effectively pretested and evaluated with a purposive sample of divergent types of people. Also, as discussed in the next section, purposive sampling is frequently used by qualitative researchers.

Example of purposive sampling:

Friedemann, Montgomery, Rice, and Farrell (1999) studied family members' involvement in the nursing home. The first stage of their sampling plan involved purposively sampling 24 nursing homes with a diversity of policies related to family involvement, based on a survey of 208 nursing homes in southern Michigan. In the second stage, all family members of residents admitted to these nursing homes during a 20-month window were invited to participate.

Evaluation of Nonprobability Sampling

Nonprobability samples are rarely representative of the target population—some segment of the population is likely to be systematically underrepresented. Only a small fraction of the characteristics in which quantitative nurse researchers are interested are sufficiently homogeneous to render sampling bias an irrelevant consideration.

Why, then, are nonprobability samples used at all in quantitative research? Clearly, the advantage of these sampling designs lies in their convenience and economy. Probability sampling requires resources and time. There may be no option but to use a nonprobability sampling plan. Researchers using a nonprobability sample out of necessity must be cautious about their conclusions, and you as reader should be alert to the possibility of sampling bias.

 CONSUMER TIP:

Research reports are not always explicit about the type of sampling approach used. This is particularly apt to be true with nonprobability sampling plans. If the sampling design is not specified, it is probably safe to assume that a sample of convenience was used. ■

PROBABILITY SAMPLING

Probability sampling involves the random selection of elements from the population. Random selection should not be confused with random assignment, which was described in Chapter 8. Random assignment is the process of allocating subjects to different treatments on a random basis in experimental designs. Random assignment has no bearing on how subjects in the experiment were selected in the first place. A **random selection** process is one in which each element in the population has an equal, independent chance of being selected. The four most commonly used probability sampling designs are simple random, stratified random, cluster, and systematic sampling.

Simple Random Sampling

Simple random sampling is the most basic probability sampling design. Because more complex probability sampling designs incorporate features of simple random sampling, the procedures are briefly described so that you can appreciate what is involved.

After the population has been defined, the researcher establishes a **sampling frame**, the technical name for the actual list of the population elements. If nursing students attending the University of Connecticut constituted the population, then a student roster would be the sampling frame. If the population were 400-bed or larger general hospitals in the United States, then a list of all those hospitals would be the sampling frame. In actual practice, a population is sometimes defined in terms of an existing sampling frame. For example, a researcher might use a telephone directory as a sampling frame. In such a case, the population would be defined as the residents of a certain community who have telephones and who have a listed number. After a listing of the population elements has been developed or located, the elements are numbered consecutively. A table of random numbers or a computer is then used to draw, at random, a sample of the desired size.

Samples selected randomly in such a fashion are not subject to researcher biases. There is no *guarantee* that the sample will be representative of the population, but random selection does guarantee that differences between the sample and the population are purely a function of chance. The probability of selecting a markedly deviant sample through random sampling is low, and this probability decreases as the sample size increases.

Simple random sampling is a laborious process. The development of the sampling frame, enumeration of all the elements, and selection of the sample elements are time-consuming chores, particularly with a large population. Moreover, it is rarely possible to get a complete listing of population elements; hence, other methods are often used.

> **Example of random sampling:**
>
> Edwardson and Dean (1999) investigated the appropriateness of self-care responses to symptoms among elderly people living in Minneapolis. The sampling frame included all people 65 years of age and older who resided on randomly selected city streets and who were listed in the City Directory. A sample of 601 noninstitutionalized, English-speaking elders was obtained.

Stratified Random Sampling

In **stratified random sampling**, the population is divided into homogeneous subsets from which elements are selected at random. As in quota sampling, the aim of stratified sampling is to enhance the sample's representativeness. The most common procedure for drawing a stratified random sample is to group together those elements that belong to a stratum and to randomly select the desired number of elements.

The researcher may sample either proportionately (in relation to the size of the stratum) or disproportionately. If an undergraduate population in a school of nursing consisted of 10% African Americans, 5% Hispanics, and 85% whites, a **proportionate sample** of 100 students, with racial background as the stratifying variable, would consist of 10, 5, and 85 students from the respective subpopulations. Researchers often use a **disproportionate sample** whenever comparisons between strata of unequal membership size are desired. In the example at hand, the researcher might select 20 African Americans, 20 Hispanics, and 60 whites to ensure a more adequate representation of the viewpoints of the two racial minorities. (When disproportionate sampling is used, however, it is necessary to make a mathematical adjustment—known as **weighting**—to the data to arrive at the best estimate of overall population values.)

By using stratified random sampling, researchers can sharpen the precision and representativeness of the final sample. Stratified sampling may, however, be impossible if information on the stratifying variables is unavailable (*e.g.,* a student roster might not include information on race and ethnicity). Furthermore, a stratified sample requires even more labor than simple random sampling because the sample must be drawn from multiple enumerated listings.

Example of stratified random sampling:

Carty and Rosenfeld (1998) conducted a survey of nursing programs to determine the status of information technology in nursing education. A stratified random sample of 347 National League for Nursing–accredited schools (proportionately stratified by program type: diploma, associate, baccalaureate, and master) was selected to participate.

Cluster Sampling

For many populations, it is impossible to obtain a listing of the elements. For example, there is no listing of all full-time nursing students in the United States. Large-scale quantitative studies rarely use simple or stratified random sampling. The most common procedure for large-scale surveys is cluster sampling.

In **cluster sampling**, there is a successive random sampling of units. The first unit to be sampled is large groupings, or clusters. For example, in drawing a sample of nursing students, the researcher might first draw a random sample of nursing schools. The usual procedure for selecting a general sample of citizens is to sample such administrative units as states, cities, census tracts, and then households, successively. Because of the successive stages of sampling, this approach is often referred to as **multistage sampling.**

For a specified number of cases, cluster sampling tends to contain more sampling error than simple or stratified random sampling. Nevertheless, cluster sampling is more economical and practical when the population is large and widely dispersed.

Example of cluster sampling:

Trent (1997) evaluated academic advisement in RN-to-BSN programs. The first stage involved random selection of geographic areas for this type of program. Then a final sample of 323 students enrolled in either a beginning, midway, or final course in the curriculum was selected.

Systematic Sampling

Systematic sampling involves the selection of every *k*th case from some list or group, such as every 10th person on a patient list. Systematic sampling designs can be applied in such a way that an essentially random sample is drawn.* First, the size of the population is divided by the size of the desired sample to obtain the sampling interval width. The **sampling interval** is the standard distance between the selected elements. For instance, if we wanted a sample of 50 from a population of 5,000, our sampling interval would be 100 (5,000 / 50 = 100). In other words, every 100th case on the sampling frame would be sampled. Next, the first case would be selected randomly, using a table of random numbers. If the random number chosen is 73, the people corresponding to numbers 73, 173, 273, 373, and so forth would be included in the sample. Systematic sampling conducted in this manner is essentially identical to simple random sampling and in most cases is preferable because the same results are obtained in a more convenient and efficient manner.

> *Example of systematic random sampling:*
>
> Youngblut and Brooten (1999) studied the effect of having had nonparental child care on the behavior of preschool children during hospitalization. A systematic random sample of 61 single-parent families of preschoolers who had been full-term infants, identified through birth records of two newborn nurseries, was selected for the study.

Evaluation of Probability Sampling

Probability sampling is the only reliable method of obtaining representative samples in quantitative studies. Probability sampling avoids the risk of conscious or unconscious biases. If all the elements in the population have an equal probability of being selected, there is a high likelihood that the sample will represent the population adequately. A further advantage is that probability sampling allows researchers to estimate the magnitude of sampling error. **Sampling error** is the difference between population values (*e.g.*, the average heart rate of the population) and sample values (*e.g.*, the average heart rate of the sample). It is rare that a sample is perfectly representative of a population and contains no sampling error; however, probability sampling permits estimates of the degree of expected error. On the other hand, probability sampling is expensive and demanding. Unless the population is narrowly defined, it is beyond the scope of most researchers to draw a probability sample.

---

*Systematic sampling is sometimes used to sample every *k*th person without a sampling frame (*e.g.*, every 10th student entering a bookstore). In these situations, the sampling is nonprobability in nature because not every student has a chance of being selected.

SAMPLE SIZE IN QUANTITATIVE STUDIES

Sample size—the number of subjects in a sample—is a major issue in conducting and evaluating quantitative research. There is no simple equation to determine how large a sample is needed, but quantitative researchers are generally advised to use the largest sample possible. The larger the sample, the more representative it is likely to be. Every time a researcher calculates a percentage or an average based on sample data, the purpose is to estimate a population value. The larger the sample, the smaller the sampling error.

Let us illustrate this notion with an example of estimating monthly aspirin consumption in a nursing home facility (Table 10-3). The population is 15 nursing home residents whose aspirin consumption averages 16 per month. Two simple random samples with sample sizes of 2, 3, 5, and 10 were drawn from the population of 15 residents. Each sample average on the right represents an estimate of the population average, which we know is 16. (Under ordinary circumstances, the population value would be unknown to us, and we would draw only one sample.) With a sample size of 2, our estimate might have been wrong by as many as 8 aspirins (sample 1B). As the sample size increases, the average gets closer to the population value, and differences in the estimates between samples A and B get smaller. As the sample size increases, the probability of getting a deviant sample diminishes because large samples provide the opportunity to counterbalance atypical values.

Advanced researchers can estimate how large the sample should be for an adequate test of the research hypotheses through **power analysis** (Cohen, 1988). A simple example can illustrate the basic principle of power analysis. Suppose a researcher were testing a new intervention to help people quit

TABLE 10-3.	Comparison of Population and Sample Values and Averages in Nursing Home Aspirin Consumption Example		
NUMBER IN GROUP	**GROUP**	**VALUES (MONTHLY NUMBER OF ASPIRINS CONSUMED)**	**AVERAGE**
15	Population	2, 4, 6, 8, 10, 12, 14, 16, 18, 20, 22, 24, 26, 28, 30	16.0
2	Sample 1A	6, 14	10.0
2	Sample 1B	20, 28	24.0
3	Sample 2A	16, 18, 8	14.0
3	Sample 2B	20, 14, 26	20.0
5	Sample 3A	26, 14, 18, 2, 28	17.6
5	Sample 3B	30, 2, 26, 10, 4	14.4
10	Sample 4A	18, 16, 24, 22, 8, 14, 28, 20, 2, 6	15.8
10	Sample 4B	14, 18, 12, 20, 6, 14, 28, 12, 24, 16	16.4

smoking; smokers would be randomly assigned to either an experimental or a control group. How many smokers should be used in the study? When using power analysis, the researcher must estimate how large the group difference will be (*e.g.,* the difference in the average number of cigarettes smoked in the week after the intervention). This estimate might be based on previous research, on the researcher's personal experience, or on other factors. When expected differences are large, it does not take a large sample to ensure that the differences will be revealed in a statistical analysis; but when small differences are predicted, large samples are needed. Cohen (1988) claims that, for new areas of research, group differences are likely to be small. In our example, if a small group difference in postintervention smoking were expected, the sample size needed to test the effectiveness of the new program, assuming standard statistical criteria, would be about 800 smokers (400 per group). If a medium-sized difference were expected, the total sample size would still be several hundred smokers.

When samples are too small, quantitative researchers run the risk of gathering data that will not confirm the study hypotheses—even when those hypotheses are correct. Large samples are no assurance of accuracy, however. With nonprobability sampling, even a large sample can harbor extensive bias. The famous example illustrating this point is the 1936 presidential poll conducted by the magazine *Literary Digest,* which predicted that Alfred M. Landon would defeat Franklin D. Roosevelt by a landslide. A large sample of about 2.5 million people participated in this poll, but biases arose because the sample was drawn from telephone directories and automobile registrations during a Depression year when only the well-to-do (who favored Landon) had a car or telephone.

A large sample cannot correct for a faulty sampling design; nevertheless, a large nonprobability sample is preferable to a small one. When critiquing quantitative studies, you must assess both the sample size and the sample selection method to judge how representative the sample likely was.

CONSUMER TIP:

The sampling plan is often one of the weakest aspects of quantitative nursing studies (this is also true of quantitative research in other disciplines). Most nursing studies use samples of convenience, and many are based on samples that are too small to provide an adequate test of the research hypotheses. Most quantitative studies are based on samples of fewer than 200 subjects, and a great many studies have fewer than 100 subjects. Power analysis is not used by many nurse researchers, and research reports typically offer no justification for the size of the study sample. (When a power analysis is performed, the minimum power that is generally considered acceptable is .80). Small samples run a high risk of leading researchers to erroneously reject their research hypotheses. Therefore, you should be especially prepared to critique the sampling plan of studies that fail to support research hypotheses. ■

SAMPLING IN QUALITATIVE RESEARCH

Qualitative studies use small, nonrandom samples. This does not mean that qualitative researchers are unconcerned with the quality of their samples, but rather that they use different criteria for selecting study participants. This section examines considerations that apply to sampling in qualitative studies.

The Logic of Qualitative Sampling

Quantitative research is concerned with measuring attributes and relationships in a population, and therefore a representative sample is needed to ensure that the measurements accurately reflect and can be generalized to the population. The aim of most qualitative studies is to discover meaning and to uncover multiple realities; therefore, generalizability, as quantitative researchers use this term, is not a guiding criterion.

The qualitative researcher asks such questions as: Who would be an information-rich data source for my study? Whom should I talk to first, or what should I observe, to maximize my understanding of the phenomenon? Clearly, with these types of question, a critical first step in qualitative sampling is the selection of a setting with high potential for "information richness."

As the study progresses, new sampling questions emerge, such as the following: Whom can I talk to or observe to confirm my understandings? Challenge or modify my understandings? Enrich my understandings? Broaden the utility of the constructs to explain different situations? Thus, as with the overall design in qualitative studies, sampling design is an emergent one that capitalizes on early learnings to guide subsequent direction.

Types of Qualitative Sampling

Qualitative researchers usually eschew probability samples. A random sample is not the best method of selecting people who will make good informants (*i.e.*, people who are knowledgeable, articulate, reflective, and willing to talk at length with the researcher).

Qualitative researchers may begin with a convenience sample (sometimes referred to in qualitative studies as a **volunteer sample**), especially if the researcher needs potential informants to come forward to identify themselves (*e.g.*, by placing notices in newspapers for people with certain experiences). Qualitative researchers also use snowball sampling, asking early informants to make referrals for other study participants.

Example of snowball sampling:

Allan (1998) did an ethnographic study of women's explanations of being overweight among African American, Euro-American, and Mexican American women. Allan used snowball sampling to make contact with and select a broad community-based sample of 120 women of varying social status and weight.

Although qualitative sampling may begin with volunteer informants and may be supplemented with new participants through snowballing, most qualitative studies eventually evolve to a purposive sampling strategy. In qualitative research, purposive sampling is often referred to as **theoretical sampling** (especially in grounded theory studies) or **purposeful sampling**. That is, regardless of how initial participants are selected, the researcher usually strives to select sample members purposefully based on the information needs emerging from the early findings. Whom to sample next depends on who has been sampled already.

> **Example of theoretical sampling:**
>
> Nardi (1998) conducted an in-depth grounded theory study that explored the nature of addiction recovery for pregnant and parenting women in an addiction treatment program. Nardi selected 17 participants for her research through theoretical sampling.

Within purposive sampling, several alternative strategies have been identified (Patton, 1990), only a few of which are mentioned here:

- Maximum variation sampling involves purposefully selecting cases with a wide range of variation on dimensions of interest
- Extreme/deviant case sampling provides opportunities for learning from the most unusual and extreme informants (e.g., outstanding successes and notable failures)
- Typical case sampling involves selection of participants who will illustrate or highlight what is typical or average

> **Example of maximum variation sampling:**
>
> Baggs and Schmitt (1997) studied perceptions of nurse–physician collaboration among intensive care nurses and medical resident physicians. They selected 10 nurses varying in age, gender, education, certification in critical care, and administrative role, and 10 physicians varying in gender and year of residency.

Maximum variation sampling is often the sampling mode of choice in qualitative research because it is useful in documenting the scope of a phenomenon and in identifying important patterns that cut across variations. Other strategies can also be used advantageously, however, depending on the nature of the research question.

> **CONSUMER TIP:**
>
> A qualitative research report will not necessary use such terms as "maximum variation sampling," but may describe the researcher's intent in selecting study participants. ∎

Sample Size

There are no firmly established criteria or rules for sample size in qualitative research. Sample size is largely a function of the purpose of the inquiry, the quality of the informants, and the type of sampling strategy used. For example, a larger sample is likely to be needed with maximum variation sampling than with typical case sampling. Patton argues that purposive samples "be judged on the basis of the purpose and rationale of each study and the sampling strategy used to achieve the study's purpose. The sample, like all other aspects of qualitative inquiry, must be judged in context. . . ." (1990, p. 185).

In qualitative research, sample size should be determined on the basis of informational needs. Hence, a guiding principle in sampling is **data saturation** (*i.e.*, sampling to the point at which no new information is obtained and redundancy is achieved). Redundancy can typically be achieved with a fairly small number of cases, if the information from each is of sufficient depth. Phenomenologic studies are typically based on samples of 10 or fewer study participants. Grounded theory or ethnographic studies are more likely to involve samples of 20 to 50 people.

 CONSUMER TIP:

The sample size adequacy of quantitative studies can be estimated by consumers after the fact through power analysis. However, sample size adequacy in a qualitative study is more difficult to judge on the basis of reading a research report because the main criterion is redundancy of information, which is difficult for consumers to judge. Some qualitative reports explicitly state that data saturation was achieved. ■

CRITIQUING THE SAMPLING PLAN

The sampling plan of a research study—particularly a quantitative study—merits particular scrutiny because, if the sample is seriously biased or too small, the findings may be misleading or just plain wrong. In critiquing a description of a sampling plan, you should consider two issues. The first is whether the researcher has adequately described the sampling plan. Ideally, a research report includes a description of the following aspects of the sample:

- The type of sampling approach used (*e.g.*, convenience, snowball, purposive, simple random)
- The population under study and the eligibility criteria for sample selection in quantitative studies; the nature of the setting and study group in a qualitative one
- The number of participants in the study and a rationale for the sample size
- A description of the main characteristics of the participants (*e.g.*, age, gender, medical condition, race, ethnicity, and so forth) and, in a quantitative study, of the population

- In quantitative studies, the number and characteristics of potential subjects who declined to participate in the study and of subjects who agreed to participate but who subsequently withdrew

If the description of the sample is inadequate, you may not be in a position to deal with the second and principal issue, which is whether the researcher made good sampling decisions.

Evaluating Quantitative Sampling Plans

We have stressed that the main criterion for assessing the adequacy of a sampling plan in quantitative research is whether the sample is representative of the population. You will never be able to know for sure, of course, but if the sampling strategy is weak or if the sample size is small, there is reason to suspect some bias. The extent of this bias depends on several factors, including the population's homogeneity. When the researcher has adopted a sampling plan in which the risk for bias is high, he or she should have taken steps to estimate the direction and degree of this bias so that readers can draw some informed conclusions.

Even with a rigorous sampling plan, the sample may contain some bias if not all people invited to participate in a research study agree to do so. If certain segments of the population refuse to cooperate, then a biased sample can result, even when probability sampling is used. The research report ideally should provide information about **response rates** (*i.e.,* the number of people participating in a study relative to the number of people sampled), and about possible **nonresponse bias**—differences between participants and those who declined to participate.

In developing the sampling plan, the researcher makes decisions regarding the specification of the population as well as the selection of the sample. If the target population is defined broadly, the researcher may have missed opportunities to control extraneous variables, and the gap between the accessible and the target population may be too great. Your job as reviewer is to come to conclusions about the reasonableness of generalizing the findings from the researcher's sample to the accessible population and from the accessible population to a broader target population. If the sampling plan is seriously flawed, it may be risky to generalize the findings at all without further replication of the results with another sample.

Box 10-1 presents some guiding questions for critiquing the sampling plan of a quantitative research report.

Evaluating Qualitative Sampling Plans

In a qualitative study, the sampling plan can be evaluated in terms of its adequacy and appropriateness (Morse, 1991). *Adequacy* refers to the sufficiency and quality of the data the sample yielded. An adequate sample provides data without any "thin" spots. When the researcher has truly obtained saturation

BOX 10-1

GUIDELINES FOR CRITIQUING QUANTITATIVE SAMPLING DESIGNS

1. Is the target or accessible population identified and described? Are eligibility criteria specified? To whom can the study results be generalized?

2. Are the sample selection procedures clearly described? What type of sampling plan was used?

3. How adequate is the sampling plan in terms of yielding a representative sample?

4. Did some factor other than the sampling plan affect the representativeness of the sample (*e.g.*, a low response rate)?

5. Are possible sample biases identified?

6. Is the sample size sufficiently large? Was the sample size justified on the basis of a power analysis or other rationale?

with a sample, informational adequacy has been achieved, and the resulting description or theory is richly textured and complete.

Appropriateness concerns the methods used to select a sample. An appropriate sample is one resulting from the identification and use of study participants who can best supply information according to the conceptual requirements of the study. The researcher must use a strategy that will yield the fullest possible understanding of the phenomenon of interest. A sampling approach that excludes negative cases or that fails to include participants with unusual experiences may not meet the information needs of the study.

Further guidance to critiquing sampling in a qualitative study is presented in Box 10-2.

BOX 10-2

GUIDELINES FOR CRITIQUING QUALITATIVE SAMPLING DESIGNS

1. Is the setting or study group adequately described? Is the setting appropriate for the research question?

2. Are the sample selection procedures described? What type of sampling strategy was used?

3. Given the information needs of the study, was the sampling approach appropriate? Were dimensions of the phenomenon under study adequately represented?

4. Is the sample size adequate? Did the researcher stipulate that information redundancy was achieved? Do the findings suggest a richly textured and comprehensive set of data without any apparent "holes" or thin areas?

RESEARCH EXAMPLES

Below, we describe at some length the sampling plans of two nursing studies, one quantitative and the other qualitative. The guidelines in Boxes 10-1 and 10-2 can be used to evaluate the research samples.

RESEARCH EXAMPLE OF A QUANTITATIVE STUDY

Levin (1999) conducted a study to identify predictors of health care workers' use of gloves when there is a potential for blood exposure. The study was designed as a test of the Fishbein and Ajzen Theory of Reasoned Action.

Research Summary

The targeted population for Levin's study was nurses and medical laboratory workers, groups that are especially likely to be exposed to human blood. Registered nurses and medical laboratory workers were randomly selected by telephone area codes for Chicago, its suburbs, and the rural areas of Illinois. The numbers were obtained from a listing of all registered nurses with active registration status through the state of Illinois, and a listing of medical laboratory workers who received certification through the American Society of Clinical Pathologists. Levin sought to obtain a sample of 450 participants, the number she had determined was needed to test her theoretical model. To achieve this sample size, Levin oversampled by 100% to account for nonresponses and ineligible respondents. The 909 potential respondents were mailed a questionnaire and a cover letter explaining the study. The response rate was nearly 70%, which included 107 respondents who had no blood contact and were ineligible. The final sample consisted of 247 nurses and 280 laboratory workers. Response rates were comparable for both groups, but response rates were significantly lower for nurses in Chicago than for nurses in other areas of Illinois.

Only 52% of the respondents reported wearing gloves every time there was potential blood contact. The analyses revealed that the Theory of Reasoned Action was a good model for predicting the use of gloves among nurses and laboratory workers. Specifically, a person's attitude toward glove use, their intention to use gloves, and their perceived degree of risk from blood-borne diseases were strongly related to their glove use behavior. Intention was the strongest predictor of glove use, and perceived control over the use of gloves was the best predictor of intentions. Health care workers were determined to wear gloves if they felt they could control whether they wore gloves or not and had a positive evaluation of gloves.

Clinical Relevance

Despite mandates for the use of gloves by health care workers, preventable blood exposures have been documented in many studies. Thus, Levin's effort to understand factors affecting blood use has considerable significance for clinical settings.

Levin used a very strong sampling strategy that ensured that nurses and laboratory workers throughout the state of Illinois would be represented in the sample. The response rate of 70% was highly respectable for a mailed survey and was achieved by mailing a follow-up reminder and a second copy of the questionnaire to all nonrespondents. Levin was able to determine that there was a bias in the sample—that is, that nurses from Chicago were less likely than nurses from other areas to complete the questionnaire. However, there were no differences in response rates of nurses and laboratory workers, and also no difference in their use of gloves.

On the basis of Levin's study, interventions for improving glove use among health care workers could be designed or refined. For example, the findings suggest that interventions designed to improve the workers' perceived control over using gloves could be profitable. Nurses could also pose the following types of questions and discuss the issue with administrators: Are glove boxes conveniently located throughout the health care facility? Are low-protein gloves available for workers who are latex sensitive? What innovative approaches can be used to ensure that during unexpected, emergency situations nurses will have gloves immediately available (*e.g.,* attaching glove packs to patient carts or to staff uniforms)?

RESEARCH EXAMPLE OF A QUALITATIVE STUDY

Ledlie (1999) conducted a grounded theory study designed to generate a substantive theory that explains how family caregivers manage the disclosure of the diagnosis of perinatally acquired HIV disease (PAHD) to a child. Two groups of families were recruited from various community agencies that offer services to HIV patients: family caregivers of a PAHD child who had disclosed the diagnosis to the child, and family caregivers of a PAHD child who had not disclosed the diagnosis. Selection of the primary participants was purposive, and then directed by the evolving theory. To maximize the theoretical scope of the inquiry, Ledlie sought participants who varied with regard to age, gender, ethnicity, race, education, type and duration of the caregiving situation, and current stage of disease. During the course of the study, the theoretical sample included 28 participants from 18 different families—8 with disclosure and 10 without disclosure.

Ledlie found that all of the caregivers in her study struggled with issues relating to disclosing a PAHD diagnosis to their child. Ledlie's analysis led her to conclude that the basic social-psychological problem was caregiver readiness to disclose the diagnosis. The basic social process adopted by family caregivers was identified as "When the Time Comes."

Clinical Relevance

PAHD has become the newest chronic illness of childhood, and many children with the disease are now living well into their school years. Thus, caregivers are confronted with their children's questions about their illness and complex treatment regimen. The question of when, how, and what to tell children about their diagnosis poses a difficult challenge for caregivers.

Ledlie used maximum variation theoretical sampling to ensure the broadest possible theoretical utility. Her sample included 18 families and appears to have been an adequate sample size for the development of her theory. Ledlie indicated that families continued to be interviewed until theoretical saturation had occurred and no new findings were obtained.

The findings indicated that caregiver readiness was critical to diagnosis disclosure and that caregivers struggle to weigh their own readiness to disclose (including their readiness to answer critical questions) with their child's readiness to know. These findings can be used in the development of protocols to help caregivers answer their children's questions and to assist them in making decisions about disclosure. In designing these interventions, nurses should be aware that caregivers' strategies are not static; they move along in a process from complete secrecy to selective telling to complete disclosure. In working with these families, nurses can first assess where caregivers are on this continuum of disclosure and then identify any catalysts or inhibitors that can influence "when the time comes" to disclose. Because the process of caregivers' disclosure is dynamic, nurses' interventions must not be static if they are to be effective in helping with disclosure decisions.

• • • • • SUMMARY POINTS

- **Sampling** is the process of selecting a portion of the **population**, which is an entire aggregate of cases.
- An **element** (the basic unit about which information is collected) can be included in a sample if it meets the researcher's **eligibility criteria**.
- Researchers usually sample from an **accessible population** rather than an entire **target population**.
- The main consideration in assessing a sample in a quantitative study is its representativeness—the extent to which the sample is similar to the population and avoids bias. **Sampling bias** refers to the systematic overrepresentation or underrepresentation of some segment of the population.
- The principal types of **nonprobability sampling** (wherein elements are selected by nonrandom methods) are convenience, quota, and purposive sampling. Nonprobability sampling designs are convenient and economical; a major disadvantage is their potential for bias.
- **Convenience sampling** (or **accidental sampling**) uses the most readily available or most convenient group of people for the sample. **Snowball sampling**

is a type of convenience sampling in which referrals for potential partici-pants are made by those already in the sample.

- **Quota sampling** divides the population into homogeneous strata (sub-groups) to ensure representation of those subgroups in the sample; within each stratum, the researcher selects participants by convenience sampling.
- In **purposive** (or **judgmental**) **sampling**, participants are hand picked to be included in the sample based on the researcher's knowledge about the pop-ulation.
- **Probability sampling** designs, which involve the random selection of ele-ments from the population, yield more representative samples than non-probability designs and permit estimates of the magnitude of **sampling error**. Probability samples, however, are expensive and inconvenient.
- **Simple random sampling** involves the selection on a random basis of ele-ments from a **sampling frame** that enumerates all the elements.
- **Stratified random sampling** divides the population into homogeneous subgroups from which elements are selected at random.
- **Cluster sampling** (**or multistage sampling**) involves the successive selec-tion of random samples from larger to smaller units by either simple ran-dom or stratified random methods.
- **Systematic sampling** is the selection of every kth case from a list. By divid-ing the population size by the desired sample size, the researcher establishes the **sampling interval**, which is the standard distance between the selected elements.
- Advanced researchers use a procedure known as **power analysis** to estimate **sample size** needs. Large samples are preferable to small ones because larger samples tend to be more representative. However, even a large sample does not guarantee representativeness.
- Qualitative researchers use the theoretical demands of the study to select articulate and reflective informants with certain types of experience in an emergent way, capitalizing on early learnings to guide subsequent sampling decisions.
- Qualitative researchers thus most often use purposive or **theoretical sam-pling** to guide them in selecting data sources that maximize information richness. Various strategies can be used to sample purposively, including sampling to maximize variation, to select typical cases, and to learn from extreme cases.
- The criteria for evaluating qualitative sampling are informational adequacy and appropriateness.

➤ ➤ ➤ ➤ *CRITICAL THINKING ACTIVITIES*

Chapter 10 of the accompanying *Study Guide to Accompany Essentials of Nurs-ing Research,* 5th edition offers various exercises and study suggestions for reinforcing the concepts presented in this chapter. In addition, you can address the following:

1. Read the introduction and method section from the two studies in the Appendix of this book and then answer relevant questions in Box 10-1 and/or 10-2.

2. Read the full research report of Levin's (1999) study, which was used as a research example in this chapter. What could the researcher have done to increase the representativeness of her research sample? What information could the researcher have provided to indicate whether the underrepresentation of nurses from Chicago resulted in any biases in the findings?

3. Based on information in Tables 1 and 2 of Ledlie's (1999) report, to what degree did the researcher successfully achieve maximum variation sampling?

For additional review, see questions 122–135 on the study CD provided with Polit: Study Guide to Accompany Essentials of Nursing Research

SUGGESTED READINGS

Methodologic References

Cohen, J. (1988). *Statistical power analysis for the behavioral sciences* (2nd. ed.). Mahwah, NJ: Erlbaum.

Levey, P. S., & Lemeshow, S. (1980). *Sampling for health professionals.* New York: Lifetime Learning.

Morse, J. M. (1991). Strategies for sampling. In J. M. Morse (Ed.), *Qualitative nursing research: A contemporary dialogue.* Newbury Park, CA: Sage.

Patton, M. Q. (1990). *Qualitative evaluation and research methods* (2nd ed.). Newbury Park, CA: Sage.

Substantive References

Allan, J. D. (1998). Explanatory models of overweight among African American, Euro-American, and Mexican American women. *Western Journal of Nursing Research, 20,* 45–66.

Baggs, J. G., & Schmitt, M. H. (1997). Nurses' and resident physicians' perceptions of the process of collaboration in the MICU. *Research in Nursing & Health, 20,* 71–80.

Brown, J. K., Whittemore, K. T., & Knapp, T. R. (2000). Is arm span an accurate measure of height in young and middle-age adults? *Clinical Nursing Research, 9,* 84–94.

Carty, B., & Rosenfeld, P. (1998). From computer technology to information technology: Findings from a national study of nursing education. *Computers in Nursing, 16,* 259–265.

Edwardson, S. R., & Dean, K. J. (1999). Appropriateness of self-care responses to symptoms among elders. *Research in Nursing & Health, 22,* 329–339.

Friedemann, M., Montgomery, R. J., Rice, C., & Farrell, L. (1999). Family involvement in the nursing home. *Western Journal of Nursing Research, 21,* 549–567.

Ledlie, S. W. (1999). Diagnosis disclosure by family caregivers to children who have perinatally acquired HIV disease. *Nursing Research, 48,* 141–149.

Levin, P. F. (1999). Test of the Fishbein and Ajzen models as predictors of health care workers' glove use. *Research in Nursing & Health, 22,* 295–307.

Nardi, D. (1998). Addiction recovery for low-income pregnant and parenting women: A process of becoming. *Archives in Psychiatric Nursing, 12,* 81–89.

Sinclair, V. G., Wallston, K. A., Dwyer, K. A., Blackburn, D. S., & Fuchs, H. (1999). Effects of a cognitive-behavioral intervention for women with rheumatoid arthritis. *Research in Nursing & Health, 21,* 315–326.

Trent, B. A. (1997). Student perceptions of academic advising in an RN-to-BSN program. *Journal of Continuing Education in Nursing, 28,* 276–283.

Wilbur, J., Miller, A. M., Montgomery, A., & Chandler, P. (1998). Women's physical activity patterns: Nursing implications. *Journal of Obstetric, Gynecologic, and Neonatal Nursing, 27,* 383–392.

Youngblut, J. M., & Brooten, D. (1999). Alternate child care, history of hospitalization, and preschool child behavior. *Nursing Research, 48,* 29–34.

PART IV

COLLECTION OF
RESEARCH DATA

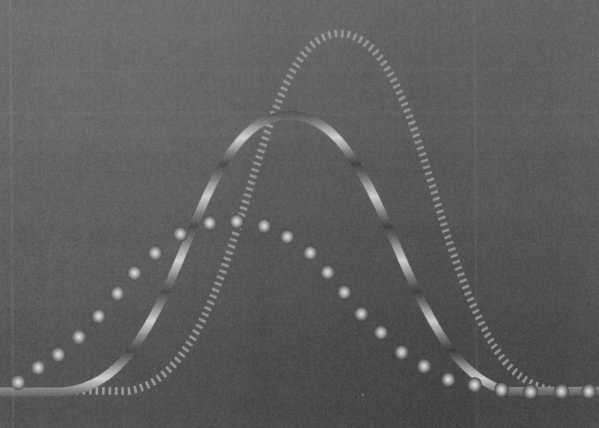

Scrutinizing Data Collection Methods

• •

Student Objectives

On completion of this chapter, the student will be able to:

○ evaluate a researcher's decision to use existing data versus collecting new data
○ discuss the four dimensions along which data collection approaches vary
○ critique a researcher's decisions regarding the data collection plan and its implementation
○ define new terms in the chapter

Self-Reports

○ distinguish between and evaluate structured and unstructured self-reports; open-ended and closed-ended questions; and interviews and questionnaires
○ identify several types of structured and unstructured self-report techniques
○ evaluate a researcher's decision to use a self-report approach

Observation

○ identify several types of phenomena that lend themselves to observation
○ distinguish between and evaluate structured and unstructured observations and describe various methods of collecting such observational data
○ identify methods of sampling observations
○ evaluate a researcher's decision to use an observational data collection approach versus an alternative approach (e.g., self-report)

Biophysiologic Measures

○ describe the major features, advantages, and disadvantages of biophysiologic measures
○ evaluate a researcher's decision to use a biophysiologic measure as well as the choice of the specific measure

• •

New Terms

Acquiescence response set bias	Diary
Biophysiologic measure	Event sampling
Bipolar adjectives	Extreme response set bias
Category system	Field notes
Checklist	Fixed-alternative question
Closed-ended question	Focus group interview
Completely unstructured interviews	Focused interview
Counterbalancing	Grand tour question
Historical research	Questionnaire
Instrument	Rating scale

Interview schedule
Reactivity
In vitro measures
In vivo measures
Item
Life history
Likert scale
Log
Methodologic notes
Mobile positioning
Moderator
Multiple positioning
Nay-sayer
Observation
Observational methods
Observational notes
Open-ended question
Participant observation
Personal notes
Pretest
Projective technique
Q sort

Records
Response alternatives
Response set biases
Scale
Secondary analysis
Self-report
Semantic differential
Semi-structured interview
Single positioning
Social desirability response set bias
Structured observation
Structured self-report
Summated rating scale
Theoretical notes
Time sampling
Topic guide
Unstructured observation
Unstructured self-report
Vignette
Visual analog scale
Yea-sayer

The phenomena in which a researcher is interested must be translated into concepts that can be measured, observed, or recorded. The task of selecting or developing methods for gathering data is among the most challenging in the research process. Without appropriate data collection methods, the validity of research conclusions is easily challenged.

OVERVIEW OF DATA COLLECTION AND DATA SOURCES

There are many alternative approaches to data collection, and these approaches vary along several dimensions. This introductory section provides an overview of some of the important dimensions.

Existing Data Versus New Data

One of the first data decisions an investigator makes concerns the use of existing data versus new data gathered specifically for the study. Most of this chapter is devoted to methods researchers use to generate new data, but they sometimes can take advantage of existing information. A meta-analysis (see Chap. 6) is one type of study that relies on available data—that is, from research reports.

Historical research typically relies on available data. Data for historical research are usually in the form of written, narrative records of the past: diaries, letters, newspapers, minutes of meetings, reports, and so forth. Nurses have used historical research methods to examine a wide range of phenomena.

Example of historical research:

Sandelowski (2000) studied the historical evolution and political/moral context of technological instruments in obstetric surveillance and diagnosis, and nurses' use of those instruments.

Sometimes researchers perform a **secondary analysis**, which is the use of data gathered in a previous study—often by other researchers—to test new hypotheses or address new research questions. A secondary analysis can be performed with both quantitative and qualitative data.

Examples of secondary analysis:

Quantitative example: Weaver, Richmond, and Narsavage (1997) used data from a previous study of patients with chronic obstructive pulmonary disease to test an explanatory model of factors affecting functional status in this disorder.

Qualitative example: Breckenridge (1997) did a secondary analysis of data from a qualitative study of clients with end-stage renal disease. The original study was designed to examine how and by whom decisions about treatment modality were made; the secondary study examined factors that influenced the decisions.

An important existing data source for nurse researchers is **records**. Hospital records, nursing charts, physicians' order sheets, and care plan statements all constitute rich data sources. Records are an economical and convenient source of information. Because the researcher was not responsible for collecting and recording information, however, he or she may be unaware of the records' limitations, biases, or incompleteness. If the records available for use are not the entire set of all possible records, the investigator must deal with the issue of the records' representativeness. Existing records have been used in both qualitative and quantitative nursing studies.

Example of a study using records:

Rich (1999) studied the medical records of 100 patients who experienced an in-hospital cardiopulmonary arrest. The purposes of the study were to identify pre-arrest physiologic changes in the patient and to explore factors that affected the resuscitation outcome.

Key Dimensions of Data Collection Methods

If existing data are not available or are unsuitable for the research question, new data must be collected. In developing a data collection plan, the investigator makes many important decisions. A primary decision concerns the basic form of data collection to use. Three types of approach have been used most frequently by nurse researchers: self-reports, observations, and biophysiologic measures. **Self-reports** are participants' responses to questions posed by the researcher, such as in an interview. Direct **observation** of people's behaviors, characteristics, and circumstances is an alternative to self-reports for certain types of research questions. Nurses are increasingly using **biophysiologic measures** to assess important clinical variables. Sections of this chapter are devoted to these three major types of data collection.

Regardless of the approach used, data collection methods vary along several important dimensions:

- *Structure.* Research data are often collected in a highly structured manner: the same information is gathered from all participants in a comparable, prespecified way. Sometimes, however, it is more appropriate to be flexible and to allow participants to reveal relevant information in a naturalistic way.
- *Quantifiability.* Data that will be analyzed statistically must be gathered in such a way that they can be quantified. On the other hand, data that are to be analyzed qualitatively are collected in narrative form. Structured data collection approaches tend to yield data that are more easily quantified.
- *Obtrusiveness.* Data collection methods differ in terms of the degree to which people are aware of their status as study participants. If participants are fully aware of their role in a study, their behavior and responses might not be normal. When data are collected unobtrusively, however, ethical problems may emerge.
- *Objectivity.* Some data collection approaches require more subjective judgment than others. Quantitative researchers generally strive for methods that are as objective as possible. In qualitative research, however, the subjective judgment of the investigator is considered a valuable tool.

Sometimes, the research question dictates where on these four dimensions the data collection method will lie. For example, questions that are best suited for a qualitative study normally use methods that are low on structure, quantifiability, obtrusiveness, and objectivity, whereas research questions appropriate for a survey tend to require methods that are high on all four dimensions. However, researchers often have latitude in selecting or designing appropriate data collection plans.

CONSUMER TIP:

Researchers describe their data collection plan in the methods section of a research report. In a report for a quantitative study, the specific data collection methods are often described in a subsection with the heading "Measures" or "Instruments." The actual steps taken to collect the data are sometimes described in a separate subsection with the heading "Procedures." ■

SELF-REPORT METHODS

In the human sciences, a good deal of information can be gathered by direct questioning of people. If, for example, we were interested in learning about patients' perceptions of hospital care, nursing home residents' fear of death, or women's knowledge about menopause, we would likely try to obtain information by posing questions to a sample of relevant people. For some research variables, alternatives to direct questioning exist, but the unique ability of humans to communicate verbally on a sophisticated level ensures that self-reports will never be eliminated from nurse researchers' repertoire of data collection techniques.

The self-report approach consists of a range of techniques that vary in the degree of structure imposed. At one extreme are loosely structured methods that do not involve a formal written set of questions. At the other extreme are tightly structured methods involving the use of formal documents such as questionnaires. Some characteristics of different self-report approaches are discussed next.

Unstructured and Semi-Structured Self-Report Techniques

Unstructured or loosely structured **self-report** methods offer flexibility. When these methods are used, the researcher does not have a set of questions that must be asked in a specific order and worded in a given way. Instead, the researcher starts with some general questions or topics and allows the respondents to tell their stories in a naturalistic, narrative fashion. In other words, unstructured or semi-structured self-reports, usually obtained in interviews, tend to be conversational in nature.

Unstructured interviews, which are used by researchers in all qualitative research traditions, encourage respondents to define the important dimensions of a phenomenon and to elaborate on what is relevant to them, rather than being guided by the investigator's a priori notions of relevance. Unstructured interviews are the mode of choice when researchers do not have a clear idea of what it is they do not know.

Types of Unstructured Self-Reports
There are several approaches to collecting unstructured self-report data. **Completely unstructured interviews** are used when the researcher has no pre-

conceived view of the content or flow of information to be gathered. Their aim is to elucidate the respondents' perceptions of the world without imposing the researcher's views. Typically, the researcher begins by posing a broad **grand tour question** such as, "What happened when you first learned that you had AIDS?" Subsequent questions are more focused and are guided by initial responses. Ethnographic and phenomenologic studies often use unstructured interviews.

Example of a study using unstructured interviews:

Leidy and Haase (1999) explored the meaning of functional performance in patients with chronic obstructive pulmonary disease. The interviews, which were tape-recorded, began by asking the 12 respondents to describe a typical day. Respondents were encouraged to self-direct the content of the interview.

Focused (or **semi-structured**) **interviews** are used when a researcher has a list of topics that must be covered in an interview. The interviewer uses a written **topic guide** to ensure that all question areas are covered. The interviewer's function is to encourage participants to talk freely about all the topics on the guide.

Example of a study using a semi-structured interview:

Strang and Haughey (1999) studied the respite experience of family caregivers of people with dementia. The interviews were loosely structured, allowing caregivers to tell their stories. However, the interviews were guided by specific questions, such as what respite meant to them, what was helpful or not helpful, how important the relief time was, and how they felt when they returned to caregiving responsibilities.

Focus group interviews are interviews with groups of about 5 to 15 people whose opinions and experiences are solicited simultaneously. The interviewer (or **moderator**) guides the discussion according to a topic guide or set of questions. The advantages of a group format are that it is efficient and can generate a lot of dialogue, but some people are uncomfortable expressing their views or describing their experiences in front of a group.

Example of a study using focus group interviews:

Kirchhoff, Spuhler, Walker, Hutton, Cole, and Clemmer (2000) studied the experiences of intensive care nurses with end-of-life care. Data were collected from four focus groups held with randomly selected nurses from four intensive care units in two hospitals.

Life histories are narrative self-disclosures about life experiences. With this approach, the researcher asks the respondents to describe, in chronologic sequence, their experiences regarding a specified theme, either orally or in writing. Some researchers have used this approach to obtain a total life health history.

⊞ | ***Example of a study using life histories:***

Smith-Battle and Leonard (1998) studied adolescent mothers' narratives of self and visions of the future as part of a longitudinal, hermeneutic study. Data consisted of the young mothers' life history accounts of their parenting experiences over a 4-year period.

Diaries have been used by some researchers, who ask participants to maintain a daily log about some aspect of their lives for a specified time period. Nurse researchers have used health diaries to collect information about how people prevent illness, maintain health, experience morbidity, or treat health problems.

⊞ | ***Example of a study using diaries:***

Musil and her colleagues (1998) studied the health problems and health actions of community-dwelling older adults. Respondents were asked to record, each day for 4 weeks, what symptoms or unusual health problems they experienced, whether they considered this to be an illness, and what health actions they had taken.

Gathering Unstructured Self-Report Data

Researchers gather unstructured self-report data to develop a construction of a phenomenon that is consistent with that of the participants. This goal requires researchers to take steps to overcome communication barriers and to enhance the flow of meaning. For example, a researcher who is studying a subgroup that uses distinctive terms should strive before going into the field to understand those terms and their nuances.

Although unstructured interviews are conversational in nature, this does not mean that researchers enter into them casually. The conversations are purposeful ones that require advance thought and preparation. For example, the wording of questions should make sense to respondents and reflect their world view. In addition to being good questioners, the researchers must be good listeners. Only by attending carefully to what the respondent is saying can the in-depth interviewer develop appropriate follow-up questions.

Unstructured interviews are typically long—sometimes lasting several hours. The issue of how best to record such abundant information is a difficult one. Some researchers take sketchy notes as the interview progresses, filling in the details after the interview is completed. Many prefer tape recording the interviews for later transcription. Although some respondents are self-conscious when their conversation is recorded, they typically forget about the presence of recording equipment after a few minutes.

Structured Self-Report Techniques

A structured approach to collecting self-report data is appropriate when researchers know in advance exactly what they need to know and can, therefore, frame appropriate questions to obtain the needed information. **Structured self-report** data are usually collected by means of a formal, written document referred to as an **instrument.** The instrument is known as the **interview schedule** when the questions are asked orally in either a face-to-face or telephone format and as the **questionnaire** when respondents complete the instrument themselves in a paper-and-pencil format. Some features of structured self-report instruments are discussed next.

Question Form

In a totally structured instrument, respondents are asked to respond to the same questions in the same order, and they are given the same set of options for their responses. **Closed-ended questions** (also referred to as **fixed-alternative questions**) are ones in which the **response alternatives** are specified by the researcher. The alternatives may range from a simple yes or no to complex expressions of opinion. The purpose of using questions with fixed alternatives is to ensure comparability of responses and to facilitate analysis.

Many structured instruments, however, also include some **open-ended questions,** which allow participants to respond to questions in their own words. When open-ended questions are included in questionnaires, respondents must write out their responses. In interviews, the interviewer writes down responses verbatim or uses a tape-recorder for later transcription. Some examples of open-ended and closed-ended questions are presented in Box 11-1.

Both open-ended and closed-ended questions have strengths and weaknesses. Closed-ended questions are more difficult to construct than open-ended ones but easier to administer and, especially, to analyze. Furthermore, closed-ended questions are more efficient: people can complete more closed-ended questions than open-ended ones in a given amount of time. Also, in questionnaires, respondents may be unwilling to compose lengthy written responses to open-ended questions.

The major drawback of closed-ended questions is that researchers might overlook some potentially important responses. Another concern is that closed-ended questions can be superficial; open-ended questions allow for richer and fuller information if the respondents are verbally expressive and cooperative. Finally, some respondents object to choosing from alternatives that do not reflect their opinions precisely.

Instrument Construction

Researchers generally begin by developing an outline of the instrument's content. Questions for the content areas are then drafted or, if possible, borrowed or adapted from other instruments. Researchers must carefully monitor the

---

BOX 11-1   ▢

EXAMPLES OF QUESTION TYPES

Open-ended

- What led to your decision to stop smoking?
- What did you do when you discovered you had AIDS?

Closed-Ended

1. Dichotomous Question

Have you ever been hospitalized?

- ❏ 1. Yes
- ❏ 2. No

2. Multiple-Choice Question

How important is it to you to avoid a pregnancy at this time?

- ❏ 1. Extremely important
- ❏ 2. Very important
- ❏ 3. Somewhat important
- ❏ 4. Not at all important

3. "Cafeteria" Question

People have different opinions about the use of estrogen-replacement therapy for women in menopause. Which of the following statements best represents your point of view?

- ❏ 1. Estrogen replacement is dangerous and should be totally banned.
- ❏ 2. Estrogen replacement may have some undesirable side effects that suggests the need for caution in its use.
- ❏ 3. I am undecided about my views on estrogen-replacement therapy.
- ❏ 4. Estrogen replacement has many beneficial effects that merit its promotion.
- ❏ 5. Estrogen replacement is a wonder cure that should be administered routinely to menopausal women.

4. Rank-Order Question

People value different things about life. Below is a list of principles or ideals that are often cited when people are asked to name things they value most. Please indicate the order of importance of these values to you by placing a 1 beside the most important, 2 beside the next most important, and so forth.

- ❏ Achievement and success
- ❏ Family relationships
- ❏ Friendships and social interaction
- ❏ Health
- ❏ Money
- ❏ Religion

(continued)

BOX 11-1   *(Continued)*

5. Forced-Choice Question

Which statement most closely represents your point of view?

   ❏ 1. What happens to me is my own doing.
   ❏ 2. Sometimes I feel I don't have enough control over my life.

6. Rating Question

On a scale from 0 to 10, where 0 means extremely dissatisfied and 10 means extremely satisfied, how satisfied are you with the nursing care you received during your hospitalization?

Extremely dissatisfied   Extremely satisfied

0   1   2   3   4   5   6   7   8   9   10

wording of each question for clarity, sensitivity to the respondent's psychological state, freedom from bias, and (in questionnaires) reading level. Questions must then be sequenced in a psychologically meaningful order that encourages cooperation and candor.

Draft instruments are usually critically reviewed by peers or colleagues and then pretested with a small sample of respondents. A **pretest** is a trial run to determine whether the instrument is clearly worded, free from major biases, and useful in generating desired information. In large studies, the development and pretesting of self-report instruments may take many months to complete.

Interviews Versus Questionnaires

Researchers using a structured self-report approach must decide whether to use an interview or a questionnaire. You should be aware of the limitations and strengths of these alternatives because the decision may affect the findings. Questionnaires, relative to interviews, have the following advantages:

- Questionnaires are less costly and require less time and effort to administer; this is a particular advantage if the sample is geographically dispersed.
- Questionnaires offer the possibility of complete anonymity, which may be crucial in obtaining information about illegal or deviant behaviors or about embarrassing characteristics.
- The absence of an interviewer ensures that there will be no biases reflecting the respondent's reaction to the interviewer rather than to the questions themselves.

Example of a study using questionnaires:

Graninger and McCool (1998) studied nurse-midwives' use of and attitudes toward epidural analgesia. Questionnaires were mailed to a stratified random national sample of over 2,500 nurse midwives. A total of 1,605 questionnaires (60.7%) were returned.

The strengths of interviews far outweigh those of questionnaires. These strengths include the following:

- The response rate tends to be high in face-to-face interviews. Respondents are less likely to refuse to talk to an interviewer than to ignore a questionnaire, especially a mailed questionnaire. Low response rates can lead to bias because respondents are rarely a random subset of those whom the researcher intended for inclusion in the study.
- Many people simply cannot fill out a questionnaire; examples include young children, the blind, and the very elderly. Interviews are feasible with most people.
- Questions are less likely to be misinterpreted by respondents because the interviewer can determine whether questions have been understood.
- Interviewers can produce additional information through observation of respondents' living situation, level of understanding, degree of cooperativeness, and so on–all of which can be useful in interpreting responses.

Most advantages of face-to-face interviews also apply to telephone interviews. Complicated or detailed instruments are not well suited to telephone interviewing, but for relatively brief instruments, the telephone interview combines relatively low costs with high response rates.

Example of a study using structured interviews:

Kurlowicz (1998) studied the relationship between postoperative functional ability and depressive symptoms in older elective surgery patients. She first conducted in-person interviews with 78 patients 4 to 5 days after surgery (96% of those invited to participate). Telephone interviews were completed with 76 sample members (97% of the initial sample) 6 weeks after surgery.

Scales and Other Special Forms of Structured Self-Reports

Several special types of structured self-report are used by nurse researchers. These include composite social-psychological scales, vignettes, projective techniques, and Q sorts.

Composite Scales

Social-psychological scales are often incorporated into a questionnaire or interview schedule. A **scale** is a device designed to assign a numeric score to people to place them on a continuum with respect to attributes being measured, like a scale for measuring weight. Social-psychological scales quantitatively discriminate among people with different attitudes, fears, motives, perceptions, personality traits, and needs.

The most common scaling technique is the Likert scale, named after social-psychologist Rensis Likert. A **Likert scale** consists of several declarative statements (or **items**) that express a viewpoint on a topic. Respondents are asked to indicate the degree to which they agree or disagree with the opinion expressed by the statement. Table 11-1 presents an illustrative, six-item Likert scale for measuring attitudes toward the mentally ill. In this example, agreement with positively worded statements and disagreement with negatively worded statements are assigned higher scores. The first statement is positively phrased; agreement indicates a favorable attitude toward the mentally ill. Because the item has five response alternatives, a score of 5 would be given to someone strongly agreeing, 4 to someone agreeing, and so forth. The responses of two hypothetical respondents are shown by a check or an X, and their item scores are shown in the right-hand columns. Person 1, who agreed with the first statement, has a score of 4, whereas person 2, who strongly disagreed, has a score of 1. The second statement is negatively worded, and so the scoring is reversed—a 1 is assigned to those who strongly agree, and so forth. This reversal is necessary so that a high score will consistently reflect positive attitudes toward the mentally ill. A person's total score is determined by summing item scores; hence, these scales are sometimes called **summated rating scales**. The total scores of the two hypothetical respondents, shown at the bottom of Table 11-1, reflect a considerably more positive attitude toward the mentally ill on the part of person 1 (score = 26) than person 2 (score = 11). The summation feature of Likert scales makes it possible to make fine discriminations among people with different points of view. A single Likert question allows people to be put into only five categories. A six-item scale, such as the one in Table 11-1, permits much finer gradation—from a minimum possible score of 6 (6 $\times$ 1) to a maximum possible score of 30 (6 $\times$ 5).

Example of a study using a Likert scale:

Harvey, Kazis, and Lee (1999) studied the association between patient preference for involvement in health-related decision making and their satisfaction with medical care. Patient satisfaction was measured with a four-item Likert scale. An example of an item is: "I am very satisfied with the medical care I receive."

Another technique for measuring attitudes is the **semantic differential** (SD). With the SD, respondents are asked to rate a concept (e.g., primary nursing, team nursing) on a series of **bipolar adjectives**, such as good/bad, strong/weak, effective/ineffective, important/unimportant. Respondents are

TABLE 11-1. Example of a Likert Scale to Measure Attitudes Toward the Mentally Ill

DIRECTION OF SCORING*		RESPONSES†					SCORE Person 1 (√)	Person 2 (X)
		SA	A	?	D	SD		
+	1. People who have had a mental illness can become normal, productive citizens after treatment.		√			X	4	1
−	2. People who have been patients in mental hospitals should not be allowed to have children.			X	√		5	3
−	3. The best way to handle patients in mental hospitals is to restrict their activity as much as possible.		X	√			4	2
+	4. Many patients in mental hospitals develop normal, healthy relationships with staff members and other patients.			√	X		3	2
+	5. There should be an expanded effort to get the mentally ill out of institutional settings and back into their communities.	√				X	5	1
−	6. Because the mentally ill cannot be trusted, they should be kept under constant guard.		X			√	5	2
						TOTAL SCORE	26	11

*Researchers would not indicate the direction of scoring on a Likert scale administered to subjects. The scoring direction is indicated in this table for illustrative purposes only.
†SA, strongly agree; A, agree; ?, uncertain; D, disagree; SD, strongly disagree.

asked to place a check at the appropriate point on a seven-point scale that extends from one extreme of the dimension to the other. An example of an SD format is shown in Figure 11-1. The SD has the advantage of being flexible and easy to construct. The concept being rated can be virtually anything—a person, concept, controversial issue, and so on. The scoring procedure for SD responses is similar to that for Likert scales. Scores from 1 to 7 are assigned to each bipolar scale response, with higher scores generally associated with the positively worded adjective. Responses are then summed across the bipolar scales to yield a total score.

NURSE PRACTITIONERS

competent	7*	6	5	4	3	2	1	incompetent

worthless	1	2	3	4	5	6	7	valuable

important								unimportant

| pleasant | | | | | | | | unpleasant |

| bad | | | | | | | | good |

| cold | | | | | | | | warm |

| responsible | | | | | | | | irresponsible |

| successful | | | | | | | | unsuccessful |

*The score values would not be printed on the form administered to actual subjects. The numbers are presented here solely for the purpose of illustrating how semantic differentials are scored.

FIGURE 11-1. Example of a semantic differential.

Example of a study using a semantic differential:

Niedz (1998) studied factors related to hospitalized patients' perceptions of nursing care quality. One of the factors examined was organizational climate, as perceived by patients. Patients rated the concept organizational climate in terms of eight bipolar adjectives, such as helpful/unhelpful, effective/ineffective, and valuable/worthless.

Another type of psychosocial measure is the **visual analog scale** (VAS), which can be used to measure subjective experiences, such as pain, fatigue, nausea, and dyspnea. The VAS is a straight line, the end anchors of which are labeled as the extreme limits of the sensation or feeling being measured. Participants are asked to mark a point on the line corresponding to the amount of sensation experienced. Traditionally, a VAS line is 100 mm in length, which facilitates the derivation of a score from 0 to 100 through simple measurement of the distance from one end of the scale to the participant's mark on the line. An example of a VAS is presented in Figure 11-2.

Example of a study using a visual analog scale:

Lee, Portillo, and Miramontes (1999) studied fatigue as a symptom experienced by women with HIV. A sample of 100 women completed the Visual Analog Scale—Fatigue scale, which consisted of 13 visual analog lines related to fatigue and five lines related to energy.

Scales permit researchers to efficiently quantify subtle gradations in the strength or intensity of individual characteristics. A good scale can be useful both for group-level comparisons (*e.g.,* comparing the stress levels of mastec-

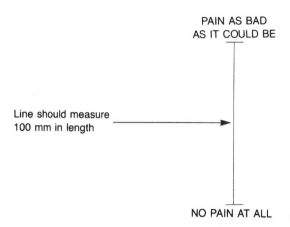

FIGURE 11-2. Example of a visual analog scale.

tomy patients before and after surgery) and for making individual comparisons (*e.g.*, predicting that patient X will not need as much emotional support as patient Y because of scores on a coping scale). Scales can be administered either verbally or in writing and are, therefore, suitable for use with most people.

Scales are susceptible to several common problems, however, the most troublesome of which are referred to as **response set biases.** The most important biases include the following:

- **Social desirability response set bias**—a tendency to misrepresent attitudes or traits by giving answers that are consistent with prevailing social views
- **Extreme response set bias**—a tendency to consistently express attitudes or feelings in extreme responses (*e.g.*, strongly agree), leading to distortions because extreme responses may not necessarily signify the greatest intensity
- **Acquiescence response set bias**—a tendency to agree with statements regardless of their content by people who are referred to as **yea-sayers.** The opposite tendency for other people (**nay-sayers**) to disagree with statements independently of the question content is less common.

These biases can be reduced through such strategies as **counterbalancing** positively and negatively worded statements, developing sensitively worded questions, creating a permissive, nonjudgmental atmosphere, and guaranteeing the confidentiality of responses.

Vignettes

Vignettes are brief descriptions of events or situations to which respondents are asked to react. The descriptions are structured to elicit information about respondents' perceptions, opinions, or knowledge about a phenomenon. The vignettes are usually written, narrative descriptions but can also be videotapes. The questions posed to respondents after the vignettes may be either open ended (*e.g.*, How would you recommend handling this situation?) or closed ended (*e.g.*, On the nine-point scale below, rate how well you believe the nurse handled the situation).

Vignettes are an economical means of eliciting information about how people might behave in situations that would be difficult to observe in daily life. For example, we might want to assess how patients would react to or feel about nurses with different personal styles of interaction. In clinical settings, it would be difficult to expose patients to many nurses, all of whom have been evaluated as having different interaction styles.

The principal problem with vignettes concerns the validity of responses. If respondents describe how they would react in a situation portrayed in the vignette, how accurate is that description of their actual behavior? Thus, although the use of vignettes can be profitable, the possibility of response biases should be recognized.

Example of a study using vignettes:

Ludwick (1999) examined the effects of patients' characteristics on nurses' clinical decisions regarding patient confusion. A sample of 100 nurses rated 30 situational vignettes on the likelihood that the patient was confused and needed restraints. Every vignette had a combination of eight patient variables (*e.g.*, age, gender, medical diagnosis). Ludwick found that older patients and patients described as less pleasant were more likely to be viewed as needing restraints.

Projective Techniques

Most self-report methods depend on a respondent's capacity for self-insight and candor. **Projective techniques** are methods for obtaining psychological measurements through verbal self-report with a minimum of participants' conscious cooperation. Projective methods give free play to the participants' imagination by providing them with ambiguous stimuli that invite personal interpretations. The rationale underlying projective techniques is that the manner in which a person reacts to unstructured stimuli is a reflection of the person's needs, motives, attitudes, or personality traits.

Projective techniques are flexible: virtually any unstructured stimulus can be used to induce projective responses. The resulting data can often be analyzed either qualitatively or quantitatively. One class of projective methods uses pictorial materials, such as the Rorschach (ink blot) test. Verbal projective techniques present participants with ambiguous verbal stimuli rather than pictorial ones. For example, word-association methods present participants with a series of words to which participants respond with the first thing that comes to mind. A third class of projective measures is expressive methods, such as play techniques, drawing and painting, and role playing. The assumption is that people express their feelings and emotions by working with or manipulating various materials.

Projective measures have been controversial among researchers. Critics point out that a high degree of inference is required in gleaning information from projective tests, and data quality depends heavily on the researcher's interpretive skill. On the other hand, some people argue that projective methods probe the unconscious mind, encompass the whole personality, and provide data of breadth and depth unattainable by more traditional methods. One useful feature of projective instruments is that they are less susceptible to faking than self-report measures. Finally, some projective techniques are particularly useful with special groups, such as children or people with speech and hearing defects.

Example of a study using projective techniques:

Polivka, Lovell, and Smith (1998) studied inner-city schoolchildren's perceptions of their neighborhoods using projective techniques. Older children did word associations with 20 descriptive words (*e.g.*, safe, dirty). Younger children drew pictures in response to three words (safe, sad, happy).

Q Sorts

In a **Q sort**, the study participant is presented with a set of cards on which words, phrases, or statements are written. The participant is asked to sort the cards along a specified bipolar dimension, such as agree/disagree. Typically, there are between 60 and 100 cards to be sorted into 9 or 11 piles, with the number of cards to be placed in each pile predetermined by the researcher.

The sorting instructions and objects to be sorted in a Q sort can vary. For example, personality can be studied by writing descriptions of personality traits on the cards; participants can then be asked to sort items on a continuum from "exactly like me" to "not at all like me." Other applications include asking patients to rate nursing behaviors on a continuum from most helpful to least helpful or asking cancer patients to rate various aspects of their treatment on a most distressing to least distressing continuum.

Q sorts can be a powerful tool, but, like other data collection techniques, they also have drawbacks. On the positive side, Q sorts are versatile and can be applied to a wide variety of problems. Requiring people to place a predetermined number of cards in each pile eliminates many response biases that can occur in Likert scales. On the other hand, it is difficult and time-consuming to administer Q sorts to a large sample of people. Some critics argue that the forced distribution of cards according to the researcher's specifications is artificial and excludes information about how the participants would ordinarily distribute their responses.

Example of a study using Q sorts:

Hillman (1997) compared the parenting behaviors of 58 parents of children diagnosed with cancer with those of 58 parents of healthy children. Child-rearing practices were measured using a 91-item Q sort. An example of one of the Q-sort statements is: "I find it difficult to punish my child."

Evaluation of Self-Report Methods

Self-report techniques—the most common method of data collection in nursing studies—are strong with respect to their directness. If researchers want to know how people feel or what they believe, the most direct approach is to ask them. Moreover, self-reports frequently yield information that would be difficult, if not impossible, to gather by other means. Behaviors can be directly *observed*, but only if people are willing to manifest them publicly. It is usually impossible for a researcher to observe such behaviors as contraceptive practices or drug usage. Furthermore, observers can only observe behaviors occurring at the time of the study; self-report instruments can gather retrospective data about activities and events occurring in the past or about behaviors in which participants plan to engage in the future. Information about feelings, values, opinions, and motives can sometimes be inferred through observation, but behaviors and feelings do not always correspond exactly. People's actions do not always indicate their state of mind. Self-report instruments can be used to measure psychological characteristics through direct communication with the participants.

Despite these advantages, self-report methods share certain weaknesses. The most serious issue is the question of the validity and accuracy of self-reports: How can we be sure that respondents feel or act the way they say they do? How can we trust the information that respondents provide, particularly if the questions could potentially require them to admit to undesirable traits? Investigators often have no alternative but to assume that most respondents have been frank. Yet, we all have a tendency to present ourselves in the best light, and this may conflict with the truth. When reading research reports, you should be alert to potential biases in self-reported data, particularly with respect to behaviors or feelings that our society judges to be controversial or wrong.

You should also be familiar with the merits of unstructured and structured self-reports. In general, unstructured interviews are of greatest utility when a new area of research is being explored. An unstructured approach allows researchers to ascertain what the basic issues are, how sensitive or controversial the topic is, how individuals conceptualize and talk about a phenomenon, and what the range is of opinions or behaviors that are relevant to the topic. Unstructured methods may also help elucidate the underlying meaning of a pattern or relationship repeatedly observed in more structured research.

Unstructured methods, however, are extremely time-consuming and demanding. Also, unstructured self-reports are not appropriate for capturing the measurable aspects of a phenomenon, such as incidence (*e.g.*, the percentage of infertile couples who elect *in vitro* fertilization), duration (*e.g.*, average time period during which pregnancy was attempted before infertility treatment was sought), or magnitude (*e.g.*, the degree of stress experienced during infertility treatment). Structured self-reports are also especially appropriate when the researcher wants to test hypotheses concerning cause-and-effect relationships.

CONSUMER TIP:

Most nursing studies reported in nursing journals use a data collection plan that is structured and quantitative, but increasing numbers of nurses are undertaking qualitative studies. Most studies that collect self-report data incorporate one or more social-psychological scale. ∎

Critiquing Self-Reports

One of the first questions you should ask is whether the researcher made the correct decision in obtaining the data by self-report rather than by an alternative method. Attention then should be paid to the adequacy of the actual methods used. Box 11-2 presents some guiding questions for critiquing self-reports.

It may be difficult to perform a thorough critique of self-report methods in studies that are reported in journals because detailed descriptions of the data collection methods are often not included. What you can expect is information about the following aspects of the self-report data collection:

- The degree of structure used in the questioning
- Whether interviews or questionnaires (or variants such as a projective method or Q sort) were used
- Whether a composite scale was administered
- How the instruments were administered (*e.g.,* by telephone, in person, by mail)
- The response rate

BOX 11-2

GUIDELINES FOR CRITIQUING SELF-REPORTS

1. Does the research question lend itself to a self-report method of data collection? Would an alternative method have been more appropriate?

2. Is the degree of structure consistent with the nature of the research question?

3. Given the research question and respondent characteristics, did the researcher use the best possible mode for collecting the data (*i.e.,* personal interviews, telephone interviews, or self-administered questionnaires)?

4. Do the questions included in the instrument or topic guide adequately cover the complexities of the problem under investigation?

5. If a composite scale was used, does its use seem appropriate? Does the scale adequately capture the target research variable?

6. If a vignette, projective technique, or Q sort was used, does its use seem appropriate?

Degree of structure is of special importance in assessing a data collection plan. The decision about an instrument's structure should be based on considerations that you can often evaluate. For example, respondents who are not very articulate are more receptive to instruments with many closed-ended questions than to questioning that forces them to compose lengthy answers. Other considerations include the amount of time available (structured instruments are more efficient); the expected sample size (open-ended questions and unstructured interviews are difficult to analyze with large samples); the status of existing information on the topic (in a new area of inquiry, a structured approach may not be warranted); and, most important, the nature of the research question.

CONSUMER TIP:

In research reports, descriptions of data collection instruments are often brief; therefore, it is not always possible to evaluate the data collection plan thoroughly. For example, if a study involved the administration of a measure of depression (*e.g.*, the Center for Epidemiological Studies Depression Scale, or CES-D), the research report most likely would not describe individual items on this scale—although the report should provide a reference to the appropriate source. Moreover, there is typically insufficient space in journals for the researcher to offer a rationale for the plan (*e.g.*, a rationale for why the CES-D was chosen instead of the Beck Depression Scale, or why depression was not measured through an approach other than structured self-report). Because of these facts, it may be difficult for you to undertake a detailed critique of the data collection plan. ■

OBSERVATIONAL METHODS

For some research questions, direct observation of people's behavior is an alternative to self-reports. Within nursing research, **observational methods** have broad applicability, particularly for clinical inquiries. Nurses are in an advantageous position to observe, relatively unobtrusively, the behaviors and activities of patients, their families, and health care staff. Observational methods can be used to gather such information as the characteristics and conditions of individuals (*e.g.*, the sleep–wake state of patients); verbal communication (*e.g.*, exchange of information at change-of-shift report); nonverbal communication (*e.g.*, facial expressions); activities (*e.g.*, geriatric patients' self-grooming activities); and environmental conditions (*e.g.*, architectural barriers in the homes of disabled people).

In observational studies, the researcher has flexibility with regard to several important dimensions:

- *The focus of the observation.* The focus can be broadly defined events (*e.g.*, patient mood swings), or it can be small, highly specific behaviors (*e.g.*, gestures, facial expressions).

- *Concealment.* As discussed in Chapter 4, researchers do not always tell people they are being observed because awareness of being observed may cause people to behave abnormally, thereby jeopardizing the validity of the observations. The problem of behavioral distortions due to the known presence of an observer is called **reactivity.**
- *Duration of observation.* Some observations can be made in a short period of time, but others, particularly those in ethnographic and other field studies, may require months or years in the field.
- *Method of recording observations.* Observations can be made through the human senses and then recorded by paper-and-pencil methods, but they can also be done with sophisticated technical equipment (*e.g.,* video equipment, specialized microphones and audio recording equipment, computers).

In summary, observational techniques can be used to measure a broad range of phenomena and are versatile along several key dimensions. Like self-report techniques, an important dimension for observational methods is degree of structure.

Unstructured Observational Methods

Qualitative researchers collect observational data with a minimum of structure and researcher-imposed constraints. Skillful **unstructured observation** permits researchers to see the world as the study participants see it, to develop a rich understanding and appreciation of the phenomena of interest, to extract meaning from events and situations, and to grasp the subtleties of cultural variation.

Naturalistic observations often are made in field settings through a technique called **participant observation.** A participant observer participates in the functioning of the group or institution under study and strives to observe and record information within the contexts, experiences, and symbols that are relevant to the participants. By assuming a participating role, the observer may have insights that would have eluded a more passive or concealed observer. Not all unstructured observational studies use participant observation, but most do, particularly in the case of ethnographic research.

Example of a nonparticipant unstructured unobservation:

Ragneskog, Gerdner, Josefsson, and Kihlgren (1998) studied antecedents to expressed agitation in nursing home patients with dementia. Their analysis was based on 60 videotaped sequences of nine patients exhibiting agitated behaviors.

The Observer-Participant Role in Participant Observation

In participant observation, the role observers play in the social group under study is important because their social position determines what they are likely to see. That is, the behaviors that are likely to be available for observation depend on the observers' position in a network of relations.

The extent of the observers' actual participation in a group is best thought of as a continuum. At one extreme of the continuum is complete immersion in the setting, with the researcher assuming full participant status; at the other extreme is complete separation, with the researcher assuming an onlooker status. The researcher may in some cases assume a fixed position on this continuum throughout the study. For example, researchers studying the stress and coping of parents whose infant has died of sudden infant death syndrome might spend time observing the parents' interactions with each other and with other family members in their homes, but they would not likely participate in the life of the family as an actual family member.

On the other hand, the researcher's role as participant may evolve over the course of the field work. The researcher may begin primarily as a bystander, with participation in group activities increasing over time. In other cases, it might be profitable to become immersed in a social setting quickly, with participation diminishing to allow more time for pure observation.

 CONSUMER TIP:

It is not unusual to find research reports that state that participant observation was used when in fact the description of the methods suggests that observation but not participation was involved. Some researchers appear to use the term "participant observation" to refer more generally to observations conducted in the field. ■

Leininger (1985) has offered the following four-phase strategy as a possible model for participant observation: (1) primarily observation; (2) primarily observation with some participation; (3) primarily participation with some observation; and (4) reflective observation. In the initial phase, the researcher observes and listens to those under study, allowing observer and participants to become acquainted and to get more comfortable in interacting. In phase 2, observation is enhanced by a modest degree of participation. As the researcher participates more actively in the social group, the reactions of people to specific researcher behaviors can be more systematically studied. In phase 3, the researcher strives to become a more active participant, learning by the experience of doing rather than just watching and listening. In phase 4, the researcher reflects on the total process of what transpired.

The observer must overcome at least two major hurdles in assuming a satisfactory role vis-à-vis participants. The first is to gain entrée into the social group under investigation; the second is to establish rapport and develop trust within that group. Without gaining entrée, the study cannot proceed; but without the trust of the group, the researcher will typically be restricted to "front stage" knowledge—that is, information distorted by the group's protective facades (Leininger, 1985). The goal of the participant observer is to "get back stage"—to learn about the true realities of the group's experiences and behaviors. On the other hand, being a fully participating member does not *necessarily* offer the best perspective for studying a phenomenon—just as being an actor in a play does not offer the most advantageous view of the performance.

Example of a participant observation:

Schnell and Kayser-Jones (1999) studied verbal and nonverbal interaction between certified nursing assistants and eating-dependent residents of a nursing home. The first phase of the study involved 6 months of general observation of life in the nursing home on all days of the week. The second 6-month phase focused on mealtime observation of 10 residents who were difficult to feed.

Gathering Unstructured Observational Data

The participant observer typically places few restrictions on the nature of the data collected, in keeping with the goal of minimizing observer-imposed meanings and structure. Nevertheless, participant observers often do have a broad plan for the types of information to be gathered. Among the aspects of an observed activity likely to be considered relevant are the following:

1. *The physical setting—"where" questions.* Where is the activity happening? What are the main features of the physical setting? What is the context within which human behavior unfolds?
2. *The participants—"who" questions.* Who is present? What are the characteristics of those present? How many people are there? What are their roles? Who is given free access to the setting—who "belongs"? What brings these people together?
3. *Activities—"what" questions.* What is going on? What are the participants doing? Is there a discernible progression of activities? How do the participants interact with one another? What methods do they use to communicate, and how frequently do they do so?
4. *Frequency and duration—"when" questions.* When did the activity begin and end? Is the activity a recurring one and, if so, how regularly does it recur? How typical of such activities is the one under observation?
5. *Process—"how" questions.* How is the activity organized? How are people interacting and communicating? How does the event unfold?
6. *Outcomes—"why" questions.* Why is the activity happening, or why is it happening in this manner? What kinds of things will ensue? What did not happen (especially if it ought to have happened) and why?

The next decision is to identify a way to sample observations and to select observational locations. Researchers generally use a combination of positioning approaches. **Single positioning** means staying in a single location for a period to observe transactions in that location. **Multiple positioning** involves moving around the site to observe behaviors from different locations. **Mobile positioning** involves following a person throughout a given activity or period.

Because participant observers cannot spend a lifetime in one site and cannot be in more than one place at a time, observation is usually supplemented with information from unstructured interviews or conversations. For example, informants may be asked to describe what went on in a meeting the observer was unable to attend, or to describe an event that occurred before the observer entered the field. In such cases, the informant functions as the observer's observer.

Recording Unstructured Observational Data

The most common forms of record keeping in participant observation studies are logs and field notes. A **log** is a daily record of events and conversations. **Field notes** may include the daily log but tend to be much broader, more analytic, and more interpretive. Field notes represent the observer's efforts to record information and also to synthesize and understand the data.

Field notes can be categorized according to their purpose. **Observational notes** are objective descriptions of events and conversations; information such as time, place, activity, and dialogue are recorded as completely as possible. **Theoretical notes** are interpretive attempts to attach meaning to observations. **Methodologic notes** are instructions or reminders about how subsequent observations will be made. **Personal notes** are comments about the researcher's own feelings during the research process.

The success of any participant observation study depends on the quality of the logs and field notes. It is clearly essential to record observations as quickly as possible, but participant observers cannot usually record information by openly carrying a clipboard or a tape-recorder because this would undermine their role as ordinary participants of the group. Observers must develop the skill of making detailed mental notes that can later be written or tape-recorded. The use of laptop computers can greatly facilitate the recording and organization of notes in the field.

Structured Observational Methods

Structured observation differs from the unstructured techniques in the specificity of behaviors selected for observation, in the advance preparation of forms, and in the kinds of activity in which observers engage. The creativity of structured observation lies not in the observation itself but rather in the formulation of a system for accurately categorizing, recording, and encoding the observations and sampling the phenomena of interest.

Categories and Checklists

One approach to making structured observations is the construction of a category system. A **category system** represents an attempt to designate in a systematic, quantitative fashion the behaviors and events transpiring within a setting. A category scheme involves listing all those behaviors or characteristics that the observer is required to observe and record.

Some category systems are constructed so that all observed behaviors within a specified domain can be classified into one (and only one) category.

Example of an exhaustive system:

Lee and Chiou (1995) developed a system for classifying nurses' postures. Their coding scheme was developed with the objective that all postures and joint positions could be categorized.

A contrasting technique is to develop a system in which only particular types of behavior are categorized. For example, if we were studying autistic children's aggressive behavior, we might develop such categories as "strikes another child," "kicks or hits walls or floor," or "throws objects around the room." In this category system, many behaviors—all that are nonaggressive— would not be classified. Nonexhaustive systems are adequate for many purposes, but one risk is that resulting data might be difficult to interpret. When a large number of behaviors are not categorized, the investigator may have difficulty placing categorized behavior into perspective.

One of the most important requirements of a category system is the careful and explicit definition of the behaviors and characteristics to be observed. Each category must be carefully explained, giving observers clear-cut criteria for assessing the occurrence of the phenomenon. Nevertheless, virtually all category systems require observer inference, to greater or lesser degree.

Examples of varying observer inference:

Low inference: Brandon and her colleagues (1999) studied the relationship between nursing care and the development of sleep–wake behaviors in high-risk preterm infants. Observers categorized sleep–wake states into six categories. For example, the "Alert" category was defined as "Eyes open and scanning."

High inference: The Abnormal Involuntary Movement Scale, which was developed by the National Institute for Mental Health and used by Grace and associates (1996) for studying tardive dyskinetic movements, contains such broad categories as "incapacitation due to abnormal movements."

Even when such categories are defined in detail, a heavy inferential burden is placed on the observer.

After a category system has been developed, the researcher constructs a **checklist**, which is the instrument used to record observed phenomena. The checklist is generally formatted with the list of behaviors from the category system on the left and space for tallying their frequency or duration on the right. The task of the observer using an exhaustive category system is to place *all* observed behaviors in one category for each integral unit of behavior (*e.g.*, a sentence in a conversation, a time interval). Checklists based on exhaustive category systems are demanding because the recording task is continuous. With nonexhaustive category systems, categories of behaviors that may or may not be manifested by participants are listed. The observer's tasks are to watch for instances of these behaviors and to record their occurrence. With this type of checklist, the observer does not classify all behaviors of the people being observed, but rather identifies the occurrence and frequency of particular behaviors.

Rating Scales

Another approach to collecting structured observational data is through the use of rating scales. A **rating scale** is a tool that requires the observer to rate some phenomena in terms of points along a descriptive continuum. The observer may be required to make ratings of behavior at intervals throughout the observation or to summarize an entire event or transaction after observation is completed.

Rating scales can be used as an extension of checklists, in which the observer records not only the occurrence of some behavior but also some qualitative aspect of it, such as its magnitude or intensity. When rating scales are coupled with a category scheme in this fashion, considerably more information about the phenomena under investigation can be obtained. The disadvantage of this approach is that it places an immense burden on the observer, particularly if there is an extensive amount of activity.

Example of an observational rating scale:

Weiss (1992) developed the Tactile Interaction Index (TII) for observing patterns of interpersonal touch. The TII category scheme comprises four dimensions: location (part of body touched); action (type of gesture used, such as grabbing, patting, and so on); duration (temporal length of touch); and intensity. Observers using the index must both classify the nature and duration of the touch and rate the intensity on a four-point scale (light, moderate, strong, and deep).

Observational Sampling

Researchers must decide how and when structured observational systems will be applied. Observational sampling methods provide a mechanism for obtaining representative examples of the behaviors being observed. One system is **time sampling**, which involves the selection of time periods during which observations will occur. The time frames may be systematically selected (*e.g.*, every 30 seconds at 2-minute intervals) or selected at random.

Event sampling selects integral behaviors or events for observation. Event sampling requires researchers to either have knowledge about the occurrence of events or be in a position to wait for or precipitate their occurrence. Examples of integral events that may be suitable for event sampling include shift changes of nurses in a hospital, cast removals of pediatric patients, and cardiac arrests in the emergency room. This sampling approach is preferable to time sampling when the events of interest are infrequent and may be missed if time sampling is used. When behaviors and events are relatively frequent, however, time sampling enhances the representativeness of the observed behaviors.

Evaluation of Observational Methods

The field of nursing is particularly well suited to observational research. Nurses are often in a position to watch people's behaviors and may, by training, be especially sensitive observers. Moreover, some nursing problems are better suited to observation than to self-reports, such as when people cannot adequately describe their own behaviors. This may be the case when people are unaware of their own behavior (*e.g.*, manifesting preoperative symptoms of anxiety), when people are embarrassed to report their activities (*e.g.*, displays of aggression or hostility), when behaviors are emotionally laden (*e.g.*, grieving behavior among the bereaved), or when people are not capable of articulating their actions (*e.g.*, young children or the mentally ill). Observational methods have an intrinsic appeal for directly capturing behaviors and events. Furthermore, virtually no other data collection method can provide the depth and variety of information as observation. With this approach, humans—the observers—are used as measuring instruments and provide a uniquely sensitive and intelligent (if fallible) tool.

Several of the shortcomings of the observational approach have already been mentioned. These include possible ethical difficulties, reactivity of the observed when the observer is conspicuous, and lack of consent to being observed. However, one of the most pervasive problems is the vulnerability of observations to bias. A number of factors interfere with objective observations, including the following:

- Emotions, prejudices, and values of the observer may result in faulty inference.
- Personal interest and commitment may color what is seen in the direction of what the observer wants to see.
- Anticipation of what is to be observed may affect what is observed.
- Hasty decisions before adequate information is collected may result in erroneous classifications or conclusions.

Observational biases probably cannot be eliminated, but they can be minimized through the careful training of observers.

As with self-reports, both unstructured and structured observational methods have advantages and disadvantages. Unstructured observational methods have the potential of yielding a richer understanding of human behaviors and social situations than is possible with structured procedures. With a skillful observer, participant observation can help the researcher "get inside" a situation and lead to a more complete understanding of its complexities. Furthermore, unstructured observational approaches are inherently flexible and, therefore, permit the observer freedom to reconceptualize the problem after becoming familiar with the situation. On the other hand, observer bias may pose a threat: once the researcher begins to participate in a group's activities, the possibility of emotional involvement becomes a salient issue. The researcher in a member role may develop a myopic view on issues of importance to the group. Another problem is that unstructured observational methods are more dependent on the observational and interpersonal skills of the observer.

Researchers generally choose an approach that matches the research problem—and their paradigmatic orientation. Unstructured observational methods are especially profitable for in-depth research in which the investigator wishes to establish an adequate conceptualization of the important issues in a social setting or to develop hypotheses. Structured observational methods are better suited to the formal testing of research hypotheses regarding measurable human behaviors.

Critiquing Observational Methods

As in the case of self-reports, the first question you should ask when critiquing an observational study is whether the data should have been collected by some other approach. The advantages and disadvantages of observational methods, discussed previously, should be helpful in considering the appropriateness of using observation.

Some additional guidelines for critiquing observational studies are presented in Box 11-3. A journal article should usually document the following aspects of the observational plan:

BOX 11-3 **GUIDELINES FOR CRITIQUING OBSERVATIONAL METHODS**

1. Does the research question lend itself to an observational approach? Would an alternative method have been more appropriate?

2. Is the degree of structure consistent with the nature of the research question?

3. To what degree were observers concealed during data collection? If there was no concealment, what effect might the observers' presence have had on the behaviors being observed?

4. What was the focus of the observation? How much inference was required on the part of the observers, and to what extend did this affect the potential for bias?

5. Where did the observations take place? To what extent did the setting influence the naturalness of the behaviors observed?

6. How were data actually recorded (*e.g.*, on field notes, checklists)? Did the recording procedure appear appropriate?

7. What was the plan by which events or behaviors were sampled? Did this plan appear appropriate?

8. What steps were taken to minimize observer biases?

- The degree of structure in the observations
- The focus of the observations
- The degree to which the observer was concealed
- For unstructured methods, how entry into the observed group was gained, the relationship between the observer and those observed, the time period over which data were collected, and the method of recording data
- For structured methods, a description of the category system or rating scales and the settings in which observations took place
- The plan for sampling events and behaviors to observe

BIOPHYSIOLOGIC MEASURES

One result of the trend toward clinical, patient-centered studies is greater use of biophysiologic and physical variables. Clinical nursing studies involve biophysiologic instruments both for creating independent variables (*e.g.*, an intervention using biofeedback equipment) and for measuring dependent variables. For the most part, our discussion focuses on the use of biophysiologic measures as dependent variables.

Uses of Biophysiologic Measures in Nursing Research

Most nursing studies in which biophysiologic measures have been used fall into one of five classes:

1. Studies of basic biophysiologic processes that have relevance for nursing care. These studies involve normal, healthy participants or a subhuman animal species.

Example:

Schneider, Correia, and Cannon (1999) studied sex differences in leukocyte invasion in injured soleus muscles of male and female mice. Leukocyte invasion was measured by counting myofibers in stained frozen muscle section slides.

2. Description of nursing actions and explorations of the ways in which nursing actions affect health outcomes. These studies do not focus on specific interventions, but rather are designed to document standard procedures or to learn how standard nursing procedures affect people.

Example:

Nick (1999) conducted a study to describe the presence of residual blood and organic matter on "clean" stethoscopes in maternal–infant units. Observation was used to measure amount of organic buildup, and a catalytic chemical test was used to detect residual blood.

3. Evaluations of a specific nursing procedure or intervention. These studies differ from the studies in the second category in that they involve the testing of a new intervention, usually in comparison with standard methods of care. Typically, these studies involve a hypothesis stating that the innovative nursing procedure will result in improved biophysiologic outcomes among patients.

Example:

Hill, Kurkowski, and Garcia (2000) used an experimental design to test the effectiveness of a nursing intervention (cheek and jaw support) on cardiopulmonary functions of preterm infants during feeding. The outcome measures included heart rate, oxygen saturation, and respiratory rate.

4. Studies to evaluate or improve the measurement and recording of biophysiologic information gathered by nurses. Clinically, the accurate measurement of biophysiologic phenomena is crucial, and therefore some studies focus on improving clinical measurements.

Example:

Fallis and Christiani (1999) conducted a study to determine whether predictive mode axillary temperature measurement is accurate in full-term newborns. Electronic thermometer predictive and monitor mode axillary temperatures were compared.

5. Studies of the correlates of physiologic functioning in patients with health problems. Researchers study possible antecedents and consequences of biophysiologic indicators to gain insight into potential treatments or modes of care.

Example:

Lewicki and coauthors (1997) studied various biophysiologic measures (*e.g.*, hemoglobin, hematocrit, and serum albumin levels) in cardiac patients in relation to their risk for pressure ulcers.

Types of Biophysiologic Measures

Biophysiologic measures include both *in vivo* and *in vitro* measures. **In vivo measures** are those performed directly within or on living organisms. Examples of *in vivo* measures include blood pressure, body temperature, and vital capacity measurement. *In vivo* instruments are available to measure all bodily functions, and technological advances continue to improve the ability to measure biophysiologic phenomena more accurately, conveniently, and rapidly.

> 🖽 ***Example of a study with in vivo measures:***
>
> Gift and Shepard (1999) studied fatigue and other symptoms in men and women with chronic obstructive pulmonary disease. Pulmonary function tests included measures of forced expiratory volume in the first second of exhalation (FEV_1), forced vital capacity (FVC), and FEV_1/FVC.

With ***in vitro* measures**, data are gathered from participants by extracting some biophysiologic material from them and subjecting it to laboratory analysis. The analysis is normally done by specialized laboratory technicians. *In vitro* measures include chemical measures (*e.g.*, the measurement of hormone, sugar, or potassium levels); microbiologic measures (*e.g.*, bacterial counts and identification); and cytologic or histologic measures (*e.g.*, tissue biopsies).

> 🖽 ***Example of a study with in vitro measures:***
>
> Allen (1999) studied changes in cholesterol levels in women 1 year after coronary artery bypass surgery. Fasting plasma lipid levels were measured in a standardized laboratory, yielding measures of total cholesterol, high-density and low-density lipoprotein cholesterol, and triglyceride levels.

Evaluation of Biophysiologic Measures

Biophysiologic measures offer a number of advantages to nurse researchers, including the following:

- Biophysiologic measures are relatively accurate and precise, especially when compared with psychological measures, such as self-report measures of anxiety, pain, and so forth.
- Biophysiologic measures are objective. Two nurses reading from the same spirometer output are likely to record the same tidal volume measurements, and two different spirometers are likely to produce identical readouts. Patients cannot easily distort measurements of biophysiologic functioning deliberately.
- Biophysiologic instrumentation provides valid measures of the targeted variables: thermometers can be depended on to measure temperature and not blood volume, and so forth. For nonbiophysiologic measures, the question of whether an instrument is really measuring the target concept is an ongoing concern.
- Because equipment for obtaining biophysiologic measurements is available in hospital settings, the cost to nurse researchers of collecting biophysiologic data may be low or nonexistent.

Biophysiologic measures also have a few disadvantages:

- The measuring tool may affect the variables it is attempting to measure. The presence of a sensing device, such as a transducer, located in a blood vessel partially blocks that vessel and, hence, alters the pressure-flow characteristics being measured.
- There are normally interferences that create artifacts in biophysiologic measures. For example, noise generated within a measuring instrument interferes with the signal being produced.
- Energy must often be applied to the organism when taking the biophysiologic measurements; extreme caution must continually be exercised to avoid damaging cells by high-energy concentrations.

In summary, biophysiologic measures are plentiful, tend to be accurate and valid, and are extremely useful in clinical nursing studies. However, care must be exercised in using them with regard to practical, ethical, medical, and technical considerations.

Critiquing Biophysiologic Measures

Biophysiologic measures offer the nurse researcher many advantages, as discussed previously, and their shortcomings are relatively minor. As always, however, the most important consideration in evaluating a data collection strategy is the appropriateness of the measures for the research question. The objectivity, accuracy, and availability of biophysiologic measures are of little significance if an alternative method would have resulted in a better measurement of the key concepts. Stress, for example, could be measured in various ways: through self-report (*e.g.,* through the use of a scale such as the State-Trait Anxiety Inventory); through direct observation of participants' behavior during exposure to stressful stimuli; or by measuring heart rate, blood pressure, or levels of adrenocorticotropic hormone in urine samples. The choice of which measure to use must be linked to the way that stress is conceptualized in the research problem.

Additional criteria for assessing the use of biophysiologic measures are presented in Box 11-4. The general questions to consider are these: Did the researcher select the correct biophysiologic measure? Was care taken in the collection of the data? Did the researcher competently interpret the data?

 CONSUMER TIP:

Many nursing studies integrate a variety of data collection approaches. In quantitative studies, structured self-reports combined with biophysiologic measures are especially common. Qualitative studies are especially likely to combine unstructured observations and self-reports. ■

> **BOX 11-4**
>
> ## GUIDELINES FOR CRITIQUING BIOPHYSIOLOGIC METHODS
>
> 1. Does the research question lend itself to a biophysiologic approach? Would an alternative method have been theoretically more appropriate?
>
> 2. Was the proper instrumentation used to obtain the biophysiologic measurements? Would an alternative instrument or method have been more appropriate?
>
> 3. Does the researcher appear to have the skills necessary for proper interpretation of the biophysiologic measures?

IMPLEMENTING THE DATA COLLECTION PLAN

In addition to selecting methods for collecting data, researchers must develop and implement a plan for gathering the data. This involves decisions that could affect the quality of the data being collected.

One important decision concerns who will collect the data. In many studies, the researcher hires assistants to collect data rather than doing it personally. This is especially likely to be the case in large-scale quantitative studies. In other studies, nurses or other health care staff are asked to assist in the collection of data. From your perspective as a consumer, the critical issues are whether the people collecting data might have introduced any biases and whether they were able to produce valid and accurate data. In any research endeavor, adequate training of data collectors is essential.

Another issue concerns the circumstances under which data were gathered. For example, it may be critical to ensure total privacy to participants. In most cases, it is important for the researcher to create a nonjudgmental atmosphere in which participants are encouraged to be candid or behave naturally. Again, you as a consumer must ask whether there is anything about the way in which the data were collected that could have introduced bias or otherwise affected data quality.

In evaluating the data collection plan of a study, then, you should critically appraise not only the actual methods chosen but also the procedures used to collect the data. Box 11-5 provides some specific guidelines for critiquing the procedures used to collect research data.

RESEARCH EXAMPLES

In this section, we present summaries of actual nursing studies. Use the guidelines presented in this chapter to evaluate the researchers' data collection plans, referring to the original articles if necessary.

BOX 11-5

GUIDELINES FOR CRITIQUING DATA COLLECTION PROCEDURES

1. Who collected the research data? Were the data collectors qualified for their role, or is there something about them (*e.g.*, their professional role, their relationship with study participants) that could undermine the collection of unbiased, high-quality data?

2. How were data collectors trained? Does the training appear adequate?

3. Where and under what circumstances were the data gathered? Were other people present during the data collection? Could the presence of others have created any distortions?

4. Did the collection of data place any undue burdens (in terms of time or stress) on participants? How might this have affected data quality?

RESEARCH EXAMPLE OF STRUCTURED SELF-REPORT AND BIOPHYSIOLOGIC MEASURES

Brooks-Brunn (2000) conducted a study to identify risk factors for the development of postoperative pulmonary complications (PPCs) after total abdominal hysterectomy. Her data sources included self-reports, chest examinations, and medical records.

Research Summary

In Brooks-Brunn's multisite study, 120 patients undergoing a total abdominal hysterectomy were included in the sample. The research design was prospective: the women were recruited into the sample preoperatively, and their PPC status was subsequently determined postoperatively.

Brooks-Brunn collected data on a wide range of risk factors that had previously been identified in the literature and that were accessible to the health care team. These included preoperative, intraoperative, and postoperative risk factors. Preoperative factors included information on the subjects' health habits, demographic characteristics, and medical history. This information was obtained through a structured interview and review of medical charts. Information about intraoperative risk factors (*e.g.*, duration of anesthesia and location, direction, and length of the incision) was obtained from charts as well. Postoperative risk factors included the presence of a nasogastric tube and the initial method of pain management. After surgery, subjects underwent a daily interview and chest examination. The dependent variable, presence or absence of PPCs, was based on a combination of biophysiologic measures, such as body temperature, abnormal breath sounds, and cough and sputum production.

In the research sample, 11% of subjects developed a PPC. Brooks-Brunn's results indicated that the patients most likely to develop a PPC were older, had a history of smoking, and had a history of cancer or congestive heart failure. Also, women at highest risk were those who had an upper (versus lower) abdominal surgical location and had a vertical incision. Factors that were not found to be reliably related to PPC risk included obesity, history of asthma, history of chronic obstructive pulmonary disease, duration of anesthesia during surgery, and type of analgesia used postoperatively.

Clinical Relevance

Postoperative pulmonary complications are relatively common and are associated with increased morbidity and mortality as well as longer hospital stay. Until Brooks-Brunn had undertaken her study, there had been little research on risk factors associated with PPCs among women undergoing gynecologic surgery.

The design for Brooks-Brunn's study was strong: prospective designs are always more reliable than retrospective designs. She also appeared to be thorough in assessing a wide variety of risk factors and drawing on several data sources. Another strength is that the sample was drawn from two sites. However, it was a relatively small sample for a correlational study; therefore, it would be unwise to generalize without further replications.

Nevertheless, the study does provide an important foundation for further identification of important risk factors. Furthermore, nurses can use the information from this study to be on the alert for patients who have the risk factors found to be correlated with PPC and, especially, for patients with multiple risk factors. When these high-risk patients are identified, nurses can then play a key role in preventing PPCs through patient education, assessment, and initiation of interventions both preoperatively and postoperatively. Nursing interventions can be designed to target risk factors that are modifiable and amenable to manipulation, such as smoking behavior. The preoperative and postoperative periods provide nurses with a "window of opportunity" to promote smoking cessation in these high-risk patients.

RESEARCH EXAMPLE OF UNSTRUCTURED SELF-REPORT AND OBSERVATION

Vivian and Wilcox (2000) conducted a study that focused on compliance communication (nurse–patient communication) in home health care. Their study combined observational and interview data.

Research Summary

In Vivian and Wilcox's (2000) study, *compliance communication* referred to communication about patient care for situations in which the patient or family had some degree of responsibility for carrying out the medical regime.

Nurse–patient communication of six registered nurses and 25 adult patients from two home care agencies was the focus of this research.

Phase I of the study involved participant observation. Each of the six nurses was accompanied on a day of rounds. A total of 25 home visits were observed, with visits ranging from 15 to 75 minutes. In the car between home visits and at the close of each day, informal unstructured interviews with the nurses were conducted. During Phase II, a semi-structured format was used to interview each of the six nurses individually. This semi-structured format focused on the topics of patient needs, nurse's role in home care, expectation for compliance, and strategies used to promote patient compliance. The in-depth interviews required between 1 and $1^1/_2$ hours to complete. In addition, the researcher and nurse spent between 15 and 30 minutes after the interview discussing patients who had been visited in Phase I. Finally, telephone interviews were held with 11 patients and eight family members.

Data analysis revealed five categories of compliance communication: (a) education of patients and family members, (b) arrangement of additional support services, (c) removal of obstacles to compliance, (d) provision of positive reinforcement or rewards, and (e) use of threats or scare tactics. Educating patients and family members emerged as the strongest theme as a primary means to promote patient compliance.

Clinical Relevance

Patient noncompliance in carrying out treatment recommendations is a significant problem in contemporary health care. Noncompliance can result in wasting of health resources, frustration to clinicians, and potential threats to patients' health.

The researchers' use of multiple data collection methods on nurse–patient compliance communication was a strength of this study. By using participant observation in Phase I, the researchers were able to make observations that sharpened the saliency of their questions in the unstructured, semi-structured, and telephone interviews they subsequently conducted. Moreover, by using both observation and interviews, the researchers were able to examine the degree of consistency between self-reports and actual behavior. Finally, through their observations, they were able to study both verbal and nonverbal forms of communication.

Results of Vivian and Wilcox's study have clinical implications for nurses in achieving the goals of home care of moving patients toward self-care and independence. Based on their findings, Vivian and Wilcox suggested the following strategies for educating patients and their families: reinforcing compliance messages by repetition and reminders; inquiring why a patient is noncompliant; offering to help a patient in complying with a treatment regimen; having a patient practice compliance; and setting short-term goals related to compliance. Although some of these strategies may be unique to home care, these "sequential influence attempts" may also have relevance to non–home care situations.

• • • • • *SUMMARY POINTS*

- Some researchers use existing data in their studies—for example, those doing **historical research**, meta-analyses, **secondary analyses**, or an analysis of **records**.
- Data collection methods vary along four dimensions: structure, quantifiability, researcher obtrusiveness, and objectivity.
- The three principal data collection methods for nurse researchers are self-reports, observations, and biophysiologic measures.
- **Self-report** data are collected by means of an oral interview or written questionnaire. Self-report methods are an indispensable means of collecting data but are susceptible to errors of reporting.
- Unstructured self-reports, used in qualitative studies, include **completely unstructured interviews**, which are conversational discussions on the topic of interest; **focused** (or **semi-structured**) **interviews**, using a broad **topic guide**; **focus group interviews**, which involve discussions with small groups; **life histories**, which encourage respondents to narrate their life experiences regarding some theme; and **diaries**, in which respondents are asked to maintain daily records about some aspects of their lives.
- Structured self-reports usually employ a formal **instrument**—a **questionnaire** or **interview schedule**—that may contain a combination of **open-ended questions** (which permit respondents to respond in their own words) and **closed-ended questions** (which offer respondents fixed alternatives from which to choose).
- Questionnaires are less costly than interviews, offer the possibility of anonymity, and run no risk of interviewer bias; however, interviews yield a higher response rate, are suitable for a wider variety of people, and provide richer data than questionnaires.
- Social-psychological **scales** are self-report tools for quantitatively measuring the intensity of such characteristics as personality traits, attitudes, needs, and perceptions.
- **Likert scales** (or **summated rating scales**) present the respondent with a series of **items** worded favorably or unfavorably toward some phenomenon; responses indicating level of agreement or disagreement with each statement are scored and summed into a composite score.
- The **semantic differential (SD)** technique consists of a series of scales with **bipolar adjectives** (*e.g.*, good/bad) along which respondents rate their reactions toward phenomena.
- A **visual analog scale (VAS)** is used to measure, along a line designating a bipolar continuum, subjective experiences, such as pain, fatigue, and nausea.
- Scales are versatile and powerful but are susceptible to **response set biases**—the tendency of some people to respond to items in characteristic ways, independently of item content.
- **Vignettes** are brief descriptions of some event, person, or situation to which respondents are asked to react.

- **Projective techniques** encompass various data collection methods that rely on the participant's projection of psychological traits or states in response to vaguely structured stimuli.
- **Q sorts** involve the sorting of a set of statements into piles according to specified criteria.
- **Observational methods**, which include both structured and unstructured procedures, are techniques for acquiring data through the direct observation of phenomena.
- One type of **unstructured observation** is **participant observation**, in which the researcher gains entrée into the social group of interest and participates to varying degrees in its functioning while making in-depth observations of activities and events. **Logs** of daily events and **field notes** of the observer's experiences and interpretations constitute the major data collection instruments.
- **Structured observations**, which dictate what the observer should observe, often involve **checklists**—tools based on **category systems** for recording the appearance, frequency, or duration of prespecified behaviors or events. Alternatively, the observer may use a **rating scale** to rate some phenomenon along a dimension of interest (*e.g.,* fast/slow).
- Most structured observations use a sampling plan (such as **time sampling** or **event sampling**) for selecting the behaviors, events, and conditions to be observed.
- Observational techniques are a versatile and important alternative to self-reports; however, various observational biases can pose a threat to the validity and accuracy of observational data.
- Data may also be derived from **biophysiologic measures**, which can be classified as either *in vivo* **measurements** (those performed within or on living organisms) or *in vitro* **measurements** (those performed outside the organism's body, such as blood tests). Biophysiologic measures have the advantage of being objective, accurate, and precise.
- In developing a data collection plan, the researcher must decide who will collect the data, how the data collectors will be trained, and what the circumstances for data collection will be.

➤ ➤ ➤ ➤ *CRITICAL THINKING ACTIVITIES*

Chapter 11 of the accompanying *Study Guide to Accompany Essentials of Nursing Research*, 5th edition offers various exercises and study suggestions for reinforcing the concepts presented in this chapter. In addition, you can address the following questions:

1. Read the Method section of one or both of the actual research studies in the Appendix of this book, paying particular attention to the data collection plan. Answer the relevant questions from Boxes 11-2 to 11-5 with regard to this study.

2. Read the Results section of the Vivian and Wilcox (2000) study that was used as a research example in this chapter. How might relevance and accuracy of the study findings have been jeopardized if only observation or only self-report had been used?

3. Read the study by Brooks-Brunn (2000), used as the quantitative research example in this chapter. Comment on the researcher's description of her data collection plan.

For additional review, see questions 136–155 on the study CD provided with Polit: Study Guide to Accompany Essentials of Nursing Research.

SUGGESTED READINGS

Methodologic References

Frank-Stromberg, M. (Ed.). (1988). *Instruments for clinical nursing research.* Norwalk, CT: Appleton & Lange.

Kerlinger, F. N. (1986). *Foundations of behavioral research* (3rd ed.). New York: Holt, Rinehart & Winston.

Leininger, M. M. (Ed.). (1985). *Qualitative research methods in nursing.* New York: Grune & Stratton.

Lofland, J., & Lofland, L. (1984). *Analyzing social settings: A guide to qualitative observation and analysis.* Belmont, CA: Wadsworth.

Polit, D. F., & Hungler, B. P. (1999). *Nursing research: Principles and methods* (6th ed.). Philadelphia: Lippincott Williams & Wilkins.

Rew, L., Bechtel, D., & Sapp, A. (1993). Self-as-instrument in qualitative research. *Nursing Research, 42,* 300–301.

Waltz, C. F., Strickland, O. L., & Lenz, E. R. (1991). *Measurement in nursing research* (2nd ed.). Philadelphia: F. A. Davis.

Substantive References

Allen, J. K. (1999). Changes in cholesterol levels in women after coronary artery bypass surgery. *Heart & Lung, 28,* 270–275.

Brandon, D. H., Holditch-Davis, D., & Beylan, M. (1999). Nursing care and the development of sleeping and waking behaviors in preterm infants. *Research in Nursing & Health, 22,* 217–229.

Breckenridge, D. M. (1997). Decisions regarding dialysis treatment modality. *Holistic Nursing Practice, 12,* 54–61.

Brooks-Brunn, J. A. (2000). Risk factors associated with postoperative pulmonary complications following total abdominal hysterectomy. *Clinical Nursing Research, 9,* 27–46.

Fallis, W. M., & Christiani, P. (1999). Neonatal axillary temperature measurement: A comparison of electronic thermometer predictive and monitor modes. *Journal of Obstetric, Gynecologic, and Neonatal Nursing, 28,* 389–394.

Gift, A. G., & Shepard, C. E. (1999). Fatigue and other symptoms in patients with chronic obstructive pulmonary disease: Do women and men differ? *Journal of Obstetric, Gynecologic, and Neonatal Nursing, 28,* 201–208.

Grace, J., Bellus, S. B., Raulin, M. L., Herz, M. I., Priest, B. L., Brenner, V., Donnelly, L., Smith, P., & Gunn, S. (1996). Long-term impact of clozapine and psychosocial treatment on psychiatric symptoms and cognitive functioning. *Psychiatric Services, 47,* 41–45.

Graninger, E. M., & McCool, W. P. (1998). Nurse-midwives' use of and attitudes toward analgesia. *Journal of Nurse-Midwifery, 43,* 250–261.

Harvey, R. M., Kazis, L., & Lee, A. F. S. (1999). Decision-making preference and opportunity in VA ambulatory care patients: Association with patient satisfaction. *Research in Nursing & Health, 22,* 39–48.

Hill, A. S., Kurkowski, T. B., & Garcia, J. (2000). Oral support measures used in feeding the preterm infant. *Nursing Research, 49,* 2–10.

Hillman, K. A. (1997). Comparing child-rearing practices in parents of children with cancer and parents of healthy children. *Journal of Pediatric Oncology Nursing, 14,* 53–67.

Kurlowicz, L. H. (1998). Perceived self-efficacy, functional ability, and depressive symptoms in older elective surgery patients. *Nursing Research, 47,* 219–226.

Kirchhoff, K. T., Spuhler, V., Walker, L., Hutton, A., Cole, B. V., & Clemmer, T. (2000). Intensive care nurses' experiences with end-of-life care. *American Journal of Critical Care, 9,* 36–42.

Lee, K. A., Portillo, C. J., & Miramontes, H. (1999). The fatigue experience for women with human immunodeficiency virus. *Journal of Obstetric, Gynecologic, and Neonatal Nursing, 28,* 193–200.

Lee, Y. H., & Chiou, W. K. (1995). Ergonomic analysis of working posture in nursing personnel: Example of modified Ovako Working Analysis System application. *Research in Nursing & Health, 18,* 67–75.

Leidy, N. K., & Haase, J. E. (1999). Functional status from the patient's perspective. *Research in Nursing & Health, 22,* 67–77.

Lewicki, L. J., Mion, L., Splane, K. G., Samstag, D., & Secic, M. (1997). Patient risk factors for pressure ulcers during cardiac surgery. *AORN Journal, 65,* 933–942.

Ludington-Hoe, S. M., Anderson, G. C., Simpson, S., Hollingsead, A., Argote, L. A., & Rey, H. (1999). Birth-related fatigue in 34–36-week preterm neonates: Rapid recovery with very early kangaroo (skin-to-skin) care. *Journal of Obstetric, Gynecologic, and Neonatal Nursing, 28,* 94–103.

Ludwick, R. (1999). Clinical decision making: Recognition of confusion and application of restraints. *Orthopaedic Nursing, 18,* 65–72.

Musil, C. M., Ahn, S., Haug, M., Warner, C., Morris, D., & Duffy, E. (1998). Health problems and health actions among community-dwelling older adults: Results of a health diary study. *Applied Nursing Research, 11,* 138–147.

Nick, J. M. (1999). Organic buildup and residual blood on infant stethoscopes in maternal-infant areas. *Journal of Obstetric, Gynecologic, and Neonatal Nursing, 28,* 143–150.

Niedz, B. A. (1998). Correlates of hospitalized patients' perceptions of service quality. *Research in Nursing & Health, 21,* 339–349.

Polivka, B. J., Lovell, M., & Smith, B. A. (1998). A qualitative assessment of inner city elementary school children's perceptions of their neighborhood. *Public Health Nursing, 15,* 171–179.

Ragneskog, H., Gerdner, L. A., Josefsson, K., & Kihlgren, M. (1998). Probable reasons for expressed agitation in persons with dementia. *Clinical Nursing Research, 7,* 189–206.

Rich, K. (1999). Inhospital cardiac arrest: Pre-event variables and nursing response. *Clinical Nurse Specialist, 13,* 147–156.

Sandelowski, M. (2000). "This most dangerous instrument": Propriety, power, and the vaginal speculum. *Journal of Obstetric, Gynecologic, and Neonatal Nursing, 29,* 73–82.

Schneider, B. S., Correia, L. A., & Cannon, J. G. (1999). Sex differences in leukocyte invasion in injured murine skeletal muscle. *Research in Nursing & Health, 22,* 243–251.

Schnell, E. S., & Kayser-Jones, J. (1999). The effect of role-taking ability on caregiver-resident mealtime interaction. *Applied Nursing Research, 12,* 38–44.

Smith-Battle, L., & Leonard, V. W. (1998). Adolescent mothers four years later: Narratives of the self and visions of the future. *Advances in Nursing Science, 20,* 36–49.

Strang, V. R., & Haughey, M. (1999). Respite: A coping strategy for family caregivers. *Western Journal of Nursing Research, 21,* 450–471.

Vivian, B. G., & Wilcox, J. R. (2000). Compliance communication in home health care: A mutually reciprocal process. *Qualitative Health Research, 10,* 103–116.

Weaver, T. E., Richmond, T. S., & Narsavage, G. L. (1997). An explanatory model of functional status in chronic obstructive pulmonary disease. *Nursing Research, 46,* 26–31.

Weiss, S. J. (1992). Measurement of the sensory qualities in tactile interaction. *Nursing Research, 41,* 82–86.

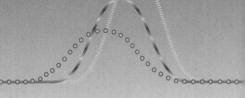

CHAPTER 12

Evaluating Measurements and Data Quality

• •

Student Objectives

On completion of this chapter, the student will be able to:

○ describe the major characteristics of measurement and identify major sources of measurement error

○ describe three aspects of reliability and specify how each aspect can be assessed

○ interpret the meaning of reliability coefficients

○ describe three different aspects of validity and specify how each aspect can be assessed

○ describe the four dimensions used in establishing the trustworthiness of qualitative data and identify methods of enhancing data quality in qualitative studies

○ evaluate the overall quality of a measuring tool or data collection approach used in a research study

○ define new terms in the chapter

• •

New Terms

Audit trail
Coefficient alpha
Concurrent validity
Confirmability
Construct validity
Content validity
Credibility
Criterion-related validity
Cronbach's alpha
Data source triangulation
Dependability
Equivalence
Error of measurement
Face validity
Factor analysis
Inquiry audit
Internal consistency
Interobserver reliability
Interrater reliability
Investigator triangulation
Known-groups technique
Measurement
Member check
Method triangulation

Negative case analysis
Obtained score
Peer debriefing
Persistent observation
Predictive validity
Prolonged engagement
Psychometric evaluation
Quantification
Reliability coefficient
Reliability
Researcher credibility
Split-half technique
Stability
Stepwise replication
Test–retest reliability
Theory triangulation
Thick description
Transferability
Triangulation
True score
Trustworthiness
Validity coefficient
Validity

Data collection methods vary in quality. An ideal data collection procedure is one that results in indicators of the constructs that are accurate, valid, and unbiased. For most concepts of interest to nurse researchers, few, if any, data collection procedures match this ideal. In this chapter, we discuss criteria for evaluating the quality of data obtained in both quantitative and qualitative research projects.

MEASUREMENT AND THE ASSESSMENT OF QUANTITATIVE DATA

In a quantitative study, data come from measures of an abstract construct. Before describing criteria for assessing quantitative measures, we briefly discuss the concept of measurement.

Measurement

Measurement involves rules for assigning numeric values to *qualities* of objects to designate the *quantity* of the attribute. No attribute inherently has a numeric value; human beings invent the rules to measure concepts. An often-quoted statement by an American psychologist, L. L. Thurstone, summarizes a position assumed by many quantitative researchers: "Whatever exists, exists in some amount and can be measured." The notion here is that attributes are not constant: they vary from day to day or from one person to another. This variability is capable of a numeric expression that signifies *how much* of an attribute is present. **Quantification** is used to communicate that amount. The purpose of assigning numbers is to differentiate among people who possess varying degrees of the critical attribute.

The definition of measurement also requires numbers to be assigned to objects according to rules rather than haphazardly. Quantification in the absence of rules would be meaningless. The rules for measuring temperature, weight, blood pressure, and other physical attributes are widely known and accepted. Rules for measuring many variables, however, have to be invented. What are the rules for measuring patient satisfaction? Pain? Depression? Whether the data are collected through observation, self-report, or some other method, the researcher must specify the criteria according to which numeric values are to be assigned.

Advantages of Measurement

A major strength of measurement is that it removes guesswork in gathering information. Consider how handicapped nurses and doctors would be in the absence of measures of body temperature, blood pressure, and so on. Because measurement is based on explicit rules, the information tends to be objective: two people measuring a person's weight using the same scale would likely get identical results. Two people scoring responses to a self-report stress scale would likely arrive at identical scores. Not all quantitative measures are completely objective, but most incorporate rules for minimizing subjectivity.

Quantitative measurement also makes it possible to obtain reasonably precise information. Instead of describing Nathan as "rather tall," for example, we can depict him as a man who is 6 feet, 2 inches tall. If we chose, or if the research required it, we could obtain even more precise height measurements. Because of the possibility for precision, the researcher can differentiate among people who possess different degrees of an attribute.

Finally, measurement is a language of communication. Numbers are less vague than words and are thus capable of communicating information to a broad audience. If a researcher reported that the average oral temperature of a sample of patients was "somewhat high," different readers might develop different conceptions about the physiologic state of the sample. If the researcher reported an average temperature of 99.6°F, however, there is no ambiguity.

Errors of Measurement

Researchers work with fallible measures. Values and scores from even the best measuring instruments have a certain amount of error. We can think of every piece of quantitative data as consisting of two parts: an error component and a true component. This can be written as an equation, as follows:

$$\text{Obtained score} = \text{True score} \pm \text{Error}$$

The **obtained** (or observed) **score** could be, for example, a patient's heart rate or score on an anxiety scale. The **true score** is the true value that would be obtained if it were possible to have an infallible measure of the target attribute. The true score is hypothetical; it can never be known because measures are not infallible. The **error of measurement**—the difference between true and obtained scores—is the result of extraneous factors that affect the measurement and result in distortions.

Many factors contribute to errors of measurement. Among the most common are the following:

- *Situational contaminants.* Measurements can be affected by the conditions under which they are produced (*e.g.,* people's awareness of an observer can affect their behavior; environmental factors, such as temperature, lighting, or time of day, can be sources of measurement error).
- *Response set biases.* A number of relatively enduring characteristics of respondents can interfere with accurate measures of an attribute (see Chap. 11).
- *Transitory personal factors.* Temporary personal factors (*e.g.,* fatigue, hunger, mood) can influence people's motivation to cooperate, act naturally, or do their best.
- *Administration variations.* Alterations in the methods of collecting data from one person to the next can affect obtained scores (*e.g.,* if some biophysiologic measures are taken before a feeding and others are taken postprandially, measurement errors might occur).
- *Item sampling.* Errors can be introduced as a result of the sampling of items used to measure an attribute. For example, a student's score on a

100-item research methods test will be influenced to a certain extent by which 100 questions are included.

This list is not exhaustive, but it illustrates that data are susceptible to measurement error from a variety of sources.

Reliability of Measuring Instruments

The **reliability** of a quantitative measure is a major criterion for assessing its quality. Reliability refers to the consistency with which an instrument measures the attribute. If a spring scale gave a reading of 120 lb for a person's weight one minute and a reading of 150 lb the next minute, we would naturally be wary of using such an unreliable scale. The less variation an instrument produces in repeated measurements of an attribute, the higher is its reliability.

Another way of defining reliability is in terms of accuracy. An instrument is reliable if its measures accurately reflect the true measures of the attribute. A reliable measure is one that maximizes the true score component and minimizes the error component of a score.

Three aspects of reliability are of interest to researchers collecting quantitative data: stability, internal consistency, and equivalence.

Stability

The **stability** of a measure is the extent to which the same scores are obtained when the instrument is used with the same people on separate occasions. Assessments of stability are derived through **test–retest reliability** procedures. The researcher administers the same measure to a sample of people on two occasions, and then compares the scores.

Suppose, for example, we were interested in the stability of a self-report scale that measured self-esteem in adolescents. Because self-esteem is a fairly stable attribute that would not change markedly from one day to the next, we would expect a reliable measure of it to yield consistent scores on two separate tests. As a check on the instrument's stability, we arrange to administer the scale 3 weeks apart to a sample of teenagers. Fictitious data for this example are presented in Table 12-1. On the whole, differences on the two tests are not large. Researchers compute a **reliability coefficient**, a numeric index of a measure's reliability, to objectively determine exactly how small the differences are. Reliability coefficients (designated as *r*) range from .00 to 1.00.[*] The higher the value, the more reliable (stable) is the measuring instrument. In the example shown in Table 12-1, the reliability coefficient is .95, which is quite high.

---

[*]Computation procedures for reliability coefficients are not presented in this textbook, but formulas can be found in the references cited at the end of this chapter. Although reliability coefficients can, technically, be negative (*i.e.*, less than .00), they are usually a positive number between .00 and 1.00.

TABLE 12-1.	Fictitious Data for Test–Retest Reliability of Self-Esteem Scale	
SUBJECT NUMBER	**TIME 1**	**TIME 2**
1	55	57
2	49	46
3	78	74
4	37	35
5	44	46
6	50	56
7	58	55
8	62	66
9	48	50
10	67	63

$r = .95$

 CONSUMER TIP:

For most purposes, reliability coefficients higher than .70 are satisfactory, but coefficients in the .85 to .95 range are far preferable. ■

The test–retest approach to estimating reliability has certain disadvantages. The major problem is that many traits of interest do change over time, independently of the instrument's stability. Attitudes, mood, knowledge, and so forth can be modified by intervening experiences between two measurements. Thus, stability indexes are most appropriate for relatively enduring characteristics, such as personality and abilities.

Example of test–retest reliability:

Stuppy (1998) tested the Wong-Baker FACES scale—a measure of pain intensity that is widely used in clinical pediatric practice—for use with mature adults. The test–retest reliability of the scale with a sample of older hospital patients (3 to 4 days between administrations) was .70.

Internal Consistency

Ideally, psychosocial scales are composed of items that all measure the same critical attribute and nothing else. On a scale to measure empathy in nurses, it would be inappropriate to include an item that is a better measure of diagnostic competence than empathy. An instrument may be said to have **internal consistency** reliability to the extent that all its subparts measure the same characteristic. This approach to reliability assesses an important source of measurement error in multi-item measures: the sampling of items.

One of the oldest methods for assessing internal consistency is the **split-half technique.** In this approach, the items comprising a test or scale are split into two groups (usually, odd versus even items) and scored, and then scores on the two half-tests are used to compute a reliability coefficient. If the two half-tests are really measuring the same attribute, the reliability coefficient will be high. More sophisticated and accurate methods of computing internal consistency estimates are now in use, most notably, **Cronbach's alpha** or **coefficient alpha.** This method gives an estimate of the split-half correlation for all possible ways of dividing the measure into two halves, not just odd versus even items. As with test–retest reliability coefficients, indexes of internal consistency range in value between .00 and 1.00. The higher the reliability coefficient, the more accurate (internally consistent) the measure.

Example of internal consistency reliability:

Stordeur, Vandenberghe, and D'hoore (2000) studied the relationship between nursing leadership style and various work outcomes. They used the Multifactor Leadership Questionnaire (MLQ), a 70-item instrument that had previously been found to have adequate reliability. In their study, which involved translating the MLQ into French, the subscale internal consistency coefficients ranged from .68 to .89.

Equivalence

The **equivalence** approach to estimating reliability—used primarily with structured observational instruments—determines the consistency or equivalence of the instrument by different observers or raters. As noted in Chapter 11, a potential weakness of direct observation is the risk for observer error. The degree of error can be assessed through **interrater** (or **interobserver**) **reliability**, which is estimated by having two or more trained observers make simultaneous, independent observations. The resulting data can then be used to calculate an index of equivalence or agreement. That is, a reliability coefficient can be computed to demonstrate the strength of the relation between the observers' ratings. When two independent observers score some phenomenon congruently, the scores are likely to be accurate and reliable.

Example of interrater reliability:

Stewart and her colleagues (1999) developed the Environment-Behavior Interaction Code (EBIC), an observational coding system to classify the behavior and environmental context of people with dementia. One version of the EBIC is a system for making ongoing observations in real time (event format); another is a global checklist developed for clinical outcome research (interval format). The mean percentages of agreement of raters were 78% for the event format and 96% for the interval format.

Interpretation of Reliability Coefficients

Reliability coefficients are an important indicator of an instrument's quality. A measure with low reliability prevents an adequate testing of a researcher's hypothesis. If data fail to confirm a research hypothesis, one possibility is that the measuring tool was unreliable—not necessarily that the expected relationships do not exist. Thus, knowledge of the reliability of an instrument is useful in interpretating research results.

Reliability estimates vary according to the procedure used to obtain them. Estimates of reliability computed by different procedures for the same instrument are not identical.

 Example of different forms of reliability:

Hess (1998) developed the Index of Professional Nursing Governance to measure the governance of hospital-based nurses. The one-month test–retest reliability was .77, and the internal consistency reliability was .97.

In addition, reliability of an instrument is related to sample heterogeneity. The more homogeneous the sample (*i.e.,* the more similar the scores), the lower the reliability coefficient will be. This is because instruments are designed to measure differences, and if sample members are similar to one another, it is more difficult for the instrument to discriminate reliably among those who possess varying degrees of the attribute.

 CONSUMER TIP:

If a research report provides information on the reliability of a quantitative scale without specifying the type of reliability measure used, it is probably safe to assume that internal consistency reliability was assessed by the Cronbach alpha method. ■

Validity of Measuring Instruments

The second important criterion for evaluating a quantitative instrument is its validity. **Validity** is the degree to which an instrument measures what it is supposed to be measuring. When a researcher develops an instrument to measure patients' perceived susceptibility to illness, he or she should take steps to ensure that the resulting scores validly reflect this variable and not something else.

The reliability and validity of an instrument are not totally independent. A measuring device that is not reliable cannot possibly be valid. An instrument cannot validly be measuring the attribute of interest if it is erratic or inaccurate. An instrument can be reliable, however, without being valid. Suppose we had the idea to measure patients' anxiety by measuring the circumference of their wrists. We could obtain highly accurate, consistent, and precise measurements of wrist circumferences, but they would not be valid indicators of anxiety. Thus, the high reliability of an instrument provides no evidence of its validity; the low reliability of a measure is evidence of low validity.

Like reliability, validity has a number of aspects and assessment approaches. One aspect is known as face validity. **Face validity** refers to whether the instrument looks as though it is measuring the appropriate construct. Although it is often useful for an instrument to have face validity, three other aspects of validity are of greater importance in assessments of an instrument: content validity, criterion-related validity, and construct validity.

 CONSUMER TIP:

In some reports, the study's focus is on data quality. That is, researchers undertake studies to examine the validity and reliability of instruments that could be used by clinicians or other nurse researchers. In these **psychometric evaluations,** information about data quality is carefully documented. ■

Content Validity

Content validity is concerned with adequacy of coverage of the content area being measured. Content validity is particularly relevant for tests of knowledge. In such a context, the validity question is: How representative are the questions on this test of the universe of all questions that might be asked on this topic?

Content validity is also relevant in measures of complex psychosocial traits. A person who wanted to develop a new instrument would begin by developing a thorough conceptualization of the construct of interest so that the measure would adequately capture the whole domain. Such a conceptualization might come from rich first-hand knowledge but is more likely to come from the results of a qualitative inquiry or from a literature review.

The content validity of an instrument is necessarily based on judgment. There are no totally objective methods for ensuring the adequate content coverage of an instrument. Experts in the content area are often called on to analyze the items' adequacy in representing the hypothetical content universe in the correct proportions. It is also possible to calculate a content validity index that indicates the extent of expert agreement, but ultimately the experts' subjective judgments must be relied on.

Example of content validity:

Leidy (1999) developed the Functional Performance Inventory, a measure of the performance dimension of functional status. Items for the scale were based on qualitative interviews with 12 patients with chronic obstructive pulmonary disease. Then, a panel of 24 experts rated the items on the scale for relevance. After Leidy revised the instrument based on feedback from the experts, the content validity was evaluated a second time by a panel of seven experts.

Criterion-Related Validity

In a **criterion-related validity** assessment, the researcher seeks to establish the relationship between scores on an instrument and some external criterion. The instrument, whatever abstract attribute it is measuring, is said to be valid if its scores correspond strongly with scores on some criterion. One difficulty of criterion-related validation is finding a reliable and valid criterion. A researcher constructing an instrument to measure nursing effectiveness might use supervisory ratings as the criterion—but how could he or she be sure that the ratings were valid and reliable? Researchers must be content with less-than-perfect criteria.

After the criterion is established, the validity can be estimated easily. A **validity coefficient** is computed by using a mathematic formula that correlates scores on the instrument with scores on the criterion variable. The magnitude of the coefficient indicates how valid the instrument is. These coefficients (r) range between .00 and 1.00, with higher values indicating greater criterion-related validity. Coefficients of .70 or higher are desirable.

Sometimes, a distinction is made between two types of criterion-related validity. **Predictive validity** refers to an instrument's ability to differentiate between people's performances or behaviors on some future criterion. When a school of nursing correlates students' incoming SAT scores with their subsequent grade-point averages, the predictive validity of the SATs for nursing school performance is being evaluated. **Concurrent validity** refers to an instrument's ability to distinguish among people who differ in their present status on some criterion. For example, a test to differentiate between patients in a mental institution who could and could not be released could be correlated with current behavioral ratings of health care personnel. The difference between predictive and concurrent validity, then, is the difference in the timing of obtaining measurements on a criterion.

Example of criterion-related validity:

Champion (1999) revised scales measuring women's perceived susceptibility to breast cancer and perceived benefits and barriers to mammography utilization. The predictive validity of the scales was established by examining scale scores in relation to actual mammography compliance.

Construct Validity

Validating an instrument in terms of **construct validity** is difficult and challenging. Construct validity is concerned with the following question: What construct is the instrument actually measuring? The more abstract the concept, the more difficult it is to establish the construct validity of the measure; at the same time, the more abstract the concept, the less suitable it is to a criterion-related validation approach. What objective criterion is there for concepts such as empathy, grief, and separation anxiety?

Construct validation is addressed in several ways, but there is always an emphasis on testing relationships predicted on the basis of theoretical considerations. Constructs are explicated in terms of other concepts; the researcher makes predictions about the manner in which the construct will function in relation to other constructs.

One approach to construct validation is the **known-groups technique.** In this procedure, groups that are expected to differ on the critical attribute are administered the instrument, and group scores are compared. For instance, in validating a measure of fear of the labor experience, the scores of primiparas and multiparas could be contrasted. Women who had never given birth would likely experience more anxiety than women who had already had children; one might question the validity of the instrument if such differences did not emerge.

Another method of construct validation consists of an examination of relationships based on theoretical predictions. A researcher might reason as follows: According to theory, construct X is related to construct Y; instrument A is a measure of construct X, and instrument B is a measure of construct Y; scores on A and B are related to each other, as predicted by the theory; therefore, it is inferred that A and B are valid measures of X and Y. This logical analysis is fallible and does not constitute proof of construct validity, but it offers important evidence.

Another approach to construct validation employs a statistical procedure known as **factor analysis**, which is a method for identifying clusters of related items on a scale. The procedure is used to identify and group together different measures of some underlying attribute and to distinguish them from measures of different attributes.

In summary, construct validation employs both logical and empirical procedures. Like content validity, construct validity requires a judgment pertaining to what the instrument is measuring. Construct validity and criterion-related validity share an empirical component, but, in the latter case, there is a pragmatic, objective criterion with which to compare a measure rather than a second measure of an abstract theoretical construct.

Example of construct validity:

Aminzadeh, Plotnikoff, and Edwards (1999) developed the Cane Use Cognitive Mediator Instrument, a tool to measure cognitive determinants of cane use among community-living older adults. They used the known-groups technique to validate the instrument; mean scores validly differentiated cane users and nonusers.

Interpretation of Validity

Like reliability, validity is not an all-or-nothing characteristic of an instrument. An instrument cannot really be said to possess or lack validity; it is a question of degree. The testing of an instrument's validity is not proved but rather is supported by an accumulation of evidence.

Strictly speaking, a researcher does not validate an instrument *per se* but rather some application of the instrument. A measure of anxiety may be valid for presurgical patients on the day before surgery but may not be valid for nursing students on the day of a final examination. Validation is a never-ending process: the more evidence that can be gathered that an instrument is measuring what it is supposed to be measuring, the greater the confidence researchers have in its validity.

 CONSUMER TIP:

In many studies involving structured self-report or observational instruments, the research report provides validity and reliability information from an earlier study, usually conducted by the researcher who developed the measure. If the sample characteristics in the original study and the new study are similar, the citation provides valuable information about data quality in the new study. Researchers may also compute new reliability coefficients for the actual research sample—typically, internal consistency or interrater reliability. ■

ASSESSMENT OF QUALITATIVE DATA

The assessment procedures described thus far cannot be meaningfully applied to such qualitative materials as responses in unstructured interviews or participant observers' field notes. This does not imply, however, that qualitative researchers are unconcerned with data quality. The central question underlying the concepts of validity and reliability is: Do the measures used by the researcher yield data reflecting the truth? Certainly, qualitative researchers are as eager as quantitative researchers to have their findings reflect the true state of phenomena.

Many qualitative nurse researchers seek to evaluate the quality of their data and their findings through procedures that have been outlined by Lincoln and Guba (1985), two proponents of the naturalistic paradigm of inquiry. These researchers have suggested four criteria for establishing the **trustworthiness** of qualitative data and the ensuing analysis: credibility, dependability, confirmability, and transferability.

 CONSUMER TIP:

Qualitative research reports are uneven in the amount of information they provide about data quality. Some do not address data quality issues at all, whereas others elaborate in detail the steps the researcher took to confirm trustworthiness. The absence of information makes it difficult for consumers to come to conclusions about the believability of qualitative findings. ■

Credibility

Careful qualitative researchers take steps to improve and evaluate data **credibility**, which refers to confidence in the truth of the data. Lincoln and Guba note that the credibility of an inquiry involves two aspects: first, carrying out the investigation in a way that believability is enhanced and, second, taking steps to *demonstrate* credibility. Lincoln and Guba suggest various techniques for improving and documenting the credibility of qualitative data. A few that are especially relevant to the evaluation of qualitative studies are mentioned here.

Prolonged Engagement and Persistent Observation

Lincoln and Guba recommend activities that increase the likelihood of producing credible data and interpretations. A first and very important step is **prolonged engagement**—the investment of sufficient time in data collection activities to have an in-depth understanding of the culture, language, or views of the group under study and to test for misinformation. Prolonged engagement is also essential for building trust and rapport with informants.

Credible data collection also involves **persistent observation**, which refers to the researcher's focus on the aspects of a situation that are relevant to the phenomena being studied. As Lincoln and Guba note, "If prolonged engagement provides scope, persistent observation provides depth" (1985, p. 304).

Triangulation

Triangulation, another technique to enhance credibility, is the use of multiple referents to draw conclusions about what constitutes the truth. Denzin (1989) has identified four types of triangulation:

1. **Data source triangulation:** using multiple data sources in a study (*e.g.,* interviewing diverse key informants about the same topic)
2. **Investigator triangulation:** using more than one person to collect, analyze, or interpret a set of data
3. **Theory triangulation:** using multiple perspectives to interpret a set of data
4. **Method triangulation:** using multiple methods to address a research problem (*e.g.,* observations plus interviews)

Triangulation provides a basis for convergence on the truth. By using multiple methods and perspectives, researchers strive to distinguish true information from information with errors.

Example of triangulation:

Maheady (1999) studied the experiences of nursing students with disabilities. The study involved data triangulation (interviews were conducted with students with physical or auditory impairments and with nursing faculty members, patients, and fellow students) and method triangulation (data were gathered through interviews, observations, and document analysis).

External Checks: Peer Debriefing and Member Checks

Two other techniques for establishing credibility involve external checks on the inquiry. **Peer debriefing** is a session held with objective peers to review and explore various aspects of the inquiry. Peer debriefing exposes the investigator to the searching questions of others who are experienced in either qualitative research or in the phenomenon being studied, or both. These sessions can also be useful to researchers interested in testing some working hypotheses or in exploring new avenues in the emergent research design.

Member checks refers to providing feedback to study participants regarding preliminary findings and interpretations and securing the participants' reactions. Member checking can be carried out both informally in an ongoing way as data are being collected and more formally after data have been collected and analyzed. Lincoln and Guba consider member checking the most important technique for establishing the credibility of qualitative data.

Example of member checking:

Strang and Haughey(1999) studied caregiver respite experiences through in-depth interviews with caregivers. Participants were given "the opportunity to validate, confirm, and reinterpret the findings, thereby ensuring that the reality of their respite experience was truthfully represented." (p. 453).

Searching for Disconfirming Evidence

Data credibility can be enhanced by the researcher's systematic search for data that challenge an emerging conceptualization or descriptive theory. The search for disconfirming evidence occurs through purposive sampling but is facilitated through other processes already described here, such as prolonged engagement and peer debriefings. The sampling of individuals who can offer conflicting viewpoints can greatly strengthen a comprehensive description of a phenomenon.

Lincoln and Guba refer to a similar activity of **negative case analysis**—a process by which researchers revise their hypotheses through the inclusion of cases that appear to disconfirm earlier hypotheses. The goal of this procedure is to refine a hypothesis or theory continuously until it accounts for all cases without exception.

Example of negative case analysis:

Coe and Neufeld (1999) explored perceptions of formal support among male caregivers of adults with cognitive impairments. Multiple in-depth interviews were conducted with 24 male caregivers. Data were analyzed through grounded theory procedures; variations and idiosyncracies were specifically sought. The "negative cases prompted further questions and led to modification in the analysis." (p. 572)

Researcher Credibility

Another aspect of credibility discussed by Patton (1990) is **researcher credibility**, the faith that can be put in the researcher. In qualitative studies, the researcher is the data collecting instrument—as well as the creator of the analytic process—and, therefore, the researcher's training, qualifications, and experience are important in establishing confidence in the data.

From your point of view as consumer, the research report should contain information about the researcher, including information about credentials and about any personal connections the researcher had to the people, topic, or community under study. For example, it is relevant for a reader of a report on AIDS patients' coping mechanisms to know that the researcher is HIV positive. Patton argues that the researcher should report "any personal and professional information that may have affected data collection, analysis and interpretation—negatively or positively. . . ." (1990, p. 472).

Dependability

The **dependability** of qualitative data refers to data stability over time and over conditions. It might be said that credibility (in qualitative studies) is to validity (in quantitative studies) what dependability is to reliability. Like the reliability–validity relationship in quantitative research, there can be no credibility in the absence of dependability.

One approach to assessing data dependability is to undertake a **stepwise replication.** This approach, which is conceptually similar to a split-half technique, involves having several researchers who can be divided into two teams. These teams deal with data sources separately and conduct, essentially, two independent inquiries through which data and conclusions can be compared.

Another technique relating to dependability is the **inquiry audit.** An inquiry audit involves a scrutiny of the data and relevant supporting documents by an external reviewer, an approach that also has a bearing on data confirmability, as we discuss next.

Example of dependability:

Gregory and her colleagues (1998) conducted a grounded theory study that explored patients' experiences with end-stage renal disease. All interview transcripts were read by two members of the team, and each member constructed independent interpretive summaries of the interview and then achieved consensus on the final version.

Confirmability

Confirmability refers to the objectivity or neutrality of the data, such that two or more independent people would agree about the data's relevance or meaning. In qualitative studies, the issue of confirmability does not focus on the characteristics of the researcher (is he or she objective and unbiased?) but rather on the characteristics of the data (*i.e.,* are the data confirmable?).

Inquiry audits can be used to establish both the dependability and confirmability of the data. In an inquiry audit, the investigator develops an **audit trail**, which is a systematic collection of documentation that allow an independent auditor to come to conclusions about the data. Six classes of records are important in creating an adequate audit trail: (1) raw data (*e.g.,* field notes, interview transcripts); (2) data reduction and analysis products (*e.g.,* theoretical notes, documentation on working hypotheses); (3) process notes (*e.g.,* methodologic notes, notes from member check sessions); (4) materials relating to intentions and dispositions (*e.g.,* personal notes on intentions); (5) instrument development information (*e.g.,* pilot forms); and (6) data reconstruction products (*e.g.,* drafts of the final report).

After the audit trail materials are assembled, the inquiry auditor proceeds to audit, in a fashion analogous to a financial audit, the trustworthiness of the data and the meanings attached to them. Although the auditing task is complex, it is an invaluable tool for persuading others that qualitative data are worthy of confidence.

Transferability

In Lincoln and Guba's framework, **transferability** refers to the extent to which the findings from the data can be transferred to other settings or groups and is thus similar to the concept of generalizability. This is, to some extent, an issue relating to sampling and design rather than to the soundness of the data *per se.* As Lincoln and Guba note, however, a researcher's responsibility is to provide sufficient descriptive data in the research report for consumers to evaluate the applicability of the data to other contexts: "Thus the naturalist cannot specify the external validity of an inquiry; he or she can provide only the thick description necessary to enable someone interested in making a transfer to reach a conclusion about whether transfer can be contemplated as a possibility" (1985, p. 316). **Thick description** refers to a rich, thorough description of the research setting, and the transactions and processes observed during the inquiry. Thus, if there is to be transferability, the burden of proof rests with researchers to provide sufficient information to permit judgments about contextual similarity.

CONSUMER TIP:

Because the process of assessing data quality in qualitative studies may be inextricably linked to data analysis, discussions of data quality are sometimes included in the results section rather than the method section of the report. In some cases, the text will not explicitly point out that data quality issues are being discussed. Readers may have to be alert to evidence of triangulation or other verification techniques in such statements as, "Informants' reports of experiences of serious illness were supported by reports of public health nurses." ∎

CRITIQUING DATA QUALITY

If data are seriously flawed, the study findings cannot be meaningful. Therefore, it is important for you as a consumer to consider whether the researcher has taken appropriate steps to collect data that accurately reflect reality. In both qualitative and quantitative studies, you have the right—indeed, the obligation—to ask: Can I trust the data? Do the data accurately reflect the true state of the phenomenon under study?

In quantitative studies, you should expect some discussion of the reliability and validity of the measures—preferably, information collected directly with the sample under study (rather than evidence from other studies). You should be wary about the results of quantitative studies when the report provides no information about data quality or when it suggests unfavorable reliability or validity. Also, data quality deserves special scrutiny when the research hypotheses are not confirmed. There may be many reasons that hypotheses are not supported by data (*e.g.*, too small a sample or a faulty theory), but the quality of the measures is an important area of concern. When hypotheses are not supported, one possibility is that the instruments were not good measures of the research constructs. Box 12-1 provides some guidelines for critiquing data quality in quantitative studies.

BOX 12-1

GUIDELINES FOR EVALUATING DATA QUALITY IN QUANTITATIVE STUDIES

1. Does there appear to be a strong congruence between the research variables as conceptualized (*i.e.*, as discussed in the introduction) and as operationalized (*i.e.*, as described in the method section)?

2. Do the rules for the measurement of the variables seem sensible? Were the data collected in such a way that measurement errors were minimized?

3. Does the report provide evidence of the reliability of the data? Does the evidence come from the research sample itself, or is it based on a prior study? If the latter, is it reasonable to believe that reliability would be similar for the research sample (*e.g.*, are the sample characteristics similar)?

4. If there is reliability information, what method of estimating reliability was used? Was this method appropriate? Is the reliability sufficiently high?

5. Does the report provide evidence of the validity of the measures? Does the evidence come from the research sample itself, or is it based on a prior study? If the latter, is it reasonable to believe that validity would be similar for the research sample (*e.g.*, are the sample characteristics similar)?

6. If there is validity information, what validity approach was used? Was this method appropriate? Does the validity of the instrument appear to be adequate?

BOX 12-2

GUIDELINES FOR EVALUATING DATA QUALITY IN QUALITATIVE STUDIES

1. Does the research report discuss efforts the researcher made to enhance or evaluate the trustworthiness of the data? If so, is the description sufficiently detailed and clear?

2. Which techniques (if any) did the researcher use to enhance and appraise the credibility of the data? Was the investigator in the field an adequate amount of time? Was triangulation used, and, if so, of what type? Did the researcher search for disconfirming evidence? Were there peer debriefings or member checks? Do the researcher's qualifications enhance the credibility of the data?

3. Which techniques (if any) did the researcher use to enhance and appraise the dependability, confirmability, and transferability of the data?

4. Were the procedures used to enhance and document data quality adequate? Given the procedures used (if any), what can you conclude about the trustworthiness of the data?

Information about data quality is equally important in qualitative studies. You should be particularly alert to information on data quality when a single researcher has been responsible for collecting, analyzing, and interpreting all the data, as is frequently the case. Some guidelines for critiquing the trustworthiness of data in qualitative studies are presented in Box 12-2.

CONSUMER TIP:

The amount of detail about data quality in a research report varies considerably. Some articles have virtually no information. In a few situations, such information may not be needed (*e.g.,* when biophysiologic instrumentation with a proven and widely known record for accuracy is used). Most research reports, however, should provide some evidence that data quality was sufficiently high to answer the research questions. Information about data quality normally is presented in the method section of the report. ■

RESEARCH EXAMPLES

In this section, we present examples of the efforts researchers took to assess data in a quantitative and a qualitative study. Use the relevant guidelines in Boxes 12-1 and 12-2 to evaluate the researchers' activities.

RESEARCH EXAMPLE OF A QUANTITATIVE STUDY

Bakas and Champion (1999) reported on the development and psychometric testing of the Bakas Caregiving Outcomes Scale (BCOS). The BCOS was designed to measure life changes when assuming the caregiving role for a family member with stroke. The researcher's efforts to develop a reliable and valid instrument for use by nurses and researchers are summarized below.

Research Summary

Items for the BCOS were developed based on theoretical definitions of social functioning, subjective well-being, and somatic health. Examples include "My future outlook" and "My physical health," which respondents answer on a 7-point scale from "changed for the best" to "changed for the worst." Content validity of the initial 48 items was assessed by five content experts. Items were retained only if 100% of the experts rated the item as relevant to the construct; 27 of the original 48 items were retained.

In the first testing of the instrument, 92 family caregivers of stroke survivors completed a questionnaire with the BCOS and other structured scales. Statistical procedures were used to eliminate items that were either redundant or of lower relevance on the BCOS. The resulting 12-item scale had an internal consistency reliability of .90. Construct validation was undertaken through factor analysis and by testing the relationship of BCOS scores with other respondent characteristics. For example, it was found that people with high scores on a scale of emotional distress had less favorable scores on the BCOS, as the researchers had predicted. Finally, criterion-related validity was tested by correlating BCOS scores with responses to a question asking how the caregiver's life had changed overall.

In a further testing of the BCOS with a second sample of 104 family caregivers, 2 other items were eliminated, and the internal consistency of the 10-item scale was computed to be .77. The second sample provided further support for the scale's construct and criterion-related validity. The authors concluded that the BCOS "is a brief, easy-to-administer instrument with evidence of internal consistency reliability, as well as content, construct, and criterion-related validity" (p. 258).

Clinical Relevance

Stroke is the most frequent cause of disability among seniors and is the second most common cause of dementia. Family caregivers of stroke survivors experience depression and other emotional problems, social confinement, and general ill health. An instrument that measures changes in social functioning, subjective well-being, and health of family caregivers of stroke patients could be used to identify caregivers in need of nursing interventions.

One of the strengths of the BCOS is its theoretical base. The items on this instrument were developed from Lazaras' transaction-based approach to stress. The acceptable levels of reliability and validity achieved in the psychometric testing of the BCOS with two predominantly Caucasian samples provide evidence of its clinical applicability. Further psychometric testing is needed, however, with minority populations.

The authors indicated that "the scale could easily be used as an assessment tool to determine family caregivers in need of intervention, as well as to document their progress over time" (p. 258). Home care nurses who have stroke survivors in their caseload could periodically assess any changes in their family caregivers using the BCOS. If any deterioration in the caregivers' social functioning, subjective well-being, or overall health is detected, nurses could then intervene to support family caregivers.

RESEARCH EXAMPLE OF A QUALITATIVE STUDY

Banister (1999) conducted an ethnographic study to explore mid-life women's perceptions of their changing bodies within the Western cultural context. The study involved in-depth interviews with 23 mid-life women. Her efforts to enhance and document data quality are summarized below.

Research Summary

Data collection in this study was carried out in two phases. The first phase involved in-depth, unstructured interviews with study participants. The second phase involved gathering the participants into groups for verification of emerging domains and further theory development.

Methods used to strengthen the data's credibility included triangulation, peer debriefing, member checks, and the maintenance of a reflective journal by the researcher, who was herself a mid-life woman. With respect to member checking, the author wrote, "To assure that the analysis accurately represented the social world of mid-life women, participants were invited to comment on the analyzed material throughout the research process and to suggest changes where they felt the materials did not reflect their experiences" (p. 525). Banister recognized that her position as a woman in mid-life could both enhance and threaten the truth value of the study. She therefore maintained a reflective journal in which she reflected on reactions in the field and ways in which they might influence her interpretation and the representation of the women's experiences.

With respect to dependability and confirmability, Banister maintained an audit trail in a research journal that documented all of her methodologic decisions. Transferability was facilitated through rich description of the women and their contexts.

The results of this rigorous qualitative study indicated that women's mid-life experience of their changing bodies is full of contradiction and change. Issues of loss, cultural influences that perpetuate ageism and sexism, lack of consistent information about menopause, questioning, redefining self, and self-care all played a central role in the women's lives during this time of transition.

Clinical Relevance

Growing proportions of women are entering mid-life, and yet there appears to be little solid information about their perceptions, their situations, and their health care needs. Banister's study makes a contribution to our understanding of mid-life women's experiences and the role that sociocultural and physiologic factors play in those experiences. Banister conducted a careful study that was strengthened by her steps to enhance and ensure data quality.

Banister found that a salient characteristic of the mid-life experience of women was their questioning about their changing bodies and critically reflecting on the cultural construction of their realities—findings that have implications for clinical practice. Educating women regarding menopause and their changing bodies is a critical nursing intervention. Women need not only facts about what is happening to their changing bodies but also opportunities to discuss the ambiguity between cultural stereotypes of mid-life women and their personal experiences. One such type of opportunity could be a support group facilitated by nurses in which cultural avoidance of issues facing mid-life women could be openly discussed. By encouraging mid-life women to reflect and question critically, health care providers can assist them to enhance the quality of their lives. The findings also suggest that nurses and other health care professionals could profitably engage in critically questioning their own assumptions and biases toward mid-life women. These biases could influence the caring they provide these women. Nurses are in an excellent position with their many interactions with women to help to demystify our society's attitudes and beliefs about the mid-life transition in women's lives.

• • • • • *SUMMARY POINTS*

- **Measurement** involves a set of rules according to which numeric values are assigned to objects to represent varying degrees of some attribute.
- Few quantitative measuring instruments are infallible. Sources of measurement error include situational contaminants, response set biases, and transitory personal factors, such as fatigue.
- **Obtained scores** from an instrument consist of a **true score** component—the value that would be obtained if it were possible to have a perfect measure of the attribute—and an error component, or **error of measurement**, that represents measurement inaccuracies.
- **Reliability** is the degree of consistency or accuracy with which an instrument measures an attribute. The higher the reliability of an instrument, the lower the amount of error in the obtained scores.
- There are different methods for assessing an instrument's reliability and for computing a **reliability coefficient**. The **stability** aspect, which concerns the extent to which the instrument yields the same results on repeated administrations, is evaluated by **test–retest procedures**.
- The **internal consistency** aspect of reliability, which refers to the extent to which all the instrument's items are measuring the same attribute, is assessed using either the **split-half reliability technique** or, more likely, **Cronbach's alpha method**.

- When the focus of a reliability assessment is on establishing **equivalence** between observers in rating or coding behaviors, estimates of **interrater** (or **interobserver**) **reliability** are obtained.
- **Validity** is the degree to which an instrument measures what it is supposed to be measuring.
- **Content validity** is concerned with the sampling adequacy of the content being measured.
- **Criterion-related validity** focuses on the correlation between the instrument and an outside criterion.
- **Construct validity** refers to the adequacy of an instrument in measuring the construct of interest. One construct validation method is the **known-groups technique**, which contrasts the scores of groups that are presumed to differ on the attribute; another is **factor analysis**, a statistical procedure for identifying unitary clusters of items or measures.
- Qualitative researchers evaluate the **trustworthiness** of their data using the criteria of credibility, dependability, confirmability, and transferability.
- **Credibility**, roughly analogous to validity in a quantitative study, refers to the believability of the data. Techniques to improve the credibility of qualitative data include **prolonged engagement**, which strives for adequate scope of data coverage, and **persistent observation**, which is aimed at achieving adequate depth.
- **Triangulation** is the process of using multiple referents to draw conclusions about what constitutes the truth. The four major forms are **data source triangulation, investigator triangulation, theoretical triangulation, and method triangulation**.
- Two important tools for establishing credibility are **peer debriefings**, wherein the researcher obtains feedback about data quality and interpretation from peers, and **member checks**, wherein informants are asked to comment on the data and the researcher's interpretations.
- **Dependability** of qualitative data refers to the stability of data over time and over conditions and is somewhat analogous to the concept of reliability in quantitative studies.
- **Confirmability** refers to the objectivity or neutrality of the data. Independent inquiry audits by external auditors can be used to assess and document dependability and confirmability.
- **Transferability** is the extent to which findings from the data can be transferred to other settings or groups. Transferability can be enhanced through **thick descriptions** of the context of the data collection.

➤ ➤ ➤ ➤ *CRITICAL THINKING ACTIVITIES*

Chapter 12 of the accompanying *Study Guide to Accompany Essentials of Nursing Research,* 5th edition offers various exercises and study suggestions for reinforcing the concepts presented in this chapter. In addition, you can consider the following:

1. Read the method section from one or both of the actual research studies in the Appendix of this book, and then answer the questions in Box 12-1 and 12-2.

2. In the example in the text illustrating test–retest reliability, Stuppy (1998) calculated the reliability coefficient as .70. Why do you think the coefficient wasn't higher?

3. In the example in the text illustrating interrater reliability, Stewart and her colleagues (1999) found that the reliability was higher in the interval format than in the event format. Why do you think this occurred?

4. Comment on the efforts that Vivian and Wilcox (2000) used to enhance data quality in their qualitative study described in the research example in Chapter 11.

For additional review, see questions 156–171 on the study CD provided with Polit: Study Guide to Accompany Essentials of Nursing Research.

SUGGESTED READINGS

Methodologic References

Brink, P. J. (1991). Issues of reliability and validity. In J. M. Morse (Ed.). *Qualitative nursing research: A contemporary dialogue.* Newbury Park, CA: Sage.

Denzin, N. K. (1989). *The research act* (3rd ed.). New York: McGraw-Hill.

Guilford, J. P. (1964). *Psychometric methods* (2nd ed.). New York: McGraw-Hill.

Kerlinger, F. N. (1986). *Foundations of behavioral research* (3rd ed). New York: Holt, Rinehart & Winston.

Lincoln, Y. S., & Guba, E. G. (1985). *Naturalistic inquiry.* Newbury Park, CA: Sage.

Nunnally, J. (1978). *Psychometric theory.* New York: McGraw-Hill.

Patton, M. Q. (1990). *Qualitative evaluation and research methods.* Newbury Park, CA: Sage.

Waltz, C. F., Strickland, O. L., & Lenz, E. R. (1991). *Measurement in nursing research* (2nd ed.). Philadelphia: F. A. Davis.

Substantive References

Aminzadeh, F., Plotnikoff, R., & Edwards, N. (1999). Development and evaluation of the Cane Use Cognitive Mediator Instrument. *Nursing Research, 48,* 269–275.

Bakas, T., & Champion, V. (1999). Development and psychometric testing of the Bakas Caregiving Outcomes Scale. *Nursing Research, 48,* 250–259.

Banister, E. M. (1999). Women's mid-life experience of their changing bodies. *Qualitative Health Research, 9,* 520–537.

Champion, V. L. (1999). Revised Susceptibility, Benefits, and Barriers Scale for mammography screening. *Research in Nursing & Health, 22,* 341–348.

Coe, M., & Neufeld, A. (1999). Male caregivers' use of formal support. *Western Journal of Nursing Research, 21,* 568–588.

Gregory, D. M., Way, C. Y., Hutchinson, T. A., Barrett, B. J., & Parfrey, P. A. (1998). Patients' perceptions of their experiences with ESRD and hemodialysis treatment. *Qualitative Health Research, 8,* 764–783.

Hess, R. G. (1998). Measuring nursing governance. *Nursing Research, 47,* 35–42.

Leidy, N. K. (1999). Psychometric properties of the Functional Performance Inventory in patients with chronic obstructive pulmonary disease. *Nursing Research, 48,* 20–28.

Maheady, D. C. (1999). Jumping through hoops, walking on egg shells: The experiences of nursing students with disabilities. *Journal of Nursing Education, 38,* 162–170.

Stewart, N. J., Hiscock, M., Morgan, D. G., Murphy, P. B., & Yamamoto, M. (1999). Development and psychometric evaluation of the Environment–Behavior Interaction Code (EBIC). *Nursing Research, 48,* 261–268.

Stordeur, S., Vandenbergue, C., & D'hoore, W. (2000). Leadership styles across hierarchical levels in nursing departments. *Nursing Research, 49,* 37–43.

Strang, V. R., & Haughey, M. (1999). Respite: A coping strategy for family caregivers. *Western Journal of Nursing Research, 21,* 450–471.

Stuppy, D. J. (1998). The FACES pain scale: Reliability and validity with mature adults. *Applied Nursing Research, 11,* 84–89.

PART V

ANALYSIS OF RESEARCH DATA

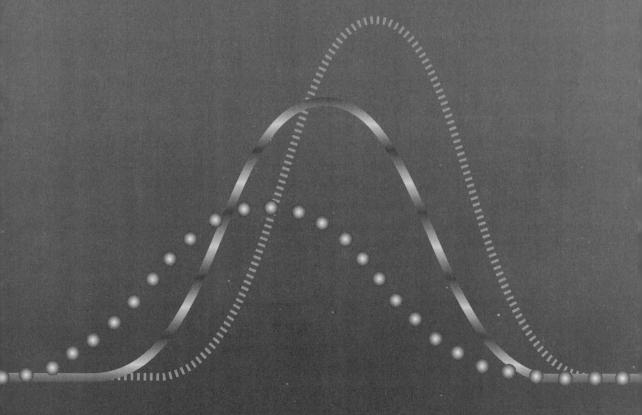

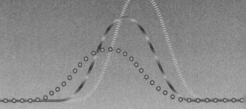

CHAPTER 13

Analyzing Quantitative Data

Student Objectives

On completion of this chapter, the student will be able to:

○ identify the four levels of measurement and describe and compare characteristics of each
○ distinguish descriptive and inferential statistics
○ describe the characteristics and shapes of frequency distributions
○ identify and compare measures of central tendency and variability and interpret these measures
○ interpret a correlation coefficient
○ describe the principle of sampling distributions
○ describe the logic and purpose of tests of statistical significance and describe hypothesis testing procedures
○ distinguish the characteristics and uses of parametric and nonparametric tests
○ specify the appropriate applications for *t*-tests, analysis of variance, chi-squared tests, and correlation coefficients and interpret the meaning of the calculated statistics
○ describe the applications and principles of multiple regression and analysis of covariance
○ understand the results of simple statistical procedures described in a research report
○ define new terms in the chapter

New Terms

Alpha
Analysis of covariance (ANCOVA)
Analysis of variance (ANOVA)
Bell-shaped curve
Bimodal distribution
Bivariate descriptive statistics
Causal modeling
Central tendency
Chi-squared test
Contingency table
Correlation
Correlation coefficient
Correlation matrix
Covariate
Cross-tabulation
Degrees of freedom
Dependent groups *t*-test
Descriptive statistics
Discriminant function analysis

Estimation procedures
F ratio
Factor analysis
Frequency distribution
Frequency polygon
Hypothesis testing
Independent groups *t*-test
Inferential statistics
Interaction effects
Interval measurement
Inverse relationship
Laws of probability
Level of significance
Level of measurement
Linear structural relations analysis (LISREL)
Logistic regression
Logit analysis
Main effects

Mean

Median

Mode

Multimodal distribution

Multiple comparison procedures

Multiple correlation analysis

Multiple correlation coefficient

Multiple regression analysis

Multivariate analysis of covariance (MANCOVA)

Multivariate analysis of variance (MANOVA)

Multivariate statistics

N

Negative relationship

Negative skew

Nominal measurement

Nonsignificant result

Normal distribution

Nonparametric test

Null hypothesis

Odds

Odds ratio

Ordinal measurement

p value

Paired t-test

Parametric test

Parameter

Path analysis

Pearson's r

Perfect relationship

Positive relationship

Positive skew

Post hoc tests

Product–moment correlation coefficient

r

R

R^2

Range

Ratio measurement

Repeated measures ANOVA

Sampling distribution of the mean

Sampling error

Skewed distribution

Spearman's rank-order correlation (Spearman's rho)

Standard deviation

Standard error of the mean

Statistic

Statistical test

Statistically significant

Symmetric distribution

Test statistic

t-test

Two-way ANOVA

Type I error

Type II error

Unimodal distribution

Univariate descriptive statistics

Variability

Variance

The data collected in a study do not by themselves answer research questions or test research hypotheses. The data need to be systematically analyzed so that trends and patterns of relationships can be detected. This chapter describes statistical procedures for analyzing quantitative data, and Chapter 14 discusses the analysis of qualitative data.

LEVELS OF MEASUREMENT

A quantitative measure can be classified according to its **level of measurement.** This classification system is important because the types of statistical analysis that can be performed depend on the measurement level employed. There are four major classes, or levels, of measurement:

1. **Nominal measurement**, the lowest level, involves using numbers simply to categorize characteristics. Examples of variables that are nominally measured include gender, blood type, and nursing specialty. The numbers assigned in nominal measurement do not convey quantitative information. If we establish a rule to code males as 1 and females as 2, the numbers have no numeric meaning. The number 2 here does not mean "more than" 1. Nominal measurement provides information only about categorical equivalence and nonequivalence; hence, the numbers cannot be treated mathematically. It is nonsensical, for example, to compute the average gender of the sample by adding the numeric values and dividing by the number of participants.

> **Example of nominal measurement:**
>
> Meek (2000) compared healthy subjects and patients with chronic obstructive pulmonary disease (COPD) in a study of the effect of attention on the perception of breathlessness. Health group status (healthy versus COPD) was a nominal variable.

2. **Ordinal measurement** ranks objects based on their relative standing on a specified attribute. If a researcher rank-orders people from heaviest to lightest, this is ordinal measurement. As another example, consider this ordinal scheme for measuring ability to perform activities of daily living: 1 = is completely dependent; 2 = needs another person's assistance; 3 = needs mechanical assistance; and 4 = is completely independent. The numbers signify incremental ability to perform the activities of daily living independently. Ordinal measurement does not, however, tell us how much greater one level of an attribute is than another level. For example, we do not know if being completely independent is twice as good as needing mechanical assistance. As with nominal measures, the mathematic operations permissible with ordinal-level data are restricted.

> **Example of ordinal measurement:**
>
> Cheever and Hardin (1999) studied the effects of traumatic events and social supports on adolescents' self-health assessments. Self-health, the dependent variable, was measured on an ordinal scale: (1) poor; (2) fair; (3) good; and (4) excellent.

3. **Interval measurement** occurs when the researcher can specify the ranking of objects on an attribute and the distance between those objects. Most educational and psychological tests (*e.g.,* the Scholastic Aptitude Test, or SAT) are based on interval scales. A score of 550 on the SAT is higher than a score of 500, which, in turn, is higher than 450. Moreover, the difference between 550 and 500 is presumed to be equivalent to the difference between 500 and 450. Interval scales expand analytic possibilities: interval-level data can be averaged mean-

ingfully, for example. Many sophisticated statistical procedures require interval measurements.

Example of interval measurement:

King (2000), in a study designed to examine gender differences on early recovery from cardiac surgery, administered several psychosocial scales that were interval measures, including a 5-item social support scale and the 12-item Duke Activity Status Index.

---

4. **Ratio measurement** is the highest level of measurement. Ratio scales, unlike interval scales, have a rational, meaningful zero and therefore provide information about the absolute magnitude of the attribute. For example, the Fahrenheit scale for measuring temperature (interval measurement) has an arbitrary zero point. Zero on the thermometer does not signify the absence of heat; it would not be appropriate to say that 60°F is twice as hot as 30°F. Many physical measures, however, are ratio measures with a rational zero. A person's weight, for example, is a ratio measure. It is perfectly acceptable to say that someone who weighs 200 lb is twice as heavy as someone who weighs 100 lb. All the statistical procedures suitable for interval data are also appropriate for ratio-level data.

Example of ratio measurement:

Hill, Kurkowski, and Garcia (2000) studied the effect of oral support on preterm infants' nutritive sucking patterns and cardiopulmonary functions. Most of their outcome measures were on a ratio scale, including number and duration of sucking bursts, number and duration of pauses, and heart beat.

Researchers generally strive to use the highest levels of measurement possible because higher levels yield more information and are amenable to more powerful analytic procedures than lower levels.

DESCRIPTIVE STATISTICS

Without statistics, quantitative data would be a chaotic mass of numbers. Statistical procedures enable the researcher to summarize, organize, interpret, and communicate numeric information. Statistics are classified as either descriptive or inferential. **Descriptive statistics** are used to describe and synthesize data. Averages and percentages are examples of descriptive statistics. When such indexes are calculated on data from a population, they are referred to as **parameters.** A descriptive index from a sample is a **statistic.** Most scientific questions are about parameters; researchers calculate statistics to estimate them.

Frequency Distributions

Data that are not analyzed or organized are overwhelming. It is not even possible to discern general trends in the data without some structure. Consider the 60 numbers in Table 13-1. Let us assume that these numbers are the scores of 60 high school students on a 30-item test of knowledge about AIDS—scores that are on an interval scale. Visual inspection of the numbers in this table provides little insight on student performance.

Frequency distributions are a method of imposing order on numeric data. A **frequency distribution** is a systematic arrangement of numeric values from the lowest to the highest, together with a count (or percentage) of the number of times each value was obtained. The 60 test scores are presented as a frequency distribution in Table 13-2. This arrangement makes it convenient to see at a glance the highest and lowest scores, the most common score, where the scores clustered, and how many students were in the sample (total sample size is typically designated as *N* in research reports). None of this was easily discernible before the data were organized.

Some researchers display frequency data graphically in a **frequency polygon** (Fig. 13-1). In frequency polygons, scores are on the horizontal line (with the lowest value on the left), and the vertical line indicates frequency counts or percentages. Data distributions are sometimes described by their shapes. **Symmetric distribution** occurs if, when folded over, the two halves of a frequency polygon would be superimposed (Fig. 13-2). In an asymmetric or **skewed distribution**, the peak is off center, and one tail is longer than the other. When the longer tail is pointed toward the right, the distribution has a **positive skew**, as in the first graph of Figure 13-3. Personal income is an example of a positively skewed attribute. Most people have moderate incomes, with only a few people with high incomes at the right end of the distribution. If the longer tail points to the left, the distribution has a **negative skew**, as in the second graph in Figure 13-3. Age at death is an example of a negatively skewed attribute. Here, the bulk of people are at the far right end of the distribution, with relatively few people dying at an early age.

Another aspect of a distribution's shape concerns how many peaks or high points it has. A **unimodal distribution** has one peak (graph A, Fig. 13-2),

TABLE 13-1.   AIDS Knowledge Test Scores

22	27	25	19	24	25	23	29	24	20
26	16	20	26	17	22	24	18	26	28
15	24	23	22	21	24	20	25	18	27
24	23	16	25	30	29	27	21	23	24
26	18	30	21	17	25	22	24	29	28
20	25	26	24	23	19	27	28	25	26

TABLE 13-2. Frequency Distribution of AIDS Knowledge Test Scores		
SCORE	FREQUENCY	PERCENTAGE
15	1	1.7
16	2	3.3
17	2	3.3
18	3	5.0
19	2	3.3
20	4	6.7
21	3	5.0
22	4	6.7
23	5	8.3
24	9	15.0
25	7	11.7
26	6	10.0
27	4	6.7
28	3	5.0
29	3	5.0
30	2	3.3
	$N = 60$	100.0

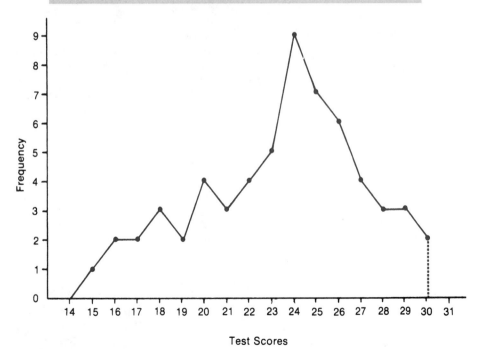

FIGURE 13-1. Frequency polygon of AIDS knowledge test scores.

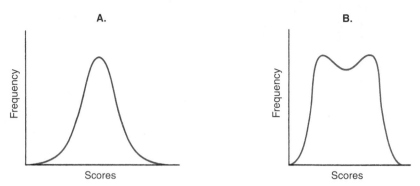

FIGURE 13-2. Examples of symmetric distributions.

whereas a **multimodal distribution** has two or more peaks—that is, two or more values of high frequency. A multimodal distribution with two peaks is a **bimodal distribution**, illustrated in graph B of Figure 13-2.

Some distributions have special names. Of particular interest is the **normal distribution** (sometimes referred to as a **bell-shaped curve**). A normal distribution is symmetric, unimodal, and not very peaked, as illustrated in graph A of Figure 13-2. Many attributes of humans (*e.g.*, height, intelligence, grip strength) have been found to approximate a normal distribution.

Example of frequency information:

Table 13-3 presents distribution information on sample characteristics from a study of the effect of relaxation therapy on preterm labor outcomes (Janke, 1999). This table shows, for selected background characteristics, both the frequency *(N)* and percentage of sample members in various categories. For example, 76 subjects (71.0%) were married and 31 (29.0%) were unmarried.

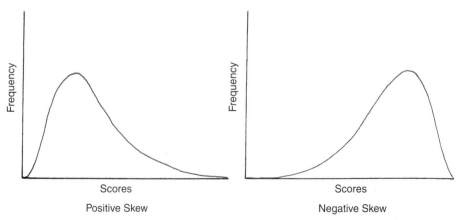

FIGURE 13-3. Examples of skewed distributions.

TABLE 13-3.	Example of Table Showing Frequency Distribution Information: Sample Characteristics in Study of the Effect of Relaxation Therapy on Preterm Labor Outcomes	
CATEGORY	**N = 107**	**PERCENTAGE**
Race/ethnicity	White: 92	86.0
	Nonwhite: 15	14.0
Marital status	Married: 76	71.0
	Unmarried: 31	29.0
Income	$25,000 or less: 33	31.4
	>$25,000 to 55,000: 36	34.3
	>$55,000: 36	34.3
Parity	Nullipara: 43	40.2
	Primipara: 44	41.1
	Multipara: 20	18.7

Adapted from Janke, J. (1999). The effect of relaxation therapy on preterm labor outcomes. *Journal of Obstetric, Gynecologic, and Neonatal Nursing, 28,* 255–263, Table 1.

Central Tendency

For variables on an interval or ratio scale, a distribution of values is usually of less interest than an overall summary. The researcher asks such questions as: What was the average postintervention blood pressure of the patients? How depressed was the typical mother after childbirth? These questions seek a single number that best represents the whole distribution. Such indexes of typicalness are measures of **central tendency.** To lay people, the term *average* is normally used to designate central tendency. There are three commonly used kinds of averages, or measures of central tendency: the mode, the median, and the mean.

- **Mode:** The mode is the number that occurs most frequently in a distribution. In the following distribution, the mode is 53:

  50 51 51 52 53 53 53 53 54 55 56

The value of 53 was obtained four times, a higher frequency than for other numbers. The mode of the AIDS knowledge test scores was 24 (see Table 13-2). The mode, in other words, identifies the most popular value. The mode is used primarily for describing typical or high-frequency values for nominal measures. For example, in the study by Janke (see Table 13-3), we could make the following statement: The typical (modal) patient was a white, married primipara with an income of more than $25,000.

- **Median:** The median is that point in a distribution above which and below which 50% of the cases fall. Consider the following set of values:

2 2 3 3 4 5 6 7 8 9

The value that divides the cases in half is midway between 4 and 5, and thus 4.5 is the median. For the AIDS knowledge test scores, the median is 24. An important characteristic of the median is that it does not take into account individual score values and is thus insensitive to extreme values. In the above set of values, if the value of 9 were changed to 99, the median would remain 4.5. Because of this property, the median is the preferred index of central tendency with highly skewed distributions and when a single typical value is of interest. In research reports, the median may be abbreviated as *Md* or *Mdn*.

- **Mean:** The mean is equal to the sum of all values divided by the number of participants—in other words, what people refer to as the average. The mean of the AIDS knowledge test scores is 23.42 (1405 ÷ 60). As another example, consider the following weights of eight people:

85 109 120 135 158 177 181 195

In this example, the mean is 145. Unlike the median, the mean is affected by the value of every score. If we were to exchange the 195-lb person for one weighing 275 lb, the mean weight would increase from 145 to 155 lb. A substitution of this kind would leave the median unchanged. In research reports, the mean is often symbolized as M or $\bar{X}$ (e.g., $\bar{X} = 145$).

For interval-level or ratio-level measurements, the mean, rather than the median or mode, is usually the statistic reported. Of the three indexes, the mean is the most stable: if repeated samples were drawn from a population, the means would fluctuate less than the modes or medians. Because of its stability, the mean generally is the best estimate of the central tendency of the population. When a distribution is highly skewed, however, the mean does not characterize the center of the distribution; in such situations, the median is preferred. For example, the median is a better central tendency measure of family income than the mean because income is positively skewed.

Variability

Two sets of data with identical means could be quite different with respect to how spread out or dispersed the data are (*i.e.,* how different the people are from one another on the attribute of interest). The **variability** of two distributions could be different even when the means are identical.

Consider the distributions in Figure 13-4, which represent hypothetical scores of students from two high schools on the SAT. Both distributions have an average score of 500, but the two groups of students are clearly dif-

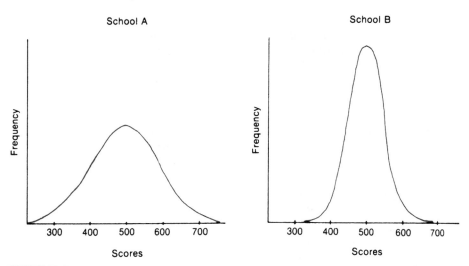

FIGURE 13-4. Two distributions of different variability.

ferent. In school A, there is a wide range of scores—from scores below 300 to some above 700. In school B, on the other hand, there are few low scorers but also few outstanding test achievers. School A is more heterogeneous (*i.e.,* more variable) than school B, whereas school B is more homogeneous than school A.

Researchers compute an index of variability to summarize the extent to which scores in a distribution differ from one another. Several such indexes have been developed, the most important of which are the range and the standard deviation.

- **Range:** The range is the highest score minus the lowest score in a distribution. In the example of the AIDS knowledge test scores, the range is 15 (30 − 15). In the distributions in Figure 13-4, the range for school A is 500 (750 − 250), whereas the range for school B is 300 (650 − 350). The chief virtue of the range is its ease of computation. Because it is based on only two scores, however, the range is unstable: from sample to sample drawn from the same population, the range tends to fluctuate considerably. Moreover, the range ignores score variations between the two extremes. In school B of Figure 13-4, if a single student obtained a score of 250 and another obtained a score of 750, the range of both schools would then be 500—despite large differences in their heterogeneity. For these reasons, the range is used largely as a gross descriptive index.
- **Standard deviation:** The most widely used variability index is the standard deviation. Like the mean, the standard deviation is calculated based on every value in a distribution. The standard deviation summarizes the average amount of deviation of values from the mean. In the

AIDS knowledge test example, the standard deviation is 3.725.* In research reports, the standard deviation is often abbreviated as *s* or *SD*. Occasionally, the standard deviation is simply shown in relation to the mean without a formal label, such as M = 4 (1.5) or M = 4 ± 1.5, where 4 is the mean and 1.5 is the standard deviation.†

A standard deviation is more difficult to interpret than the range. With regard to the AIDS knowledge test, you might well ask, 3.725 *what?* What does the number mean? We will try to answer these questions from several angles. First, as discussed, the SD is an index of how variable scores in a distribution are. If two groups of students had means of 23 on the AIDS knowledge test, but one group had an SD of 7 and the other had an SD of 3, we would immediately know that the second group was more homogeneous (*i.e.,* their scores were more similar to one another).

The standard deviation represents the average of deviations from the mean. The mean tells us the single best point for summarizing an entire distribution, and a standard deviation tells us how much, on average, the scores deviate from that mean. In the AIDS test example, they deviated by an average of just under 4 points. A standard deviation might thus be interpreted as an indication of our degree of error when we use a mean to describe an entire data set.

In normal and near-normal distributions, there are roughly three standard deviations above and below the mean. Suppose we had a normal distribution with a mean of 50 and an SD of 10 (Fig. 13-5). In such a distribution, a fixed percentage of cases fall within certain distances from the mean. Sixty-eight percent of all cases fall within 1 SD above and below the mean. Thus, in this example, nearly 7 of 10 scores are between 40 and 60. Ninety-five percent of the scores in a normal distribution fall within 2 SDs from the mean. Only a handful of cases—about 2% at each extreme—lie more than 2 SDs from the mean. Using this figure, we can see that a person who obtained a score of 70 achieved a higher score than about 98% of the sample.

Example of means and SDs:

Some measures of central tendency and variability from an actual nursing study are presented in Table 13-4. This study (Picot, Zauszniewski, Debanne, & Holston, 1999) examined the mood and blood pressure responses of black female caregivers and noncaregivers. The table shows the means and standard

---

*Formulas for computing the standard deviation, as well as other statistics discussed in this chapter, are not shown in this textbook. The emphasis here is on helping readers to understand the statistics and their applications. References at the end of the chapter can be consulted for computation formulas.

†Occasionally, a research report will make a reference to an index of variability known as the **variance**. The variance is simply the value of the standard deviation squared. In the example of the AIDS knowledge test scores, the variance is 3.725^2, or 13.876.

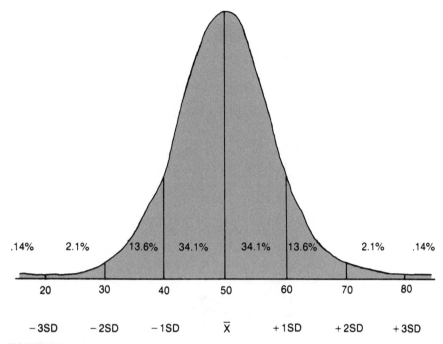

.14%   2.1%   13.6%   34.1%   34.1%   13.6%   2.1%   .14%

20   30   40   50   60   70   80

−3SD   −2SD   −1SD $\overline{X}$ +1SD   +2SD   +3SD

FIGURE 13-5. Standard deviations in a normal distribution.

deviations of the two groups of women on five dependent variables: three mood states (anger, anxiety, and sadness) and diastolic and systolic blood pressure. The table indicates that caregivers had higher scores than noncaregivers on all outcomes except for diastolic blood pressure. Moreover, for every outcome, the caregivers were more heterogeneous than the noncaregivers, as can be seen by comparing the standard deviations in parentheses.

TABLE 13-4. Example of Table Showing Central Tendency and Variability: Study of Mood and Blood Pressure Responses in Black Female Caregivers and Noncaregivers

CHARACTERISTICS	NONCAREGIVERS ($n = 38$) $\overline{X}$(SD)	CAREGIVERS ($n = 37$) $\overline{X}$(SD)
Anger	2.10 (1.38)	2.71 (1.45)
Anxiety	2.65 (1.66)	3.21 (1.57)
Sadness	3.53 (1.72)	3.96 (1.80)
Diastolic blood pressure	81.37 (9.32)	78.96 (10.63)
Systolic blood pressure	130.48 (14.24)	131.18 (17.51)

Adapted from Picot, S.F., Zauszniewski, J.A., Debanne, S.M., & Holston, E.C. (1999). Mood and blood pressure responses in black female caregivers and noncaregivers. *Nursing Research, 48*, 62–70, Table 2.

Bivariate Descriptive Statistics

So far, our discussion has focused on descriptive indexes of single variables—**univariate** (one-variable) **descriptive statistics.** The mean, mode, standard deviation, and so forth are used to describe one variable at a time. Research usually is concerned, however, with relationships. **Bivariate** (two-variable) **descriptive statistics** describe relationships between two variables.

Contingency Tables

A **contingency table** is a two-dimensional frequency distribution in which the frequencies of two variables are **cross-tabulated.** Suppose we have data on patients' gender and whether they are nonsmokers, light smokers (≤1 pack of cigarettes a day), or heavy smokers (>1 pack a day). Here, the question is whether there is a tendency for men to smoke more heavily than women or *vice versa.* Some fictitious data on these two variables are shown in a contingency table in Table 13-5. Six cells are created by placing one variable (gender) along the vertical dimension and the other variable (smoking status) along the horizontal dimension. After all subjects are allocated to the appropriate cells, percentages can be computed. This simple procedure allows us to see at a glance that, in this sample, women were more likely than men to be nonsmokers (45.4% versus 27.3%) and less likely to be heavy smokers (18.2% versus 36.4%). Contingency tables usually are used with nominal data or ordinal data that have few levels or ranks. In the present example, gender is a nominal measure, and smoking status is an ordinal measure.

> *Example of a contingency table:*
>
> Table 13-6 presents a cross-tabulation table from an actual study that examined the presence of dyspnea in emergency department visits among patients with

TABLE 13-5. Contingency Table for Gender and Smoking Status Relationship

| | GENDER | | | | | |
| | Female | | Male | | Total | |
SMOKING STATUS	*N*	%	*N*	%	*N*	%
Nonsmoker	JHI IHI 10	45.4	JHI I 6	27.3	16	36.4
Light smoker	JHI III 8	36.4	JHI III 8	36.4	16	36.4
Heavy smoker	IIII 4	18.2	JHI III 8	36.4	12	27.3
TOTAL	22	50.0	22	50.0	44	100.0

TABLE 13-6. **Example of a Contingency Table: Study of Dyspnea in Relation to Diagnoses and Dispositions**

DIAGNOSIS	DYSPNEA %	DYSPNEA n	NO DYSPNEA %	NO DYSPNEA n	TOTAL n
COPD	78.2	187	21.8	52	239
Asthma	87.6	346	12.4	49	395
Mixed COPD and asthma	66.7	12	33.3	6	18
Restrictive	71.4	10	28.6	4	14
Congestive heart failure	61.6	197	38.4	123	320
TOTAL	76.3	752	23.7	234	986

COPD, chronic obstructive pulmonary disease.
Adapted from Parshall M.B. (1999). Adult emergency visits for chronic cardiorespiratory disease: Does dyspnea matter? *Nursing Research, 48,* 62–70, Table 2.

chronic cardiorespiratory diseases (Parshall, 1999). The table shows, for patients with different diseases, whether there was a dyspnea complaint. Overall, 76.3% of the sample reported dyspnea. Asthmatic patients were especially likely to report dyspnea: 87.6% of the asthmatic patients, compared with 61.6% of those with congestive heart failure, reported dyspnea.

A comparison of Tables 13-5 and 13-6 illustrates that cross-tabulated data can be presented in one of two ways: cell percentages can be computed on the basis of either row totals or column totals. In Table 13-5, the number 10 in the first cell (female nonsmokers) was divided by the column total (*i.e.,* by the total number of females—22) to arrive at the percentage (45%) of females who were nonsmokers. (The table might well have shown 63% in this cell—the percentage of nonsmokers who were female). In Table 13-6, the number 187 in the first cell (COPD patients with dyspnea) was divided by the row total (*i.e.,* by the total number of COPD patients—239) to yield the percentage of 78.2%. Computed the other way, the researcher would have gotten 24.9%— the percentage of patients with dyspnea who had a COPD diagnosis. Either approach is acceptable, although the former is generally preferred because then the percentages in a column add up to 100%.

 CONSUMER TIP:

You may need to spend an extra minute when examining cross-tabulation tables to determine which total—row or column—was used as the basis for calculating percentages. ■

Correlation

The most common method of describing the relationship between two variables is through **correlation** procedures. The correlation question is: To what extent are two variables related to each other? For example, to what degree are anxiety test scores and blood pressure measures related? This question can be answered quantitatively by calculating a **correlation coefficient**, which describes the *intensity* and *direction* of a relationship.

Two variables that are related are height and weight: tall people tend to weigh more than short people. The relationship between height and weight would be a **perfect relationship** if the tallest person in a population was the heaviest, the second tallest person was the second heaviest, and so on. The correlation coefficient summarizes how "perfect" a relationship is. The possible values for a correlation coefficient range from −1.00 through .00 to +1.00. If height and weight were perfectly correlated, the correlation coefficient expressing this would be 1.00 (the actual correlation coefficient is in the vicinity of .50 to .60 for a general population). Height and weight have a **positive relationship** because greater height tends to be associated with greater weight.

When two variables are unrelated, the correlation coefficient is zero. One might anticipate that a woman's dress size is unrelated to her intelligence. Large women are as likely to perform well on tests of mental ability as small women. The correlation coefficient summarizing such a relationship would presumably be in the vicinity of .00.

Correlation coefficients running between .00 and −1.00 express a **negative**, or **inverse, relationship.** When two variables are inversely related, increments in one variable are associated with decrements in the second. For example, there is a negative correlation between depression and self-esteem. This means that, on average, people with *high* self-esteem tend to be *low* on depression. If the relationship were perfect (*i.e.*, if the person with the highest self-esteem score had the lowest depression score and so on), then the correlation coefficient would be −1.00. In actuality, the relationship between depression and self-esteem is usually moderate—in the vicinity of −.40 or −.50. Note that the higher the *absolute value* of the coefficient (*i.e.*, the value disregarding the sign), the stronger the relationship. A correlation of −.80, for instance, is much stronger than a correlation of +.20.

The most commonly used correlation index is the **product–moment correlation coefficient** (also referred to as **Pearson's** r), which is computed with interval or ratio measures. The correlation index generally used for ordinal measures is **Spearman's rank-order correlation** (r_s), sometimes referred to as **Spearman's rho.**

It is difficult to offer guidelines on what should be interpreted as strong or weak relationships. This determination depends on the nature of the variables. If we were to measure patients' body temperature both orally and rectally, a correlation *(r)* of .70 between the two measurements would be low. For most psychosocial variables (*e.g.*, stress and severity of illness), however, an r

of .70 would be rather high. Perfect correlations (+1.00 and −1.00) are extremely rare.

In research reports, correlation coefficients are often reported in tables displaying a two-dimensional **correlation matrix**, in which every variable is displayed in both a row and a column. To read a correlation matrix, one finds the row for one variable and reads across until the row intersects with the column for the second variable.

Example of a correlation matrix:

Table 13-7 presents a correlation matrix from a study that examined relationships among adverse patient outcomes and amount of nursing care (Blegen, Goode, and Reed, 1998). The table lists, on the left, the seven variables in the matrix: two staffing variables (hours of all nursing care; proportion of RN care, relative to care by nursing assistants/LPNs) and five patient outcome variables. The numbers in the top row, from 1 to 7, correspond to the 7 variables: 1 is hours of all nursing care, 2 is proportion of RN care, and so on. At the intersection of row 1 and column 1, we find the value 1.00, which simply indicates that the variable "hours of nursing care" is perfectly correlated with itself. The next entry represents the correlation between hours of nursing care and proportion of RN care. The value of .59 indicates a moderately strong, positive relationship between these two variables: As nursing care (relative to patient days) increases, so does the proportion of care given by RNs. The table indicates that staffing increases with certain adverse outcomes. For example, patient death is fairly strongly correlated with hours of care (.64). On the other hand, greater hours of care is also correlated to some degree with better outcomes—for example, with fewer patient falls (−.26). The weakest correlation in the matrix is between patient falls and infections (−.02), and the strongest is between death and decubitus (.82).

INTRODUCTION TO INFERENTIAL STATISTICS

Descriptive statistics are useful for summarizing data, but usually researchers do more than simply describe. **Inferential statistics,** which are based on the **laws of probability,** provide a means for drawing conclusions about a population, given data from a sample.

Sampling Distributions

When estimating population characteristics, it is important to obtain representative samples, and probability (random) sampling is best suited to securing such samples. Inferential statistical procedures are based on the assumption of random sampling from populations, although this assumption is widely violated.

Even with random sampling, however, sample characteristics are seldom identical to those of the population. Suppose we had a population of 30,000

TABLE 13-7.	Example of a Correlation Matrix: Study of Nurse Staffing and Patient Outcomes						
	1	**2**	**3**	**4**	**5**	**6**	**7**
1. Hours of all nursing care	1.0	.59	−.12	−.26	.56	.57	.64
2. Proportion of RN care		1.00	−.15	−.31	.16	.18	.35
3. Medication errors			1.00	.19	−.35	−.05	−.14
4. Patient falls				1.00	−.02	−.21	−.21
5. Infections					1.00	.74	.67
6. Decubiti						1.00	.82
7. Death							1.00

Adapted from Blegen, M.A., Good, C.J., & Reed, L. (1998). Nurse staffing and patient outcomes. *Nursing Research, 47,* 43–50, Table 2.

nursing school applicants. The mean SAT score for the population is 500 and the standard deviation is 100. Now suppose that we do not know these parameters but that we must estimate them based on scores from a random sample of 25 students. Should we expect a mean of exactly 500 and a standard deviation of 100 for this sample? It would be improbable to obtain identical values. Let us say that, instead, we calculated a mean of 505. If a completely new random sample of 25 students were drawn and another mean computed, we might obtain a value such as 497. Sample statistics fluctuate and are unequal to the corresponding population parameter because of **sampling error.** The challenge for a researcher is to determine whether sample values are good estimates of population parameters.

A researcher works with only one sample, but to understand the logic of inferential statistics, we must perform a mental exercise. Consider drawing a sample of 25 students from the population of applicants, calculating a mean, replacing the 25 students, and drawing a new sample. Each mean is considered a separate datum. If we drew 5000 samples, we would have 5000 means (data points) that could be used to construct a frequency polygon, as shown in Figure 13-6. This kind of distribution is called a **sampling distribution of the mean.** A sampling distribution is a theoretical rather than an actual distribution because in practice no one draws consecutive samples from a population and plots their means. Statisticians have demonstrated that (1) sampling distributions of means follow a normal distribution and (2) the mean of a sampling distribution composed of an infinite number of sample means is equal to the population mean. In the present example, the mean of the sampling distribution is 500, the same value as the mean of the population.

Remember that when scores are normally distributed, 68% of the cases fall between +1 SD and −1 SD from the mean. Because a sampling distribution of means is normally distributed, the probability is 68 out of 100 that any

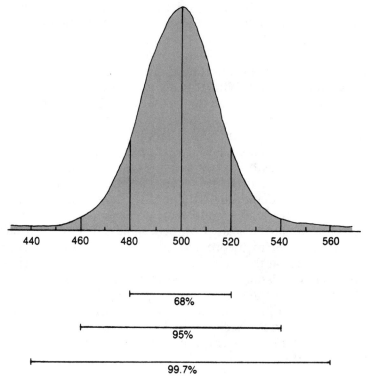

FIGURE 13-6. Sampling distribution of a mean.

randomly drawn sample mean lies within the range of values between +1 SD and −1 SD of the mean. The problem, then, is to determine the value of the standard deviation of the sampling distribution—which is called the **standard error of the mean** (or SEM). The word *error* signifies that the sample means comprising the distribution contain some error in their estimates of the population mean. The smaller the standard error (*i.e.*, the less variable the sample means), the more accurate are the means as estimates of the population value.

Because no one actually constructs a sampling distribution, how can its standard deviation be computed? Fortunately, there is a formula for estimating the standard error of the mean from data from a single sample, using two pieces of information: the sample's standard deviation and sample size. In the present example, the SEM has been calculated as 20, as shown in Figure 13-6. This statistic is an estimate of how much sampling error there would be from one sample mean to another in an infinite number of samples of 25 students.

We can now estimate the probability of drawing a sample with a certain mean. With a sample size of 25 and a population mean of 500, the chances are about 95 out of 100 that a sample mean would fall between the values of 460 and 540—2 SDs above and below the mean. Only 5 times out of 100 would the mean of a randomly selected sample exceed 540 or be less than

460. In other words, only 5 times out of 100 would we be likely to draw a sample whose mean deviates from the population mean by more than 40 points.

Because the SEM is partly a function of sample size, we need only increase sample size to increase the accuracy of our estimate. Suppose that instead of using a sample of 25 applicants to estimate the population's average SAT score, we use a sample of 100. With this many students, the standard error of the mean would be 10 rather than 20. In this situation, the probability of obtaining a sample whose mean is greater than 520 or less than 480 would be about 5 in 100. The chances of drawing a sample with a mean very different from that of the population are reduced as sample size increases because large numbers promote the likelihood that extreme cases will cancel each other out.

You may be wondering why you need to learn about these abstract statistical notions. Consider, though, that what we are talking about concerns how likely it is that a researcher's results are accurate. As an intelligent consumer, you need to evaluate critically how believable research results are so that you can decide whether to incorporate the findings into nursing practice. The concepts underlying the standard error are important in such an evaluation and are related to issues we stressed in Chapter 10 on sampling. First, the more homogeneous the population is on the critical attribute (*i.e.*, the smaller the standard deviation), the more likely it is that results calculated from a sample will be accurate. Second, the larger the sample size, the greater is the likelihood of accuracy. The concepts discussed in this section are the basis for statistical hypothesis testing.

Hypothesis Testing

Statistical inference consists of two major techniques: estimation of parameters and hypothesis testing. **Estimation procedures** are used to estimate a single population characteristic, such as a mean value (*e.g.,* the mean temperature of appendicitis patients). Estimation procedures, however, are not common because researchers typically are more interested in relationships between variables than in estimating the accuracy of a single sample value. For this reason, we focus on hypothesis testing.

Statistical **hypothesis testing** provides objective criteria for deciding whether hypotheses should be accepted as true or rejected as false. Suppose a nurse researcher hypothesizes that maternity patients exposed to a teaching film on breastfeeding will breastfeed longer than mothers who do not see the film. The researcher subsequently learns that the mean number of days of breastfeeding is 131.5 for 25 experimental subjects and 125.1 for 25 control subjects. Should the researcher conclude that the hypothesis has been supported? True, the group differences are in the predicted direction, but the results might simply be due to sampling fluctuations. The two groups might *happen* to be different by chance, regardless of exposure to the film; perhaps in another sample, the group means would be nearly identical. Hypothesis testing helps researchers to make objective decisions about study results. Researchers need such a mechanism to help them decide which results are likely to reflect chance differences and which are likely to reflect true hypothesized effects.

The procedures used in testing hypotheses are based on rules of negative inference. In the above example, the researcher found that those who had seen the teaching film breastfed longer, on average, than those who had not. There are two possible explanations for this outcome: (1) the experimental treatment was successful in encouraging breastfeeding or (2) the difference was due to chance factors (*e.g.,* differences in the characteristics of the two groups even before the film was shown).

The first explanation is the researcher's **scientific hypothesis**, and the second is the **null hypothesis.** The null hypothesis, it may be recalled, states that there is no relationship between the independent and dependent variables. Statistical hypothesis testing is basically a process of disproof or rejection. It cannot be demonstrated directly that the scientific hypothesis is correct. But it is possible to show, using theoretical sampling distributions, that the null hypothesis has a high probability of being incorrect, and such evidence lends support to the scientific hypothesis.

The rejection of the null hypothesis, then, is what the researcher seeks to accomplish through **statistical tests.** Although null hypotheses are accepted or rejected on the basis of sample data, the hypothesis is made about population values. The real interest in testing hypotheses, as in all statistical inference, is to use a sample to draw conclusions about a population.

Type I and Type II Errors

Researchers decide whether to accept or reject the null hypothesis by determining how probable it is that observed group differences are due to chance. Because information about the population is not available, it cannot be asserted flatly that the null hypothesis is or is not true. The researcher must be content to say that the hypothesis is either probably true or probably false. Statistical inferences are based on incomplete information; hence, there is always a risk of making an error.

	The actual situation is that the null hypothesis is:	
	True	False
True (Null accepted)	Correct decision	Type II error
False (Null rejected)	Type I error	Correct decision

The researcher calculates a test statistic and decides that the null hypothesis is:

FIGURE 13-7. Outcomes of statistical decision making.

A researcher can make two types of error: (1) rejection of a true null hypothesis or (2) acceptance of a false null hypothesis. Figure 13-7 summarizes the possible outcomes of a researcher's decision. An investigator makes a **Type I error** by rejecting the null hypothesis when it is, in fact, true. For instance, if we concluded that the experimental treatment was effective in promoting breastfeeding when, in fact, group differences were due to sampling error, we would have made a Type I error. In the reverse situation, we might conclude that observed differences in breastfeeding were due to random sampling fluctuations when, in fact, the experimental treatment did have an effect. Acceptance of a false null hypothesis is called a **Type II error.**

 CONSUMER TIP:

Type II errors are especially likely to occur when small samples are used to estimate population values. If a research report indicates that a research hypothesis was not supported by the data, consider whether a Type II error might have occurred as a result of inadequate sample size. ■

Level of Significance

The researcher does not know when an error in statistical decision making has been committed. The validity of a null hypothesis could only be ascertained by collecting data from the population, in which case there would be no need for statistical inference.

The degree of risk in making a Type I error is controlled by the researcher, who selects a **level of significance.** Level of significance is the phrase used to signify the probability of making a Type I error. The two most frequently used levels of significance (referred to as **alpha** or α) are .05 and .01. With a .05 significance level, we accept the risk that out of 100 samples, a true null hypothesis would be rejected 5 times. In 95 out of 100 cases, however, a true null hypothesis would be correctly accepted. With a .01 significance level, the risk of making a Type I error is lower: In only one sample out of 100 would we erroneously reject the null hypothesis. By convention, the minimal acceptable alpha level for scientific research is .05.

Naturally, researchers would like to reduce the risk of committing both types of error. Unfortunately, lowering the risk of a Type I error increases the risk of a Type II error. The stricter the criterion for rejecting a null hypothesis, the greater the probability of accepting a false null hypothesis. However, researchers can reduce the risk of a Type II error simply by increasing their sample size.*

Tests of Statistical Significance

Within a hypothesis testing framework, the researcher uses study data to compute a **test statistic.** For every test statistic, there is a related theoretical sam-

---

*The risk of committing a Type II error can be estimated through power analysis. In many nursing studies, the risk of a Type II error is high because of small sample size, suggesting a need for greater use of power analysis among nurse researchers.

pling distribution, analogous to the sampling distribution of means. Hypothesis testing uses theoretical distributions to establish probable and improbable values for the test statistics, which are, in turn, used as a basis for accepting or rejecting the null hypothesis.

A simple example will illustrate the process. Suppose we wanted to test the hypothesis that the average SAT score for students applying to nursing schools is higher than that for all other students taking the SAT, whose mean score is 500. The null hypothesis is that there is no difference in the mean population scores of students who do or do not apply to nursing school. Let us say that the mean score for a sample of 100 nursing school applicants is 525, with a standard deviation of 100. Using statistical procedures, we can test the null hypothesis that the mean of 525 is a chance fluctuation from the population mean of 500.

In hypothesis testing, researchers assume that the null hypothesis is true and then gather evidence to disprove it. Assuming a mean of 500 for the nursing school applicant population, a sampling distribution can be constructed with a mean of 500 and a standard deviation equal to 10. In this example, 10 is the standard error of the mean, calculated from a formula that used the sample standard deviation of 100 for a sample of 100 students. This is shown in Figure 13-8. Based on normal distribution characteristics, we can determine probable and improbable values of sample means from the nursing school applicant population. If, as is assumed, the population mean is actually 500,

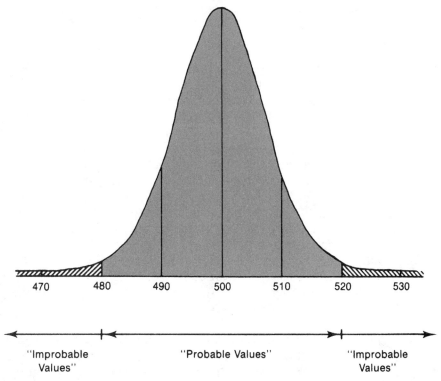

| "Improbable Values" | "Probable Values" | "Improbable Values" |

FIGURE 13-8. Sampling distribution for hypothesis testing example of SAT scores.

95% of all sample means would fall between 480 and 520 because 95% of the cases are within 2 SDs of the mean. The obtained sample mean of 525 lies in the region considered improbable if the null hypothesis is correct, assuming that our criterion of improbability is an alpha level of .05. The improbable range beyond 2 SDs corresponds to only 5% (100% − 95%) of the sampling distribution. We would thus reject the null hypothesis that the mean of the nursing school applicant population equals 500. We would not be justified in saying that we have proved the research hypothesis because the possibility of having made a Type I error remains.

Researchers reporting the results of hypothesis tests state that their findings are **statistically significant.** The word *significant* should not be read as important or meaningful. In statistics, the term *significant* means that obtained results are not likely to have been due to chance, at some specified level of probability. A **nonsignificant result** means that any observed difference or relationship could have been the result of a chance fluctuation.

 CONSUMER TIP:

Inferential statistics are usually more difficult to understand than descriptive statistics. It may help to keep in mind that inferential statistics are just a tool to help us evaluate whether the results are likely to be real and replicable, or simply spurious. As recommended in Chapter 3, you can overcome much of the abstruseness of the results section by translating the basic thrust of the research findings into everyday language. ■

Parametric and Nonparametric Tests

The bulk of the tests that we discuss in this chapter—and also most tests used by researchers—are **parametric tests.** Parametric tests are characterized by three attributes: (1) they focus on population parameters; (2) they require measurements on at least an interval scale; and (3) they involve other assumptions about the variables under consideration, such as the assumption that the variables are normally distributed in the population.

Nonparametric tests, by contrast, are not based on the estimation of parameters and involve less restrictive assumptions about the shape of the distribution of the critical variables. Nonparametric tests are usually applied when the data have been measured on a nominal or ordinal scale.

Parametric tests are more powerful than nonparametric tests and are generally preferred when variables are measured on at least the interval scale. Nonparametric tests are most useful when the data under consideration cannot in any manner be construed as interval measures or when the data distribution is markedly nonnormal.

Overview of Hypothesis Testing Procedures

In the next section, various statistical procedures for testing research hypotheses are discussed. The emphasis is on explaining applications of statistical tests and on interpreting their meaning rather than on computations.

Each statistical test described in this chapter has a particular application and can be used only with particular kinds of data; however, the overall process of testing hypotheses is basically the same for all tests. The steps that a researcher takes are the following:

1. *Determining which test statistic to use.* The researcher must consider such factors as whether a parametric test is justified, which levels of measurement were used for the measures, and, if relevant, how many groups are being compared.
2. *Selecting the level of significance.* An α level of .05 is usually acceptable, but, in some cases, the level is set more stringently at .01 or .001.
3. *Computing a test statistic.* The researcher then calculates a test statistic based on the collected data, using appropriate computation formulas.
4. *Calculating degrees of freedom.* The term **degrees of freedom** *(df)* is used throughout hypothesis testing to refer to the number of observations free to vary about a parameter. The concept is too complex for full elaboration here, but the computation of degrees of freedom is easy.
5. *Comparing the test statistic to a tabled value.* Theoretical distributions have been developed for all test statistics, and values for these distributions are available in tables. The tabled values enable the researcher to determine whether the computed test statistic value is beyond what is probable if the null hypothesis is true. The researcher examines a table for the test used, obtains a tabled value corresponding to the relevant degrees of freedom and significance level, and compares the tabled value to the computed test statistic. If the tabled value is smaller than the absolute value of the test statistic, the results are statistically significant; if the tabled value is larger, the results are nonsignificant.

When a computer is used for the analysis, the researcher follows only the first step and then gives the necessary commands to the computer. The computer calculates the test statistic, degrees of freedom, and the *actual* probability that the relationship being tested is due to chance. For example, the computer may print that the probability (p) of an experimental group doing better on a measure of postoperative recovery than the control group on the basis of chance alone is .025. This means that fewer than 3 times out of 100 (or only 25 times out of 1000) would a group difference of the size observed occur by chance. This computed probability can then be compared with the desired level of significance. In the present example, if the significance level were .05, the results would be significant because .025 is more stringent than .05. If .01 was the significance level, the results would be nonsignificant (sometimes abbreviated *NS*). Any computed probability level greater than .05 (*e.g.*, .20) indicates a nonsignificant relationship (*i.e.*, one that could have occurred on the basis of chance in more than 5 out of 100 samples). In the section that follows, several specific statistical tests and their applications are described.

BIVARIATE STATISTICAL TESTS

You will find that researchers use a wide variety of statistical tests to make inferences about the validity of their hypotheses. Some of the most frequently used bivariate tests are briefly described and illustrated below.

t-*Tests*

A common research situation is the comparison of two groups of people on a dependent variable. The appropriate procedure for testing the statistical significance of a difference between the means of two groups is the parametric test known as the *t*-test.

Suppose a researcher wanted to test the effect of early discharge of maternity patients on their perceived maternal competence. The researcher administers a scale of perceived maternal competence 1 week after delivery to 10 primiparas who were discharged early (*i.e.*, within 24 hours of delivery) and to 10 others who remained in the hospital for longer periods. Some hypothetical data for this example are presented in Table 13-8. The mean scores for the two groups are 19.0 and 25.0, respectively. Is this difference a true population difference—is it likely to be replicated in other samples of early-discharge and later-discharge mothers? Or is the group difference just the result of chance fluctuations? The 20 scores—10 for each group—vary from one person to another. Some variability reflects individual differences in perceived maternal competence. Some of the variability could also be due to measurement error (unreliability of the researcher's scale), some could be the result of the participants' moods on that particular day, and so forth. The research

TABLE 13-8. Fictitious Data for *t*-Test Example: Scores on a Perceived Maternal Competence Scale for Two Groups of Mothers	
REGULAR-DISCHARGE MOTHERS	**EARLY-DISCHARGE MOTHERS**
30	23
27	17
25	22
20	18
24	20
32	26
17	16
18	13
28	21
29	14
Mean = 25.0	Mean = 19.0
$t = 2.86$; $df = 18$; $p < .05$	

question is: Can a significant portion of the variability be attributed to the independent variable—time of discharge from the hospital? The *t*-test allows the researcher to answer this question objectively.

The formula for the *t* statistic uses group means, sample size, and variability to calculate a value for *t*. In the present example, the computed value of *t* is 2.86. Next, degrees of freedom are calculated. Here, the degrees of freedom are equal to the total sample size minus 2 ($df = 20 - 2 = 18$). Then, the tabled value for *t* with 18 degrees of freedom is determined. For an level of .05, the tabled value of *t* is 2.10. *This value establishes an upper limit to what is probable if the null hypothesis is true.* Thus, the calculated *t* of 2.86, which is larger than the tabled value of the statistic, is improbable (*i.e.,* statistically significant). We are now in a position to say that the primiparas discharged early had significantly lower perceptions of maternal competence than those who were not discharged early. The group difference in perceived maternal competence is sufficiently large that it is unlikely to reflect merely chance fluctuations. In fewer than 5 out of 100 samples would a difference this great be found by chance alone.

The situation we just described calls for an **independent groups *t*-test**: The study participants in the two groups were different people, independent of each other. There are certain situations for which this type of *t*-test is not appropriate. For example, if means for a single group of people measured before and after an intervention were being compared, the researcher would compute a **paired *t*-test** (also known as a **dependent groups *t*-test**), using a different formula.

⊞ *Example of a t-test:*

Table 13-9 presents the results of three independent *t*-tests from a study that evaluated the effectiveness of a nurse-managed smoking cessation intervention among pregnant women who smoked (Gebauer, Kwo, Haynes, & Wewers, 1998). The two groups of women did not differ significantly in terms of preintervention smoking—both groups smoked about 13 cigarettes per day, on average. However, at follow-up, women in the experimental group smoked significantly fewer cigarettes than women in the control group ($p = .008$).

TABLE 13-9. Example of a Table with *t*-Tests: Smoking History for Experimental and Control Group Women

VARIABLE	EXPERIMENTAL	CONTROL	*t*	*p*	*N*
Mean smoking rate per day at initial visit	13.3	12.5	0.52	.602	162
Mean smoking rate per day at follow-up	7.8	13.7	2.76	.008	129

Adapted from Gebauer, C., Kwo, C., Haynes, E. F., & Wewers, M. E. et al. (1998). A nurse-managed smoking cessation Intervention during pregnancy. *Journal of Obstetric, Gynecologic, and Neonatal Nursing, 27,* 47–53, Table 4.

Analysis of Variance

Analysis of variance (ANOVA) is a parametric procedure used to test mean group differences of three or more groups. The statistic computed in an ANOVA is the **F ratio**. ANOVA decomposes the total variability of a dependent variable into two components: variability attributable to the independent variable and variability due to all other sources (*e.g.*, individual differences, measurement error). Variation between groups is contrasted with variation within groups to yield an *F* ratio.

Suppose we wanted to compare the effectiveness of different instructional techniques to teach high school students about AIDS. One group of students is exposed to a film on AIDS, a second group is given a special lecture, and a third control group receives no special instruction. The dependent variable is the student's score on the AIDS knowledge test the day after the intervention. The null hypothesis is that the group population means for AIDS knowledge test scores are the same, whereas the research hypothesis predicts that they are different.

The 60 test scores shown in Table 13-1 are reproduced in Table 13-10, according to treatment group. As this table shows, there is variation from one student to the next within a group, and there are also group differences. The mean test scores are 25.35, 24.75, and 20.35 for groups A, B, and C, respectively. These means are different, but are they significantly different? Or do the differences reflect random fluctuations?

An ANOVA applied to these data yields an *F* ratio of 18.64. In ANOVA, two types of degree of freedom are calculated: between groups (the number of

TABLE 13-10.	Fictitious Data for One-Way ANOVA: Instructional Mode Effects on AIDS Knowledge Test Scores				
FILM GROUP (A)		**LECTURE GROUP (B)**		**CONTROL GROUP (C)**	
26	25	22	24	15	22
20	29	24	25	26	19
16	30	27	21	24	20
25	27	23	27	18	22
25	29	23	25	20	18
23	28	26	21	20	24
26	26	22	24	19	18
25	25	24	29	21	23
24	27	24	28	17	20
23	28	30	26	17	24
Mean 25.35		24.75		20.35	

$F = 18.64$; $df = 2, 57$; $p < .001$.

groups minus 1) and within groups (the total number of subjects minus the number of groups). In this example, then, $df = 2$ and 57. In a table of values for a theoretical F distribution, we would find that the value of F for 2 and 57 df, for an alpha of .05, is 3.16. Because our obtained F value of 18.64 exceeds 3.16, we reject the null hypothesis that the population means are equal. The observed group differences in mean test scores would be obtained by chance in fewer than 5 samples out of 100. (Actually, the probability of achieving an F of 18.64 by chance is less than 1 in 1000.) In research reports, tables displaying ANOVA results are usually organized in a format similar to that used in Table 13-9 for t-tests, with descriptive statistics on the dependent variables for the groups being compared, followed by the value of the test statistic (F) and the probability level.

The data in our example support the hypothesis that the instructional interventions affect students' knowledge about AIDS, but we cannot tell from these results whether treatment A was significantly more effective than treatment B. Statistical analyses known as **multiple comparison procedures** (also called *post hoc* **tests**) are needed. The function of these procedures is to isolate the comparisons between group means that are responsible for rejecting the overall ANOVA null hypothesis. Note that it is *not* appropriate to use a series of t-tests (Group A versus B, A versus C, and B versus C) in this situation because this would increase the risk of a Type I error.

ANOVA also can be used to test the effect of two (or more) independent variables on a dependent variable (*e.g.*, when a factorial experimental design has been used). Suppose we wanted to determine whether the two instructional techniques discussed previously were equally effective in helping freshmen and sophomore high school students acquire knowledge about AIDS. We could set up a design in which freshmen and sophomores would be randomly assigned, separately, to the two modes of instruction. Some hypothetical data, shown in Table 13-11, reveal the following about two **main effects:** On average, people in the film group scored higher than those in the lecture group (25.35 versus 24.75); and sophomore students scored higher than freshmen (26.20 versus 23.90). In addition, there is an **interaction effect:** Freshmen scored higher when exposed to the lecture, whereas sophomores scored higher when exposed to the film. By performing a **two-way ANOVA** on these data, it would be possible to ascertain the statistical significance of these differences.

A type of ANOVA known as **repeated measures ANOVA** is often used when the means being compared are means at different points in time (*e.g.*, mean blood pressure at 2, 4, and 6 hours after surgery). This is analogous to a dependent groups t-test, extended to three or more points of data collection, because it is the same people being measured multiple times. When two or more groups are measured several times, a repeated measures ANOVA provides information about a main effect for time (do the measures differ significantly over time?); a main effect for groups (do the group means differ significantly?); and an interaction effect (do the groups differ more at certain times?).

TABLE 13-11. Fictitious Data for Two-Way (2 x 2) ANOVA Example: Instructional Mode and Year in School in Relation to Test Scores						
	INSTRUCTIONAL MODE					
YEAR IN SCHOOL	**Film**			**Lecture**		
Freshman	26 20	$\bar{X} = 23.3$		22 24	$\bar{X} = 24.5$	Freshmen mean = 23.90
	16 25			27 33		
	25 23			23 26		
	26 25			22 24		
	24 23			24 30		
Sophomore	25 29	$\bar{X} = 27.4$		24 25	$\bar{X} = 25.0$	Sophomore mean = 26.20
	30 27			21 27		
	29 28			27 25		
	26 25			21 24		
	27 28			28 26		
Film group mean	25.35	Lecture group mean		24.75		Grand mean = 25.05

 Example of an ANOVA:

Pressler and her colleagues (1999) compared the behavioral responses of newborns of insulin-dependent diabetic mothers with newborns of nondiabetic, healthy mothers. The outcome measures were scores on the Neonatal Behavioral Assessment Scale, measured on the first and second day after birth. The results indicated a significant effect for time on several scales. For example, for all newborns, mean scores on reflex functioning was significantly better on Day 2 than on Day 1 ($F = 33.83$; $df = 1, 39$; $p < .01$). There was also a significant effect on this same scale for groups ($F = 30.81$; $df = 1, 39$; $p < .01$): Infants of diabetic mothers performed significantly worse than their matched controls. There were no time–maternal health status interactions.

CONSUMER TIP:

Experimental repeated measures designs (see Chap. 8) call for either a dependent groups *t*-test or a repeated measures ANOVA because the same people are measured more than once after being randomly assigned to a different ordering of treatments. However, repeated measures ANOVA can also be used in studies that do not involve an experimental repeated measures design if outcomes are measured more than once. ∎

Chi-Squared Test

The **chi-squared** (χ^2) **test** is a nonparametric procedure used to test hypotheses about the proportion of cases that fall into various categories, as when a contingency table has been created. Consider the following example. A researcher is interested in studying the effect of planned nursing instruction on patients' compliance with a self-medication regimen. The experimental group is instructed by nurses who are implementing a new instructional approach based on Orem's Self-Care Model. A second (control) group of patients is cared for by nurses who continue their usual mode of instruction. The research hypothesis is that a higher proportion of people in the experimental than in the control group will comply with the regimen. Some hypothetical data for this example are presented in Table 13-12.

The chi-squared statistic is computed by summing differences between the observed frequencies in each cell and frequencies that would be expected if there were no relationship between the independent and dependent variable. In this example, the value of the computed χ^2 statistic is 18.18, which we can compare with the value from a theoretical chi-squared distribution. For the chi-squared statistic, the degrees of freedom are equal to the number of rows minus 1 times the number of columns minus 1. In the present case, df = 1×1, or 1. With one degree of freedom, the value that must be exceeded to establish significance at the .05 level is 3.84. The obtained value of 18.18 is substantially larger than would be expected by chance. Thus, we can conclude that a significantly larger proportion of patients in the experimental group (60%) than in the control group (30%) were compliant.

Example of a chi-squared test.

Mikhail (1999) compared perceived impediments to prenatal care among three groups of low-income women with different levels of prenatal care: inadequate, intermediate, and adequate. The findings indicated that the groups differed significantly with regard to several perceived impediments, such as fear of a medical examination; 30.2% of the women with inadequate care, compared with 6.2% of those with adequate care, reported this problem ($\chi^2 = 9.03$; $df = 2$; $p < .02$).

Correlation Coefficients

Pearson's r is both descriptive and inferential. As a descriptive statistic, r summarizes the magnitude and direction of a relationship between two variables.

TABLE 13-12. **Observed Frequencies for a Chi-Squared Example on Patient Compliance**

	EXPERIMENTAL	CONTROL	TOTAL
Compliance	60	30	90
Noncompliance	40	70	110
TOTAL	100	100	200

$\chi^2 = 18.18$; $df = 1$; $p < .001$.

As an inferential statistic, r is used to test hypotheses about population correlations. The null hypothesis is that there is no relationship between two variables of interest.

Suppose we were studying the relationship between patients' self-reported level of stress (higher scores imply more stress) and the pH level of their saliva. With a sample of 50 patients, we find that $r = -.29$. This value indicates a tendency for people with high stress scores to have lower pH levels than those with low stress scores. But we need to ask whether this finding can be generalized to the population. Does the coefficient of $-.29$ reflect a random fluctuation, observed only in this particular sample, or is the relationship significant? Degrees of freedom for correlation coefficients are equal to the number of participants minus 2, or 48 in this example. In a statistical table for correlation coefficients, the tabled value for r with $df = 48$ and a .05 significance level is .282. Because the absolute value of the calculated r is .29 and thus larger than .282, the null hypothesis can be rejected. There is a significant, modest relationship between patients' self-reported level of stress and the acidity of their saliva.

Example of correlation coefficients:

Wolff and Ratner (1999) hypothesized that a person's sense of coherence (SOC) is inversely related to stress and recent traumatic life events. They found, in a national sample of Canadians, that SOC was significantly correlated with chronic stress ($r = -.53$; $p < .01$) and with recent stressful life events ($r = -.33$; $p < .01$), supporting their hypotheses.

Guide to Bivariate Statistical Tests

The selection and use of a statistical test depends on several factors, such as the number of groups and the levels of measurement of the research variables. To aid you in evaluating the appropriateness of statistical procedures used in studies, a chart summarizing the major features of several tests is presented in Table 13-13. This table does not include every test you may encounter in research reports, but it does include the bivariate statistical tests most often used by nurse researchers.

MULTIVARIATE STATISTICAL ANALYSIS

Nurse researchers have become increasingly sophisticated, and many now use complex **multivariate statistics** to analyze their data. We use the term *multivariate* to refer to analyses dealing with at least three—but usually many more—variables simultaneously. This evolution has resulted in increased rigor in nursing studies, but one unfortunate side effect is that it is becoming more challenging for novice consumers to understand research reports.

TABLE 13-13.	Guide to Widely Used Bivariate Statistical Tests			

NAME	TEST STATISTIC	PURPOSE	MEASUREMENT LEVEL* IV	MEASUREMENT LEVEL* DV
PARAMETRIC TESTS				
t-test for independent groups	*t*	To test the difference between two independent group means	Nominal	Interval, ratio
t-test for dependent groups	*t*	To test the difference between two dependent group means	Nominal	Interval, ratio
Analysis of variance (ANOVA)	*F*	To test the difference among the means of three or more independent groups, or of more than one independent variable	Nominal	Interval, ratio
Repeated measures ANOVA	*F*	To test the difference among means of three or more related groups or sets of scores	Nominal	Interval, ratio
Pearson's *r*	*r*	To test the existence of a relationship between two variables	Interval, ratio	Interval, ratio
NONPARAMETRIC TESTS				
Chi-squared test	χ^2	To test the difference in proportions in two or more independent groups	Nominal	Nominal
Mann-Whitney *U*-test	*U*	To test the difference in ranks of scores on two independent groups	Nominal	Ordinal
Kruskal-Wallis test	*H*	To test the difference in ranks of scores of three or more independent groups	Nominal	Ordinal
Wilcoxon signed ranks test	*T (Z)*	To test the difference in ranks of scores of two related groups	Nominal	Ordinal
Friedman test	χ^2	To test the difference in ranks of scores of three or more related groups	Nominal	Ordinal
Phi coefficient	ϕ	To test the magnitude of a relationship between two dichotomous variables	Nominal	Nominal
Spearman's rank-order correlation	r_s	To test the existence of a relationship between two variables	Ordinal	Ordinal

*Measurement level of the independent variable (IV) and dependent variable (DV).

Given the introductory nature of this text and the fact that many of you are not proficient with even basic statistical procedures, it is not possible to describe in detail the complex analytic procedures that now appear in nursing journals. However, we present some basic information that might assist you in reading reports in which two commonly used multivariate statistics are used: multiple regression and analysis of covariance (ANCOVA).

Multiple Regression

Correlations enable researchers to make predictions. For example, if the correlation between SAT scores and grades in a nursing program were .60, nursing school administrators could make predictions—albeit imperfect predictions—about applicants' future academic performance. Because two variables are rarely perfectly correlated, researchers often strive to improve their ability to predict a dependent variable by including more than one independent variable in the analysis. For example, a researcher might predict that an infant's birth weight is related to the amount of prenatal care the mother received. The researcher could collect data on birth weight and number of prenatal visits and then compute a correlation coefficient to determine whether a significant relationship between the two variables exists (*i.e.,* whether prenatal care could help predict infant birth weight). Birth weight is affected by many other factors, however, such as gestational period and mothers' nutritional practices during the pregnancy and their smoking behavior. Many researchers, therefore, perform an analysis called **multiple regression analysis** (or **multiple correlation analysis**) that allows them to use more than one independent variable to explain or predict a dependent variable. (In multiple regression, the dependent variables are interval- or ratio-level variables. Independent variables are either interval- or ratio-level variables or dichotomous nominal-level variables, such as male/female.)

When several independent variables are used to predict a dependent variable, the resulting statistic is the **multiple correlation coefficient**, symbolized as R. Unlike the bivariate correlation coefficient r, R does not have negative values. R varies from .00 to 1.00, showing the *strength* of the relationship between several independent variables and a dependent variable, but not *direction*.

There are several ways of evaluating R. One is to determine whether R is statistically significant—that is, whether the overall relationship between the independent variables and the dependent variable is likely to be real or the result of chance sampling fluctuations. This is done through the computation of an F statistic that can be compared with tabled F values.

A second way of evaluating R is to determine whether the addition of new independent variables adds further predictive power. For example, a researcher might find that the R between infant birth weight on the one hand and maternal weight and prenatal care on the other is .30. By adding a third independent variable—let's say maternal smoking behavior—R might increase to .36. Is the increase from .30 to .36 statistically significant? In other words, does knowing whether the mother smoked during her pregnancy improve our understanding of the birth-weight outcome, or does the increased R value simply reflect a relationship peculiar to this sample of women? Multiple regression procedures provide a way of answering this question.

The magnitude of the *R* statistic is also informative. Researchers would like to predict a dependent variable perfectly. In the birth-weight example, if it were possible to identify all the factors that lead to differences in infants' weight, the researcher could collect the relevant data to obtain an *R* of 1.00. Usually, the value of *R* in a nursing research study is much smaller—seldom higher than .60. An interesting feature of the *R* statistic is that, when squared, it can be interpreted as the proportion of the variability in the dependent variable accounted for by the independent variables. If a researcher predicting infant birth weight achieved an *R* of .80 (R^2 = .64), we could say that the independent variables accounted for nearly two thirds (64%) of the variability in infants' birth weights. One third of the variability, however, is caused by factors not identified or measured. Researchers usually report multiple correlation results in terms of $\boldsymbol{R^2}$ rather than *R*.

Multiple regressions yield information about how each independent variable is related to the dependent variable. Although it is beyond our scope to explain how to read multiple regression tables, you should recognize that multiple regression analysis indicates whether an independent variable is significantly related to the dependent variable *even when* the other independent variables are controlled. Let us assume that our birth-weight researcher used 10 independent variables to predict or explain infant birth weight. If the amount of prenatal care received during pregnancy continued to be significantly related to the birth-weight outcome, this would mean that prenatal care was truly correlated with birth weight even with the other nine variables (which might be the extraneous variables) controlled. The example in the next section explains this concept in greater detail.

Example of multiple regression:

In the previously cited study by Wolff and Ratner (1999), multiple regression was used to predict sense of coherence (SOC) from stress, life events, social support, and other independent variables. The value of R was .57. Thus, the independent variables accounted for 32% of the variability in SOC scores (*i.e.*, R^2 = .32).

Analysis of Covariance

Analysis of covariance (ANCOVA), which is essentially a combination of ANOVA and multiple regression, is used to control extraneous variables statistically. This approach can be especially valuable in certain types of research situations, such as when a nonequivalent control group design is used. The initial equivalence of the experimental and comparison groups in these studies is always questionable; thus, the researcher must consider whether the results were influenced by preexisting group differences. When experimental control through randomization is lacking, ANCOVA offers the possibility of *post hoc* statistical control.

Because the concept of statistical control may mystify you, we will explain the underlying principle with a simple illustration. Suppose we were interested in testing the effectiveness of a special training program on physical fitness, using as subjects the employees of two companies. Employees of one company receive the experimental physical fitness intervention, and those of the second company do not. The employees' score on a physical fitness test is the dependent variable. The research question is: Can some of the individual differences in performance on the physical fitness test be attributed to participation in the special program? Physical fitness is also related to other, extraneous characteristics of the study participants (*e.g.,* their age)—characteristics that might differ between the two intact groups.

Figure 13-9 illustrates how ANCOVA works. The large circles represent total variability (*i.e.,* the total extent of individual differences) in physical fitness scores for both groups. A certain amount of variability can be explained by age differences: Younger people tend to perform better on the test than older ones. This relationship is represented by the overlapping small circle on the left in part A of Figure 13-9. Another part of the variability can be explained by participation in the physical fitness program, represented here by the overlapping small circle on the right. In part A, the fact that the two small circles (age and program participation) themselves overlap indicates that there is a relationship between these two variables. In other words, people in the experimental group are, on average, either older or younger than those in the comparison group. Because of this relationship, which could distort the results of the study, age should be controlled.

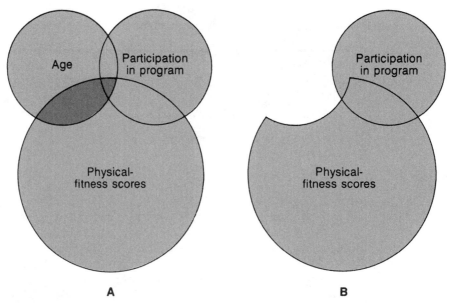

A   B

FIGURE 13-9. Schematic diagram illustrating the principle of analysis of covariance.

ANCOVA can accomplish this by statistically removing the effect of the extraneous variable (age) on physical fitness. This is designated in part A of Figure 13-9 by the darkened area of the large circle. Part B illustrates that the analysis would examine the effect of program participation on fitness scores *after* removing the effect of age (called a **covariate** in ANCOVA). With the variability associated with age removed, we get a more precise estimate of the training program's effect on physical fitness. Note that even after removing variability resulting from age, there is still individual variability not associated with program participation (the bottom half of the large circle) that is not explained. This means that analytic precision could be further enhanced by controlling additional extraneous variables (for example, nutritional habits, smoking status). ANCOVA can accommodate multiple extraneous variables.

Analysis of covariance tests the significance of differences between group means after adjusting scores on the dependent variable to eliminate the effect of the covariates. This adjustment uses multiple regression procedures. The ANCOVA procedure produces *F* statistics—one for evaluating the significance of the covariates and another for evaluating the significance of group differences—that can be compared with tabled values of *F* to determine whether to accept or reject the null hypothesis. ANCOVA, like multiple regression analysis, is an extremely powerful and useful analytic technique for controlling extraneous or confounding influences on dependent measures.

Example of ANCOVA:

Munet-Vilaró, Folkman, and Gregorich (1999) studied depression in three Latino groups: Mexicans in Mexico City, Latino immigrants in San Francisco, and Puerto Ricans living in southern Puerto Rico. ANCOVA was used to control group differences with respect to such extraneous characteristics as age, education, and gender. The analysis revealed that depression differed significantly among the three groups even after adjusting for covariates. The Latino immigrant group had the highest mean depression scores.

Other Multivariate Techniques

Several other related multivariate techniques increasingly are being used in nursing studies. We mention these techniques briefly to acquaint you with terms you might encounter in the research literature.

Discriminant Function Analysis

In multiple regression analysis, the dependent variable is a measure on either the interval or ratio scale. **Discriminant function analysis** is used to make predictions about membership in groups—that is, about a dependent variable measured on the nominal scale. For example, a researcher might wish to use several independent variables to predict membership in such groups as: complying versus noncomplying cancer patients; overweight versus normal-weight people; or normal pregnancies versus those terminating in a miscarriage. In discriminant function analysis, as in multiple regression, the independent variables are either interval- or ratio-level measures or dichotomous nominal variables (*e.g.,* smoker versus nonsmoker).

Logistic Regression

Logistic regression (or **logit analysis**) analyzes the relationships between multiple independent variables and a nominal-level dependent variable. It is thus used in situations similar to discriminant function analysis, but it employs a different statistical estimation procedure that many prefer for nominal-level dependent variables. Logistic regression transforms the probability of an event occurring (*e.g.,* that a woman will practice breast self-examination or not) into its **odds** (*i.e.,* into the ratio of one event's probability relative to the probability of a second event). After further transformations, the analysis examines the relationship of the independent variables to the transformed dependent variable. For each predictor, the logistic regression yields an **odds ratio**, which is the factor by which the odds change for a unit change in the predictors.

Example of logistic regression:

Mentes, Culp, Maas, and Rantz (1999) used logistic regression to assess possible risk factors that could be used to predict acute confusion in long-term care settings. Their analysis revealed that variables that significantly differentiated the presence or absence of acute confusion included inadequate fluid intake, a recent fall, and a diagnosis of dementia. The odds ratio for fluid intake was 3.4 ($p < .0001$), indicating that acute confusion was nearly $3\frac{1}{2}$ times more likely among those with insufficient hydration.

Factor Analysis

Factor analysis is widely used by researchers seeking to develop, refine, or validate complex instruments. The major purpose of factor analysis is to reduce a large set of variables into a smaller, more manageable set. Factor analysis disentangles complex interrelationships among variables and identifies which variables go together as unified concepts or factors. For example, suppose a researcher has prepared 50 Likert statements aimed at measuring women's attitudes toward menopause. It would not be appropriate to combine all 50 items to form a scale score because there are various dimensions, or themes, to women's attitudes toward menopause. One dimension may relate to the issue of aging, another may concern the loss of ability to reproduce, and so on. These various dimensions should serve as the basis for scale construction, and factor analysis offers an objective, empirical method for doing so.

🔡 *Example of factor analysis:*

Anderson and her colleagues (1999) explored methods of combining nursing home resident assessment data into a case mix index. Ten resident outcomes were selected, and factor analysis was used to reduce the 10 indicators into a smaller number of outcomes. Four factors were identified: Behavior Problems, Fracture, Complications of Immobility, and Use of Physical Restraints.

Multivariate Analysis of Variance

Multivariance analysis of variance (MANOVA) is the extension of ANOVA to more than one dependent variable. This procedure is used to test the significance of differences between the means of two or more groups on two or more dependent variables, considered simultaneously. For instance, if a researcher wanted to examine the effect of two methods of exercise treatment on both diastolic and systolic blood pressure, then a MANOVA would be appropriate. Covariates can also be included, in which case the analysis would be called a **multivariate analysis of covariance (MANCOVA)**.

Causal Modeling

Causal modeling involves the development and statistical testing of a hypothesized explanation of the causes of a phenomenon. **Path analysis**, which is based on multiple regression, is a widely used approach to causal modeling. Alternative methods of testing causal models are also being used by nurse researchers, the most important of which is **linear structural relations analysis**, more widely known as **LISREL**. Both LISREL and path analysis are highly complex statistical techniques whose utility relies on a sound underlying causal theory.

Guide to Multivariate Statistical Analyses

In selecting a multivariate analysis, the researcher must attend to such issues as the number of independent variables, the number of dependent variables, the measurement level of all variables, and the desirability of controlling extraneous variables. Table 13-14 is an aid to help you evaluate the appropriateness of multivariate statistics used in research reports. This chart includes the major multivariate analyses used by nurse researchers.

READING AND INTERPRETING STATISTICAL INFORMATION

Statistical findings are communicated in the results section of a research report and are reported in the text as well as in tables (or, less frequently, figures). This section provides some assistance in reading and interpreting statistical information.

TABLE 13-14. Guide to Widely Used Multivariate Statistical Analyses

| NAME | PURPOSE | MEASUREMENT LEVEL* | | | NUMBER OF: | | |
		IV	DV	COV	IVs	DVs	COVs
Multiple correlation, regression	To test the relationship between two or more IVs and 1 DV; to predict a DV from two or more IVs	N, I, R	I, R		2+	1	
Analysis of covariance (ANCOVA)	To test the difference between the means of two or more groups, while controlling for one or more covariate	N	I, R	N, I, R	1+	1	1+
Multivariate analysis of variance (MANOVA)	To test the difference between the means of two or more groups for two or more DVs simultaneously	N	I, R		1+	2+	
Multivariate analysis of covariance (MANCOVA)	To test the difference between the means of two or more groups for two or more DVs simultaneously, while controlling for one or more covariate	N	I, R	N, I, R	1+	2+	1+
Factor analysis	To determine the dimensionality or structure of a set of variables						
Discriminant analysis	To test the relationship between two or more IVs and one DV; to predict group membership; to classify cases into groups	N, I, R	N		2+	1	
Logistic regression	To test the relationship betweenDS two or more IVs and one DV; to predict the probability of an event; to estimate relative risk (odds ratios)	N, I, R	N		2+	1	

*Measurement level of the independent variable (IV), dependent variable (DV), and covariates (Cov): N = nominal, I = interval, R = ratio.

Tips on Reading Text With Statistical Information

There are usually three types of information reported in the results section. First, there are descriptive statistics (such as those shown in Table 13-4), which typically provide readers with a basic overview of the participants' characteristics and their performance on the dependent variables. Information about the subjects' background characteristics enables readers to draw conclusions about the groups to which the findings might be generalized. Second, some researchers provide statistical information that enables readers to evaluate the extent of any biases. For example, researchers sometimes compare the characteristics of people who did and did not agree to participate in the study (*e.g.*, using *t*-tests). Or, in a quasi-experimental design, evidence of the preintervention comparability of the experimental and comparison groups might be presented so that readers can evaluate the study's internal validity. Finally, inferential statistics relating to the research questions or hypotheses are presented. If the findings do not support the researcher's hypotheses, further analyses might be undertaken to help unravel the meaning of the results.

The text of research reports normally tells the readers certain facts about the statistical tests that were performed, including (1) what test was used, (2) the actual value of the calculated statistic, (3) the degrees of freedom, and (4) the level of statistical significance. Examples of how the results of various statistical tests would likely be reported in the text are shown below.

1. *t*-test: $t = 1.68$; $df = 160$; $p = .09$
2. Chi-squared: $\chi^2 = 6.65$; $df = 2$; $p < .05$
3. Pearson's *r:* $r = .26$; $df = 100$; $p < .01$
4. ANOVA: $F = 0.18$; $df = 1, 69$, NS

Note that the significance level is sometimes reported as the actual computed probability that the null hypothesis is correct, as in example 1. In this case, the observed group differences could be found by chance in 9 out of 100 samples; thus, this result is not statistically significant because the differences have an unacceptably high chance of being spurious. The probability level is sometimes reported simply as falling below or above the researchers' significance criterion, as in examples 2 and 3. In both cases, the results are statistically significant because the probability of obtaining such results by chance alone is less than 5 (or 1) in 100. Note that you need to be careful to read the symbol that follows the **p value** (the probability value) correctly: The symbol $<$ means less than—that is, the results are statistically significant; the symbol $>$ means greater than—that is, the results are not statistically significant. When results do not achieve statistical significance at the desired level, researchers simply may indicate that the results were not significant (NS), as in example 4.

Statistical information is normally noted parenthetically following a sentence describing the findings, as in the following example: The patients in the experimental group had a significantly lower rate of infection than those in the control group ($\chi^2 = 7.99$, $df = 1$, $p < .01$). In reading a research report, it is not important to absorb numeric information regarding the actual statistical test. For example, the actual value of χ^2 has no inherent interest. What is important is to grasp whether the statistical tests indicate that the research hypotheses are supported (as demonstrated by significant results) or not supported (as demonstrated by nonsignificant results).

Tips on Reading Statistical Tables

The use of tables in the results section allows the researcher to condense a considerable amount of statistical information into a compact space and also prevents redundancy. Consider, for example, putting information from a correlation matrix (see Table 13-7) into the text: "The correlation between hours of nursing care and medication errors was $-.12$; the correlation between hours of nursing care and number of patient falls was $-.26$. . . ."

Unfortunately, although tables are efficient, they may be daunting and difficult to decipher. Part of the problem is the lack of standardization in table preparation. There is no universally accepted method of presenting *t*-test information, for example, and so each table may present a new challenge. Another problem is that some researchers try to include an enormous amount of information in their tables; we deliberately used tables of relative simplicity and clarity as examples in this chapter.

We know of no magic solution for helping you to comprehend tables in research reports, but we have a few suggestions. First, read the text and the tables simultaneously because the text may help to unravel what the table is trying to communicate. Second, before trying to understand the numbers in a table, try to glean as much information as possible from the accompanying words. Table titles and footnotes often communicate critical pieces of information. The table headings should be carefully reviewed because these indicate what the variables in the analyses were (often listed in the far left-hand column of the table as row labels) and what statistical information is included (usually specified in the top row as the column headings). Third, you may find it helpful to consult the glossary of symbols in Box 13-1 at the end of this chapter to determine the meaning of a statistical symbol included in a report table. Note that not all symbols in Box 13-1 were described in this chapter; therefore, it may be necessary to refer to a statistics textbook, such as that of Polit (1996), for further information. We recommend that you devote some extra time to making sure you have grasped what the tables are conveying and that, for each table, you write out a sentence or two that summarizes some of the tabular information in "plain English."

BOX 13-1   GLOSSARY OF SELECTED STATISTICAL SYMBOLS

This list contains some commonly used symbols in statistics. The list is in approximate alphabetical order, with English and Greek letters intermixed. Nonletter symbols have been placed at the end.

a — Regression constant, the intercept

α — Greek alpha; significance level in hypothesis testing, probability of Type I error

b — Regression coefficient, slope of the line

β — Greek beta, probability of a Type II error; also, a standardized regression coefficient (beta weights)

χ^2 — Greek chi squared, a test statistic for several nonparametric tests

CI — Confidence interval around estimate of a population parameter

df — Degrees of freedom

η^2 — Greek eta squared, index of variance accounted for in ANOVA context

f — Frequency (count) for a score value

F — Test statistic used in ANOVA, ANCOVA and other tests

H_0 — Null hypothesis

H_1 — Alternative hypothesis; research hypothesis

λ — Greek lambda, a test statistic used in several multivariate analyses (Wilks' lambda)

μ — Greek mu, the population mean

M — Sample mean (alternative symbol for $\bar{X}$)

MS — Mean square, variance estimate in ANOVA

n — Number of cases in a subgroup of the sample

N — Total number of cases or sample members

p — Probability that observed data are consistent with null hypothesis

r — Sample Pearson's product–moment correlation coefficient

r_S — Spearman's rank-order correlation coefficient

R — Multiple correlation coefficient

R^2 — Coefficient of determination, proportion of variance in *dependent variable* attributable to *independent variables*

R_C — Canonical correlation coefficient

ρ — Greek rho, population correlation coefficient

SD — Sample standard deviation

(continued)

BOX 13-1   *(Continued)*

SEM	Standard error of the mean
σ	Greek sigma (lowercase), population standard deviation
Σ	Greek sigma (uppercase), sum of
SS	Sum of squares
t	Test statistics used in *t*-tests (sometimes called Student's *t*)
U	Test statistic for the Mann-Whitney *U*-test
$\bar{X}$	Sample mean
x	Deviation score
Y'	Predicted value of Y, dependent variable in regression analysis
z	Standard score in a normal distribution
$\|$	Absolute value
$\leq$	Less than or equal to
$\geq$	Greater than or equal to
$\neq$	Not equal to

Lattavo, K. Britt, J. & Dobal, M. (1995). Agreement between measures of pulmonary artery and tympanic temperatures. *Research in Nursing & Health*, 18, 365–370. Reprinted by permission for Wiley-Liss, Inc., a subsidiary of John Wiley & Sons, Inc.

CONSUMER TIP:

In tables, probability levels associated with the significance tests are sometimes presented directly, as in Table 13-9. Here, the actual significance of each t-test is indicated in the next-to-last column, headed "*p*." However, researchers often indicate significance levels in tables through asterisks placed next to the value of the test statistic. By convention, one asterisk signifies p < .05, two asterisks signify $p < .01$, and three asterisks signify $p < .001$ (there is usually a key at the bottom of the table that indicates what the asterisks mean). Thus, if this system had been used in Table 13-9, the first t would have nothing next to it (implying nonsignificance), whereas the second would be presented as 2.76**. ■

CRITIQUING QUANTITATIVE ANALYSES

For novice research consumers, it is often difficult to critique statistical analyses. We hope this chapter has helped to demystify what statistics are all about, but we also recognize the limited scope of this presentation.

Although it would be unreasonable to expect you to now be adept at evaluating statistical analyses, there are certain things you should routinely look for in reviewing research reports. Some specific guidelines are presented in Box 13-2.

The first issue is whether the data and the research problem lend themselves to quantitative analysis. Not all information collected in research projects is quantitative, nor should it necessarily be converted to numbers. In Chapter 14, we discuss how researchers go about analyzing qualitative information.

Another aspect of the critique should focus on the decisions about what analyses to include in the report. Researchers generally perform many more analyses than can be reported in a short journal article. You should determine whether the reported statistical information adequately describes the sample and important research variables and reports the results of statistical tests for all hypotheses. You might also wish to consider whether the author included

---

BOX 13-2

GUIDELINES FOR CRITIQUING QUANTITATIVE ANALYSES

1. Does the report include any descriptive statistics? Do these statistics sufficiently describe the major characteristics of the researcher's data set?

2. Were the correct descriptive statistics used? (*e.g.*, were percentages reported when a mean would have been more informative?)

3. Does the report include any inferential statistical tests? If not, should it have (*e.g.*, were groups compared without information on the statistical significance of group differences)?

4. Was a statistical test performed for each of the hypotheses or research questions?

5. Do the selected statistical tests appear to be appropriate (*e.g.*, are the tests appropriate for the level of measurement of key variables)?

6. Were any multivariate procedures used? If not, should multivariate analyses have been conducted—would the use of a multivariate procedure strengthen the internal validity of the study?

7. Were the results of any statistical tests significant? Nonsignificant? What do the tests tell you about the plausibility of the research hypotheses?

8. Was an appropriate amount of statistical information reported? Were important analyses omitted, or were unimportant analyses included?

9. Were tables used judiciously to summarize statistical information? Is information in the text and tables totally redundant? Are the tables clear, with a good title and carefully labeled headings?

10. Is the researcher sufficiently objective in reporting the results?

statistical information that was not really needed, given the stated aims of the study. Another presentational issue concerns the researcher's judicious use of tables to summarize statistical information.

A thorough critique also addresses whether the researcher used the appropriate statistical procedures. Tables 13-13 and 13-14 provide summaries of the most frequently used statistical tests—although we do not expect that you will readily be able to determine the appropriateness of the tests used in a study without further statistical instruction. The major issues to consider are the number of independent and dependent variables, the levels of measurement of the research variables, the number of groups (if any) being compared, and the appropriateness of using a parametric test. When the researcher has not used a multivariate technique, you might consider whether the bivariate analysis adequately tests the relationship between the independent and dependent variables. For example, if a *t*-test or ANOVA was used, could the internal validity of the study have been enhanced through the statistical control of extraneous variables, using ANCOVA?

Finally, you can be alert to possible exaggerations or subjectivity in the reported results. The researcher should never claim that the data proved, verified, confirmed, or demonstrated that the hypotheses were correct or incorrect. Hypotheses should be described as being *supported* or *not supported, accepted* or *rejected.*

The main task for beginning consumers in reading a results section of a research report is to understand the meaning of the statistical tests. What do the quantitative results indicate about the researcher's hypothesis? How believable are the findings? The answer to such questions form the basis for interpreting the research results, a topic discussed in Chapter 15.

RESEARCH EXAMPLES

The statistical techniques described in this chapter are widely used methods of statistical analysis. Two research examples are described below. Use the guidelines in Box 13-2 to appraise the analytic decisions made by the researchers, referring to the original studies as needed.

RESEARCH EXAMPLE OF BIVARIATE INFERENTIAL STATISTICS

Research Summary

Lattavo, Britt, and Dobal (1995) conducted a study designed to compare pulmonary artery (PA), oral, axillary, and two tympanic temperatures. A primary goal of the research was to investigate whether tympanic and core PA temperatures are interchangeable (*i.e.,* whether tympanic temperature is a reliable substitute for pulmonary artery temperature). The research sample consisted of 32 patients from a medical-surgical unit of an urban community hospital.

The researchers began by computing correlation coefficients between core PA temperature and all other temperature measures. The correlations ranged from a low of .68 (for axillary temperature) to a high of .84 (for tympanic temperature as measured by the IVAC Core-Check™ tympanic thermometer). All correlations were significant at $p < .01$. However, the researchers reasoned that if the various measures are equally reliable in measuring the same phenomenon (body temperature), the r^2s (amount of shared variance) should be at least .80 (*i.e.*, the rs should be about .90 or better). Because none of the measures met this criterion, the authors questioned using alternative temperature measurements as a substitute for core PA temperature.

As a further corroboration, the researchers performed a series of paired t-tests. If the PA and tympanic measures were truly comparable, there should be no significant differences between measures made on the same patients. However, most of the t-tests were statistically significant, indicating true (not spurious) differences between the measures. For example, the mean difference between core PA temperature and IVAC Core-Check™ tympanic temperature was 0.58°F ($t = 3.58$; $df = 31$; $p < .01$). The researchers reached the following conclusion: "Based on these data, the tympanic temperature measurements are not ideal substitutes for the PA temperature measurements" (p. 369).

Clinical Relevance

Detecting and treating fever in the immunocompromised patient requires accurate and reliable temperature readings so that effective clinical decisions can be made that increase comfort, conserve energy, and enhance the immune response. Lattavo and her colleagues conducted a strong study designed to examine whether tympanic measurements are adequate. The researchers used strategies to decrease inconsistencies in temperature measurement techniques, such as having only two people collect the data. A pilot study was conducted to examine interrater reliability between the two data collectors and to ensure the reliability was of an acceptable level. The researchers' wisely used both t-tests and correlations to examine the comparability of tympanic and core PA measures.

The authors suggest several implications for clinical practice based on the findings of their study. When taking a patient's temperature using a tympanic thermometer, the nurse should hold the thermometer at the same angle as the mandible. The researchers found that holding the tympanic thermometer this way increased interrater reliability significantly. Health care agencies also need to develop policies and procedures for standard use of thermometers using new technology. The authors recommend that a single temperature site be used for as long as possible with patients to maximize the detection of subtle changes in body temperature.

RESEARCH EXAMPLE OF MULTIVARIATE STATISTICAL ANALYSIS

Research Summary

Johnson and her colleagues (1999) conducted an evaluation of a nurse-delivered smoking cessation intervention for hospitalized patients with cardiac disease. The research design was a nonequivalent control group before–after design, using smokers admitted to two inpatient cardiac units in a large Canadian hospital. Patients in one unit received the intervention, which involved two in-hospital contacts followed by 3 months of telephone support. Patients in the other unit received no special intervention.

The main outcome measures in the study were (1) self-reported smoking status 6 months after enrollment, and (2) self-reported smoking cessation self-efficacy, measured using the Smoking Abstinence Self-Efficacy Scale. When factor analyzed, this 20-item Likert scale revealed three factors that were used to form three subscales: a positive/social subscale, a negative/affective subscale, and a habit/addictive subscale.

Using t-tests and chi-squared tests, the researchers compared the baseline characteristics of the experimental and comparison group in terms of age, gender, marital status, education, and other demographic characteristics. Although the two groups were found to be similar in most respects, the experimental group was found to be significantly more affluent and significantly less likely to have been admitted for cardiac surgery. The groups were similar in terms of smoking histories.

Six months after enrollment in the study, 30.8% of control subjects and 46.0% of experimental subjects reported they were not smoking. A chi-squared test indicated that, although sizable, this difference was not statistically significant. The researchers then conducted a logistic regression to predict smoking abstinence based on group assignment, while controlling for important covariates (*e.g.,* income, surgical status, prior smoking history). They found that those in the control group were about three times as likely as those in the experimental group to resume smoking, net of background factors (odds ratio = 3.18), which was significant at the .05 level.

Multiple regression was used to predict scores on the three subscales of the self-efficacy scale. These analyses revealed that, with background variables controlled, being in the treatment group was a significant predictor of scores on the positive/social and habit/addictive subscales. The total amounts of variance accounted for in these regression analyses were 33% and 39%, respectively. The researchers concluded that the results of the study were encouraging.

Clinical Relevance

Scientific evidence supports a strong association between smoking and morbidity and mortality rates from respiratory and cardiovascular diseases.

Smoking cessation, however, can decrease these morbidity and mortality rates. A brief smoking cessation intervention designed to be implemented by nurses working on a hospital unit has considerable appeal.

Caution should be used, however, in applying the results of this study to clinical practice for a number of reasons. First, the researchers used a quasi-experimental design. Their analytic strategy, which controlled for a number of background characteristics, did, however, strengthen the internal validity of the study. Second, only 50 subjects were enrolled in the experimental group and 52 in the control group. No power analysis had been done to determine whether this sample size yielded an acceptable level of power to detect significant differences. Third, smoking status was measured solely by self-report. The subject's report of smoking status was not biochemically validated.

The findings of this study have more implications for future research than for immediate clinical practice. Because of the encouraging effectiveness of the nurse-delivered smoking cessation intervention, further research is indicated using a more rigorous design.

• • • • • *SUMMARY POINTS*

- There are four major **levels of measurement:** (1) **nominal measurement**—the classification of characteristics into mutually exclusive categories; (2) **ordinal measurement**—the ranking of objects based on their relative standing to each other on an attribute; (3) **interval measurement**—indicating not only the ranking of objects but also the amount of distance between them; and (4) **ratio measurement**—distinguished from interval measurement by having a rational zero point.
- **Descriptive statistics** enable the researcher to synthesize and summarize quantitative data.
- In a **frequency distribution**, a method of imposing order on raw data, numeric values are ordered from lowest to highest, accompanied by a count of the number (or percentage) of times each value was obtained; **frequency polygons** display frequency information graphically.
- A set of data may be completely described in terms of the shape of the distribution, central tendency, and variability.
- The shape may be **symmetric or skewed**, with one tail longer than the other; it may also be **unimodal** with one peak (*i.e.*, one value of high frequency), or **multimodal** with more than one peak.
- A **normal distribution** (bell-shaped curve) is symmetric, unimodal, and not too peaked.
- Measures of **central tendency** represent the average or typical value of a measure. The **mode** is the value that occurs most frequently in the distribution; the **median** is the point on a scale above which and below which 50% of the cases fall; and the **mean** is the arithmetic average of all the

scores. The mean is usually the preferred measure of central tendency because of its stability.

- Measures of **variability**—how spread out the data are—include the range and standard deviation. The range is the distance between the highest and lowest scores, and the **standard deviation** indicates how much, on average, the scores deviate from the mean.

- **Bivariate descriptive statistics** describe the degree and magnitude of relationships between two variables.

- A **contingency table** is a two-dimensional frequency distribution in which the frequencies of two nominal- or ordinal-level variables are **cross-tabulated**.

- **Correlation coefficients** describe the direction and magnitude of a relationship between two variables. The values range from -1.00 for a perfect negative correlation, to .00 for no relationship, to $+1.00$ for a perfect positive correlation. The most frequently used correlation coefficient is the **product–moment correlation coefficient (Pearson's r)**, used with interval- or ratio-level variables.

- **Inferential statistics**, which are based on the **laws of probability**, allow researchers to make inferences about a population based on data from a sample; they offer a framework for deciding whether the **sampling error** that results from sampling fluctuation is too high to provide reliable population estimates.

- The **sampling distribution of the mean** is a theoretical distribution of the means of many different samples drawn from the same population. Sampling distributions are the basis for inferential statistics.

- The **standard error of the mean**—the standard deviation of this theoretical distribution—indicates the degree of average error of a sample mean; the smaller the standard error, the more accurate are the estimates of the population value based on the mean of a sample.

- **Hypothesis testing** through statistical procedures enables researchers to make objective decisions about the results of their studies.

- The **null hypothesis** states that no relationship exists between the variables and that any observed relationship is due to chance or sampling fluctuations; rejection of the null hypothesis lends support to the research hypothesis.

- A **Type II error** occurs when a null hypothesis that should be rejected is accepted. If a null hypothesis is incorrectly rejected, this is a **Type I error.**

- Researchers control the risk of making a Type I error by establishing a **level of significance** (or **alpha** level), which specifies the probability that such an error will occur. The .05 level means that in only 5 out of 100 samples would the null hypothesis be rejected when it should have been accepted.

- Results from hypothesis tests are either significant or nonsignificant; statistically significant means that the obtained results are not likely to be due to chance fluctuations at a given probability level (p **level**).

- **Parametric statistical tests** involve the estimation of at least one parameter, the use of interval- or ratio-level data, and assumptions of normally distributed variables; nonparametric tests are used when the data are nominal or ordinal and the normality of the distribution cannot be assumed.

- Two common statistical tests are the *t*-test and **analysis of variance (ANOVA)**, both of which can be used to test the significance of the difference between group means; ANOVA is used when there are more than two groups.
- The most frequently used nonparametric test is the **chi-squared test**, which is used to test hypotheses relating to differences in proportions.
- Pearson's *r* can be used to test whether a correlation is significantly different from zero.
- **Multivariate statistical procedures** are increasingly being used in nursing research to untangle complex relationships among three or more variables.
- **Multiple regression**, or **multiple correlation**, is a method for understanding the effects of two or more independent variables on a dependent variable. The **multiple correlation coefficient (R)**, can be squared to estimate the proportion of variability in the dependent variable accounted for by the independent variables.
- **Analysis of covariance (ANCOVA)** permits the researcher to control extraneous variables (called **covariates**) before determining whether group differences are statistically significant.
- Other multivariate procedures used by nurse researchers include **discriminant function analysis, logistic regression, factor analysis, multivariate analysis of variance (MANOVA), multivariate analysis of covariance (MANCOVA), path analysis,** and **LISREL**.

➤➤➤➤ *CRITICAL THINKING ACTIVITIES*

Chapter 13 of the accompanying *Study Guide to Accompany Essentials of Nursing Research,* 5th edition offers various exercises and study suggestions for reinforcing the concepts presented in this chapter. In addition, you can address the following:

1. Read the method section from the quantitative research study in the Appendix of this book, and then answer the questions in Box 13-2.

2. What is the level of measurement of the two variables in Table 13-6?

3. Write a paragraph summarizing the main features of the correlation matrix in Table 13-7.

For additional review, see questions 172–197 on the study CD provided with Polit: Study Guide to Accompany Essentials of Nursing Research.

SUGGESTED READINGS

Methodologic References

Jaccard, J., & Becker, M. A. (1990). *Statistics for the behavioral sciences.* Belmont, CA: Wadsworth.

McCall, R. B. (1997). *Fundamental statistics for behavioral sciences* (7th ed.). Pacific Grove, CA: Brooks-Cole.

Polit, D. F. (1996). *Data analysis and statistics for nursing research.* Stamford, CT: Appleton & Lange.

Welkowitz, J., Ewen, R. B., & Cohen, J. (1991). *Introductory statistics for the behavioral sciences* (4th ed.). New York: Academic Press.

Substantive References

Anderson, R. A., Su, H. F., Hsieh, P. C., Allred, C. A., Owensby, S., & Joiner-Rogers, G. (1999). Case mix adjustment in nursing systems research: The case of resident outcomes in nursing homes. *Research in Nursing & Health, 22,* 271–283.

Blegen, M. A., Goode, C. J., & Reed, L. (1998). Nurse staffing and patient outcomes. *Nursing Research, 47,* 43–50.

Cheever, K. H., & Hardin, S. B. (1999). Effects of traumatic events, social support, and self-efficacy on adolescents' self-health assessment. *Western Journal of Nursing Research, 21,* 673–684.

Gebauer, C., Kwo, C., Haynes, E. F., & Wewers, M. E. (1998). A nurse-managed smoking cessation intervention during pregnancy. *Journal of Obstetric, Gynecologic, and Neonatal Nursing, 27,* 47–53.

Hill, A. S., Kurkowski, T. B., & Garcia, J. (2000). Oral support measures used in feeding the preterm infant. *Nursing Research, 49,* 2–10.

Janke, J. (1999). The effect of relaxation therapy on preterm labor outcomes. *Journal of Obstetric, Gynecologic, and Neonatal Nursing, 28,* 255–263.

Johnson, J. L., Budz, B., Mackay, M., & Miller, C. (1999). Evaluation of a nurse-delivered smoking cessation intervention for hospitalized patients with cardiac disease. *Heart & Lung, 28,* 55–64.

King, K. M. (2000). Gender and short-term recovery from cardiac surgery. *Nursing Research, 49,* 29–36.

Lattavo, K., Britt, J., & Dobal, M. (1995). Agreement between measures of pulmonary artery and tympanic temperatures. *Research in Nursing and Health, 18,* 365–370.

Meek, P. M. (2000). Influence of attention and judgment on perception of breathlessness in healthy individuals and patients with chronic obstructive pulmonary disease. *Nursing Research, 49,* 11–19.

Mentes, J., Culp, K., Maas, M., & Rantz, M. (1999). Acute confusion indicators: Risk factors and prevalence using MDS data. *Research in Nursing & Health, 22,* 95–105.

Mikhail, B. I. (1999). Perceived impediments to prenatal care among low-income women. *Western Journal of Nursing Research, 21,* 335–355.

Munet-Vilaró, F., Folkman, S., & Gregorich, S. (1999). Depressive symptomatology in three Latino groups. *Western Journal of Nursing Research, 21,* 209–224.

Parshall, M. B. (1999). Adult emergency visits for chronic cardiorespiratory disease: Does dyspnea matter? *Nursing Research, 48,* 62–70.

Picot, S. F., Zauszniewski, J. A., Debanne, S. M., & Holston, E. C. (1999). Mood and blood pressure responses in black female caregivers and noncaregivers. *Nursing Research, 48,* 150–161.

Pressler, J. L., Hepworth, J. T., LaMontagne, L. L., Sevcik, R. H., & Hesselink, L. F. (1999). Behavioral responses of newborns of insulin-dependent and nondiabetic, health mothers. *Clinical Nursing Research, 8,* 103–118.

Wolff, A. C., & Ratner, P. A. (1999). Stress, social support, and sense of coherence. *Western Journal of Nursing Research, 21,* 182–197.

CHAPTER 14

Analyzing Qualitative Data

Student Objectives

On completion of this chapter, the student will be able to:

○ distinguish four prototypical qualitative analysis styles
○ describe the four intellectual processes that typically play a role in qualitative analysis
○ describe activities that qualitative researchers perform to manage and organize their data
○ discuss the procedures used to analyze qualitative data, including both general procedures and those used in the grounded theory approach
○ assess the adequacy of the researcher's description of the steps used to analyze the data
○ evaluate the steps a qualitative analyst took to validate the understandings gleaned from thematic analysis
○ define new terms in the chapter

New Terms

Basic social process (BSP)
Categorization scheme
Conceptual files
Constant comparison
Core variable
Detailed approach to analysis
Editing analysis style
Holistic approach to analysis
Immersion/crystallization
   analysis style
Manifest content analysis
Memos

Open coding
Qualitative content analysis
Quasi-statistical analysis style
Quasi-statistics
Recontextualization
Selective approach to analysis
Selective coding
Substantive coding
Template
Template analysis style
Theme
Theoretical coding

Qualitative data take the form of loosely structured, narrative materials, such as verbatim transcripts from an in-depth interview, field notes from participant observation, or personal diaries. This chapter describes methods for analyzing such qualitative data.

INTRODUCTION TO QUALITATIVE ANALYSIS

Qualitative analysis is a labor-intensive activity that requires creativity, conceptual sensitivity, and sheer hard work. Qualitative analysis does not proceed in a linear fashion and is more complex and difficult than quantitative analysis because it is less formulaic. In this section, we discuss some general considerations relating to qualitative analysis.

Qualitative Analysis: General Considerations

The purpose of data analysis, regardless of the type of data or the underlying research tradition, is to organize, provide structure to, and elicit meaning from research data. The data analysis task is particularly challenging for qualitative researchers, for three major reasons. First, there are no systematic rules for analyzing and presenting qualitative data. The absence of systematic analytic procedures makes it difficult to present findings in such a way that their validity is patently clear. Some of the procedures described in Chapter 12 (*e.g.,* member checking and investigator triangulation) are important tools for enhancing the trustworthiness not only of the data themselves but also of the analyses and interpretation of those data.

The second challenge of qualitative analysis is the enormous amount of work required. The qualitative analyst must organize and make sense of pages and pages of narrative materials. In a recent multimethod study by one of the authors (Polit), the qualitative data consisted of transcribed, unstructured interviews with about 120 low-income women discussing life stressors and health problems. The transcriptions ranged from 30 to 50 pages in length, resulting in more than 3000 pages that had to be read and reread and then organized, integrated, and interpreted.

The final challenge comes in reducing the data for reporting purposes. Quantitative results can often be summarized in two or three tables. However, if a researcher summarized the findings of a qualitative analysis without including numerous supporting excerpts from the narrative materials, the richness of the original data would disappear—and readers would have no basis for challenging the researcher's interpretation. As a consequence, it is sometimes difficult to do a thorough presentation of the results of qualitative research in a format that is compatible with space limitations in professional journals.

 CONSUMER TIP:

Qualitative analyses are often more difficult to do than quantitative ones, but qualitative findings are generally easier to understand than quantitative findings because the stories are often told in everyday language. The readability of the qualitative reports is usually enhanced by the inclusion of verbatim excerpts taken directly from the narrative data. However, qualitative analyses are often harder to evaluate critically than quantitative analyses because the person reading the report cannot know first-hand whether the researcher adequately captured thematic patterns in the data. ■

Analysis Styles

Crabtree and Miller (1992) observed that there are nearly as many qualitative analysis strategies as there are qualitative researchers. However, they have identified four major analysis styles or patterns that fall along a continuum. At one extreme is a style that is more objective, systematic, and standardized, and at the other extreme is a style that is more intuitive, subjective, and interpretive. The four prototypical styles they described are as follows:

Quasi-statistical analysis style. The researcher using a quasi-statistical style typically begins with some preconceived ideas about the analysis and uses those ideas to sort the data. This approach is sometimes referred to as **manifest content analysis**—the researcher reviews the content of the narrative data, searching for particular words or themes that have been specified in advance. The result of the search is information that can be analyzed statistically, and hence the name **quasi-statistics.** For example, the analyst can count the frequency of occurrence of specific themes, or can cross-tabulate the occurrence of certain words.

Template analysis style. In this style, the researcher develops a **template** or analysis guide to which the narrative data are applied. The units for the template are typically behaviors, events, or linguistic expressions (*e.g.,* words). A template is more adaptable than a codebook in the quasi-statistical style. Although the researcher may begin with a rudimentary template before collecting any data, it undergoes constant revision as more data are gathered. The analysis of the resulting data, once sorted according to the template, is interpretive and not statistical. This type of style is most likely to be adopted by researchers whose research tradition is ethnography, ethology, discourse analysis, or ethnoscience.

Editing analysis style. The researcher using the editing style acts as an interpreter who reads through the data in search of meaningful segments. Once segments are identified and reviewed, the interpreter develops a **categorization scheme** and corresponding codes that can be used to sort and organize the data. The researcher then searches for the patterns and structure that connect the thematic categories. The grounded theory approach typically incorporates this type of style. Researchers whose research tradition is phenomenology, hermeneutics, or ethnomethodology use procedures that fall within the editing analysis pattern.

Immersion/crystallization analysis style. This style involves the analyst's total immersion in and reflection of the text materials, resulting in an intuitive crystallization of the data. This interpretive and subjective style is exemplified in personal case reports of a semianecdotal nature and is less frequently encountered in the nursing research literature than the other three styles.

Nurse researchers are especially likely to use an analytic strategy that can best be characterized as an editing style. Most of the remainder of this chapter describes analytic activities that are consistent with that style.

 CONSUMER TIP:

In an actual research report, the researcher is unlikely to use terms like template analysis style or editing style; these terms are post hoc characterizations of styles that are often adopted. However, if a study was done within a qualitative research tradition such as ethnography or grounded theory, this fact is likely to be reported, thereby providing readers with a sense of the overall analytic strategy. ∎

The Qualitative Analysis Process

The analysis of qualitative data typically is an active and interactive process. Qualitative researchers typically scrutinize their data carefully and deliberatively. Insights and theories cannot spring forth from the data unless the researcher is completely familiar with those data. Qualitative researchers often read their narrative data over and over in search of meaning and deeper understandings. Morse and Field (1995) note that qualitative analysis is "a process of fitting data together, of making the invisible obvious, of linking and attributing consequences to antecedents. It is a process of conjecture and verification, of correction and modification, of suggestion and defense" (p. 126). Morse and Field identified four intellectual processes that play a role in qualitative analysis:

- *Comprehending.* Early in the analytic process, qualitative researchers strive to make sense of the data and to learn "what is going on." When comprehension is achieved, the researcher is able to prepare a thorough and rich description of the phenomenon under study, and new data do not add much to that description. Thus, comprehension is completed when saturation has been attained.
- *Synthesizing.* Synthesizing involves a "sifting" of the data and putting pieces together. At this stage, the researcher gets a sense of what is typical with regard to the phenomenon and of what variation is like. At the end of the synthesis process, the researcher can make some generalized statements about the phenomenon and about the study participants.
- *Theorizing.* Theorizing involves a systematic sorting of the data. During the theorizing process, the researcher develops alternative explanations of the phenomenon under study and then holds these explanations up to determine their "fit" with the data. The theorizing process continues to evolve until the best and most parsimonious explanation is obtained.
- *Recontextualizing.* The process of **recontextualization** involves the further development of the theory such that its applicability to other settings or groups is explored. In qualitative inquiries whose ultimate goal

is theory development, it is the theory that must be recontextualized and generalized.

Although the intellectual processes in qualitative analysis are not linear in the same sense that quantitative analysis is, it is nevertheless true that these four processes follow a rough progression over the course of the study. Comprehension occurs primarily while in the field. Synthesis begins in the field but may continue well after the fieldwork has been completed. Theorizing and recontextualizing are processes that are difficult to undertake before synthesis has been completed.

QUALITATIVE DATA MANAGEMENT AND ORGANIZATION

The intellectual processes of qualitative analysis are supported and facilitated by tasks that help to organize and manage the masses of narrative data.

Developing a Categorization Scheme

The first step in analyzing qualitative data is to organize them, and the main organizational task is developing a method to classify and index the materials. The researcher must design a mechanism for gaining access to parts of the data, without having to repeatedly reread the data set in its entirety. This phase of data analysis is essentially reductionist—data must be converted to smaller, more manageable units that can be retrieved and reviewed.

The most widely used procedure is to develop a categorization scheme and to then code the data according to the categories. A categorization system is sometimes prepared (at least in a preliminary version) before data collection, but more typically the qualitative analyst develops categories based on a scrutiny of the actual data.

There are, unfortunately, no straightforward or easy guidelines for this task. The development of a high-quality categorization scheme for qualitative data involves a careful reading of the data, with an eye to identifying underlying concepts and clusters of concepts. Depending on the aims of the study, the nature of the categories may vary in level of detail or specificity as well as in level of abstraction.

Researchers whose aims are primarily descriptive tend to use concrete categories. For example, the category scheme may focus on actions or events or on different phases in a chronologic unfolding of an experience. In developing a category scheme, related concepts are often grouped together to facilitate the coding process.

Example of developing a category scheme:

The coding scheme used by Polit, London, and Martinez (2000) to categorize data relating to food insecurity and hunger in low-income families (Fig. 14-1) is an example of a category system that is fairly concrete and descriptive. For

A. Use of Food Services/Programs

1. Food stamps
2. WIC
3. Food pantries
4. Soup kitchens
5. Free lunch programs

B. Food Inadequacy

1. Problems feeding family, having enough food
2. Having to eat undesirable food
3. Hunger

C. Strategies to Avoid Hunger

1. Bargain shopping
2. Borrowing money
3. Getting food from friends, relatives
4. Eating old or unsafe food
5. Doubling up to share food costs
6. Stretching food, smaller portions
7. Smoking in lieu of eating
8. Illegal activities, fraud

D. Special Issues

1. Mothers sacrificing for children
2. Effects of welfare reform on hunger
3. Stigma

FIGURE 14-1. Polit et al.'s (2000) Coding Scheme for Food Insecurity and Hunger in Low-Income Families.

example, it allows the coders to code discussions about the use of specific resources and food assistance programs. The coding system involved four major category clusters, each with subcodes. For example, an excerpt that described a mother's purchase of day-old bread would be coded under category C.4.

Studies designed to develop a theory are more likely to develop abstract and conceptual categories. In designing conceptual categories, the researcher must break the data into segments, closely examine them, and compare them to other segments for similarities and dissimilarities to determine what type of phenomena are reflected in them and what the meaning of those phenomena are. (This is part of the process referred to as **constant comparison** by grounded theory researchers.) The researcher asks questions about discrete events, incidents, or thoughts that are indicated in an observation or statement, such as the following:

What is this?
What is going on?
What does it stand for?
What else is like this?
What is this distinct from?

Important concepts that emerge from close examination of the data are then given a label that forms the basis for a categorization scheme. These category names are necessarily abstractions, but the labels are generally sufficiently graphic that the nature of the material to which it refers is clear—and often provocative. Strauss and Corbin (1990) advise qualitative researchers as follows: "The important thing is to name a category, so that you can remember it, think about it, and most of all begin to develop it analytically" (pp. 67–68).

Coding Qualitative Data

Once a categorization scheme has been developed, all of the data are then reviewed for content and coded for correspondence to or exemplification of the identified categories. The process of coding qualitative material is seldom an easy one, for several reasons. First, the researcher may have difficulty in deciding which code is most appropriate or may not fully comprehend the underlying meaning of some aspect of the data. It may take a second or third reading of the material to grasp its nuances.

Second, the researcher often discovers in going through the data that the initial category system was incomplete or inadequate. It is not unusual for some themes to emerge that were not initially conceptualized. When this happens, it is risky to assume that the topic failed to appear in previously coded materials. That is, a concept might not be identified as salient until it has emerged three or four times in the data. In such a case, it would be necessary to reread all previously coded material to have a truly complete grasp of that category.

Another issue is that narrative materials are generally not linear. For example, paragraphs from transcribed interviews may contain elements relating to three or four different categories, embedded in a complex fashion.

Example of coding qualitative data:

An example of a multitopic segment of an interview from Polit and colleagues' (2000) study of hunger in low-income families is shown in Figure 14-2. The codes in the margin represent codes from the scheme presented in Figure 14-1.

Manual Methods of Organizing Qualitative Data

A variety of procedures have traditionally been used to organize and manage qualitative data. Before the advent of computer programs for managing qualitative data, the most usual procedure was the development of **conceptual files.** In this approach, a physical file is developed for each category, and all of the materials relating to that topic, based on the codes, are cut out and

B1   I hate being on welfare, it is a pain in the butt. I   A1
don't need their cash, but the food stamps, they
help a lot because it is hard, it is really hard. I got
to live day by day for food for my kids. I have to
call down to the shelter to get them to send you   A3
food, and you hate doing that because it is
embarrassing, but I have to live day by day. I   D3
have to do things so my kids can eat. I don't
worry about me, just for my kids because I can go
a day without eating, but as long as my kids eat.
D1   But I never have to worry about my kids starving
because I have family.   C3

FIGURE 14-2. Coded Excerpt from Polit et al. (2000) Study

inserted into the file. In this fashion, all of the content on a particular topic can be retrieved by going to the applicable file folder.

The creation of such conceptual files is clearly a cumbersome and labor-intensive task. This is particularly true when segments of the narrative materials have multiple codes (*e.g.,* the excerpt shown in Fig. 14-2). In such a situation, there would need to be six copies of the paragraph—one for each file corresponding to the six codes. The researcher must also be sensitive to the need to provide enough context that the cut-up material can be understood. Thus, it might be necessary to include material preceding or following the directly relevant materials.

Computer Programs for Managing Qualitative Data

The traditional manual methods of organizing qualitative data have a long and respected history, but sophisticated computer programs for managing qualitative data are now widely used. These programs permit the entire data file to be entered onto the computer, each portion of an interview or observational record coded, and then portions of the text corresponding to specified codes retrieved and printed (or shown on a screen) for analysis. The current generation of programs also has features that go beyond simple indexing and retrieval—they offer possibilities for actual analysis and integration of the data.

Computer programs remove the drudgery of cutting and pasting pages and pages of narrative material. However, some people prefer manual indexing because it allows the researcher to get closer to the data. Others have raised concerns about using programs for the analysis of qualitative data, objecting to having a process that is basically cognitive turned into an activity that is mechanical and technical. Despite these issues, many qualitative researchers have switched to computerized data management because it frees up their time and permits them to pay greater attention to more important conceptual issues.

CONSUMER TIP:

A good coding system is of little utility if the actual coding is not done with care. There is, of course, no way for you as a reader to know whether coding was diligently performed. However, you can have more confidence if the report mentions that two or more people were involved in coding the data, or at least portions of it, to ensure intercoder reliability. ■

ANALYTIC PROCEDURES

Data *management* tasks in qualitative research are typically reductionist in nature because they convert large masses of data into smaller, more manageable segments. By contrast, qualitative data *analysis* tasks are constructionist: they involve putting segments together into a meaningful conceptual pattern. Although there are several approaches to qualitative data analysis, some elements are common to several of them. We provide some general guidelines, followed by a description of the procedures used by grounded theory researchers and phenomenologists.

CONSUMER TIP:

Research reports vary in the amount of detail provided about qualitative analytic procedures. At one extreme are researchers who say little more than that their data were analyzed qualitatively. At the other extreme are researchers who describe the steps they took to analyze their data and validate the emerging themes. Most studies fall between the two extremes, but limited detail is more prevalent than abundant detail. ■

A General Analytic Overview

The analysis of qualitative materials generally begins with a search for **themes** or recurring regularities. Themes often develop within categories of data (*i.e.,* within categories of the coding scheme used for indexing materials) but sometimes cut across them. For example, in Polit and colleagues' (2000) study (see Fig. 14-1), one theme that emerged was that the mothers took tremendous pride in their ability to provide food for their families, including their resourcefulness in accessing food services (A codes) and in using a variety of strategies to avoid hunger (C codes).

The search for themes involves not only the discovery of commonalities across participants but also a search for natural variation. Themes that emerge are never universal. The researcher must attend not only to what themes arise but also to how they are patterned. Does the theme apply only to certain subgroups? In certain types of communities or organizations? In certain contexts? At certain periods? What are the conditions that precede the observed phenomenon, and what are the apparent consequences of it?

In other words, the qualitative analyst must be sensitive to *relationships* within the data.

✓ CONSUMER TIP:

Major themes are often the subheadings used by qualitative researchers in the results section of their reports. For example, Caliandro and Hughes (1998) studied the experience of being a grandmother with primary responsibility for an HIV-positive grandchild. They identified the following four themes, which were used to organize their results section: "Upholding the primacy of the family," "Being strong as mature women," "Living in the child-centered present," and "Living within a constricting environment." ■

A further step involves validation—that is, whether the themes inferred are an accurate representation of the phenomenon. Several validation procedures can be used, as discussed in Chapter 12. If more than one researcher is working on the study, sessions in which the themes are reviewed and specific cases discussed can be highly productive. Investigator triangulation cannot ensure thematic validity, but it can minimize idiosyncratic biases. It is also useful to undertake member checks—that is, to present the preliminary thematic analysis to some informants, who can be encouraged to offer comments to support or contradict the analysis.

At this point, some researchers introduce quasi-statistics—a tabulation of the frequency with which certain themes, relations, or insights are supported by the data. The frequencies cannot be interpreted in the same way as frequencies generated in survey studies because of imprecision in the sampling of cases and enumeration of the themes. Nevertheless, as Becker (1970) pointed out,

> Quasi-statistics may allow the investigator to dispose of certain troublesome null hypotheses. A simple frequency count of the number of times a given phenomenon appears may make untenable the null hypothesis that the phenomenon is infrequent. A comparison of the number of such instances with the number of negative cases—instances in which some alternative phenomenon that would not be predicted by his theory appears—may make possible a stronger conclusion, especially if the theory was developed early enough in the observational period to allow a systematic search for negative cases. (p. 81)

⊞ Example of tabulating qualitative data:

Barroso (1999) studied the experiences and perceptions of people who are long-term nonprogressors with HIV disease. She tabulated various strategies that her sample members used to adapt to their situation. For example, many sample members did a variety of things to take care of their physical health: eating a healthy diet (80%); decreasing drug, alcohol, and cigarette use (79%); and getting adequate rest and exercise (68%).

In the final analysis stage, the researcher strives to weave the thematic pieces together into an integrated whole. The various themes need to be inter-related to provide an overall structure (such as a theory or integrated descrip-tion) to the data. The integration task is a difficult one because it demands creativity and intellectual rigor if it is to be successful.

Grounded Theory Analysis

The general analytic procedures just described provide an overview of how qualitative researchers make sense of their data and distill from them insights into processes and behaviors operating in naturalistic settings. However, vari-ations in the goals and philosophies of qualitative researchers also lead to variations in analytic strategies. A widely used analytic approach among nurse researchers is Glaser and Strauss' (1967) grounded theory method of generating theories from data. Because of its popularity, we describe here some of the specific analytic techniques of grounded theory.

Grounded theory uses the constant comparative method of data analysis. With this method, the researcher simultaneously collects, codes, and analyzes data. Coding is a process used to conceptualize data into patterns or concepts. The empirical substance of the topic being studied is conceptualized by **sub-stantive codes**, whereas **theoretical codes** conceptualize how the substantive codes relate to each other.

There are two kinds of substantive codes: open and selective. **Open cod-ing** is used in the first stage of the constant comparative analysis to capture what is going on in the data. Open codes may be the actual words used by the participants. Through open coding, data are broken down into incidents, and their similarities and differences are examined. When coding at this level, the researcher asks, "What category or property of a category does this incident indicate?" (Glaser, 1978, p.57). Open coding ends when the core variable is discovered, and then selective coding begins.

The **core variable** is a pattern of behavior that is relevant or problematic for study participants. In **selective coding**, the researcher codes only those variables that are related to the core variable. One kind of core variable can be a **basic social process (BSP)** which evolves over time in two or more phases. All BSPs are core variables, but not all core variables have to be BSPs.

Theoretical codes help the grounded theorist to weave the broken pieces of data back together again. Glaser (1978) identified 18 families of theoretical codes that researchers can use to help determine how the substantive codes relate to each other. Examples of these coding families are as follows:

- Cutting point family includes boundaries, critical junctures
- Strategy family focuses on tactics, strategies, and techniques

Throughout the coding and analysis process, grounded theory analysts document their ideas about the data, themes, and the emerging conceptual scheme in the form of memos. **Memos** preserve ideas that may initially not seem productive but may later prove valuable once further developed. Memos also encourage the researcher to reflect on and describe patterns in the data, relationships between categories, and emergent conceptualizations.

The grounded theory method is concerned with the generation of categories, properties, and hypotheses rather than testing them. The product of the typical grounded theory analysis is a conceptual or theoretical model that endeavors to explain a pattern of behavior that is both relevant and problematic for the people in the study. Once the basic problem emerges, the grounded theorist then goes on to discover the process these participants go through to cope or resolve this problem.

Example of grounded theory analysis:

Figure 14-3 presents the model developed by King and Jensen (1994) in their grounded theory study that conceptualized the process of women's "preserving the self" during cardiac surgery. According to this model, the process involved five phases: waiting, getting there, surviving, being there, and moving on. The strategies used by the women in preserving the self through the phases were: relating, making sense of, managing, and normalizing what was happening to them.

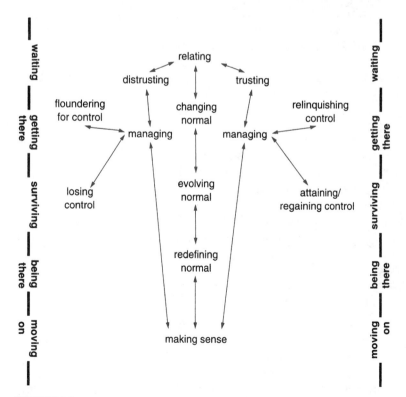

FIGURE 14-3. King and Jensen's (1994) model of preserving the self during cardiac surgery (reprinted with permission).

Phenomenological Analysis

Schools of phenomenology have developed different approaches for data analysis. In nursing, three frequently used methods of data analysis for descriptive phenomenology are the methods of Colaizzi (1978), Giorgi (1985), and Van Kaam (1966), all of whom are from the Duquesne school of phenomenology, based on Husserl's philosophy. Table 14-1 presents a comparison of the steps involved in these three methods of analysis. The basic outcome of all three methods is the description of the meaning of an experience, often through the identification of essential themes. The phenomenologist searches for common patterns shared by particular instances. However, there are some important differences among these three approaches. Colaizzi's method, for example, is the only one that calls for a final validation of the results by returning to study participants. Giorgi's analysis relies solely on the researcher. His view is that it is inappropriate to either return to the participants to validate the findings or to use external judges to review the analysis. Van Kaam's method requires that intersubjective agreement be reached with other expert judges.

A second school of phenomenolgy is the Utrecht School. Phenomenologists using this Dutch approach combine characteristics of descriptive and interpretive phenomenology. Van Manen's (1990) method is an example of this combined approach in which the researcher tries to grasp the essential meaning of the experience being studied. In reflecting on lived experience, the researcher analyzes the thematic aspects of that experience. According to Van Manen, themes can be uncovered or isolated from participants' descriptions of an experience by three different means: (1) the holistic approach, (2) the selective or highlighting approach, and the (3) detailed or line-by-line approach. In the **holistic approach**, the researcher views the text as a whole and tries to capture its meanings. In the **selective approach**, the researcher underlines, highlights, or pulls out statements or phrases that seem essential to the experience under study. In the **detailed approach**, the researcher analyzes every sentence. Once the themes have been identified, they become the objects of reflecting and interpreting through follow-up interviews with participants. Through this process, the essential themes are discovered.

A third school of phenomenology is an interpretive approach called Heideggerian hermeneutics. Diekelmann, Allen, and Tanner (1989) have described a seven-stage process of data analysis. Its outcome is to describe shared practices and common meanings. Diekelmann and colleagues' stages include the following:

1. Reading all of the interviews or texts for an overall understanding
2. Preparation of interpretive summaries of each interview
3. Analysis of selected transcribed interviews or texts by a team of researchers.
4. Resolution of any disagreements on interpretation by going back to the text.

TABLE 14-1.   Comparison of Three Phenomenological Methods

COLAIZZI (1978)	GIORGI (1985)	VAN KAAM (1966)
1. Read all protocols to acquire a feeling for them.	1. Read the entire set of protocols to get a sense of the whole.	1. List and group preliminarily the descriptive expressions that must be agreed upon by expert
of these	judges. Final listing presents	percentages
		categories in that particular sample.
2. Review each protocol and extract significant statements.	2. Discriminate units from participants' description of phenomenon being studied.	2. Reduce the concrete, vague, and overlapping expressions of the participants to more descriptive terms. (Intersubjective agreement among judges needed.)
3. Spell out the meaning of each significant statement (*i.e.,* formulate meanings).	3. Articulate the psychological insight in each of the meaning units.	3. Eliminate elements not inherent in the phenomenon being studied or that represent blending of two related phenomena.
4. Organize the formulated meanings into clusters of themes. a. Refer these clusters back to the original protocols to validate them. b. Note discrepancies among and/or between the various clusters, avoiding temptation of ignoring data or themes that do not fit.	4. Synthesize all of the transformed meaning units into a consistent statement regarding participants' experiences (referred to as the "structure of the experience"); can be expressed on a specific or general level.	4. Write a hypothetical identification and description of the phenomenon being studied.
5. Integrate results into an exhaustive description of the phenomenon under study.		5. Apply hypothetical description to randomly selected cases from the sample. If necessary, revise the hypothesized description, which must then be tested again on a new random sample.
6. Formulate an exhaustive description of the phenomenon under study in as unequivocal a statement of identification as possible.		6. Consider the hypothesized identification as a valid identification and description once preceding operations have been carried out successfully.
7. Ask participants about the findings thus far as a final validating step.		

5. Identification of common meaning by comparing and contrasting the text's shared practices.
6. Emergence of relationships among themes
7. Presentation of a draft of the themes, along with exemplars from texts, to the team; responses and suggestions are incorporated into the final draft

> **CONSUMER TIP:**
>
> Qualitative researchers who conduct studies that are not based in a formal research tradition often say that a content analysis was performed. Qualitative content analysis is the analysis of the content of narrative data to identify prominent themes and patterns among the themes—primarily using an analysis style that can be characterized as either template analysis or editing analysis. ∎

CRITIQUING QUALITATIVE ANALYSES

The task of evaluating a qualitative analysis is not an easy one, even for researchers with experience in doing qualitative research. The problem stems, in part, from the lack of standardized procedures for data analysis, but the difficulty lies mainly in the fact that readers must accept largely on faith that the researcher exercised good judgment and critical insight in coding the narrative materials, developing a thematic analysis, and integrating the materials into a meaningful whole. This is because the researcher is seldom able to include more than a handful of examples of actual data in a research report published in a journal and because the process of inductively abstracting meaning from the data is difficult to describe.

In quantitative analysis, the research can be evaluated in terms of the adequacy of specific analytic decisions (*e.g.,* did the researcher use the appropriate statistical test?). In a critique of qualitative analysis, however, the primary task is usually determining whether the researcher took sufficient steps to validate inferences and conclusions. A major focus of a critique of qualitative analyses, then, is whether the researcher has adequately documented the analytic process. Some guidelines that may be helpful in evaluating qualitative analyses are presented in Box 14-1.

RESEARCH EXAMPLES

The number of qualitative studies that have been published in nursing journals during the past decade has risen dramatically. Three research examples are described below.

BOX 14-1

GUIDELINES FOR CRITIQUING QUALITATIVE ANALYSES

1. Based on information in the report regarding either the analysis strategy or the research tradition, what type of analysis style appears to have been used?

2. Is the initial categorization scheme described? If so, does the scheme appear logical and complete? Was the scheme validated in any way (*e.g.,* did more than one person develop it collaboratively)?

3. Who coded the data—the researcher or assistants? Did the report indicate that efforts were made to determine interrater reliability of the coding?

4. Does the report describe the process by which an integrated thematic analysis was performed? What major themes emerged? If excerpts from the data are provided, do the themes appear to capture the meaning of the narratives (*i.e.,* does it appear that the researcher adequately interpreted the data and conceptualized the themes)?

5. Is the analysis parsimonious—could two or more themes be collapsed into a broader and perhaps more useful conceptualization?

6. What evidence does the report provide that the researcher's analysis is accurate and replicable?

7. Were data displayed in a manner that allows you to verify the researcher's conclusions? Was a conceptual map, model, or diagram effectively displayed to communicate important processes?

8. Was the context of the phenomenon adequately described? Does the report give you a clear picture of the social or emotional world of the study participants?

9. If the result of the study is an emergent theory or conceptualization, does it seem trivial or obvious? Does the scheme yield a meaningful and insightful picture of the phenomenon under study?

RESEARCH EXAMPLE OF A GROUNDED THEORY ANALYSIS

Research Summary

Durham (1999) conducted a grounded theory study of women's home management of preterm labor. Her purpose was to study how women managed this treatment, especially bed rest, within the context of their everyday life. In-depth interviews were conducted with 25 women being treated at home for preterm labor. The interviews, which lasted from 1 to 4 hours, were audiotaped. All of the interviews took place in the women's homes, which provided an opportunity to observe the women in their natural environments.

Constant comparison was used to analyze the data. Durham simultaneously collected, coded, and analyzed the data to provide direction for what data to collect next. Codes were collapsed into categories, and memos were written linking the categories together. The developing grounded theory was confirmed and verified by the women in subsequent interviews.

The grounded theory analysis revealed that activity restriction was the most salient aspect of the women's home management. The process by which women coped with this basic social-psychological problem involved three phases: (a) the diagnostic phase; (b) the negotiation phase; and (c) the preparation for parenthood phase.

The diagnostic phase centered on the diagnosis and realization that the women were at risk for delivering preterm. The following quote captures the drastic change in lifestyle that accompanied the news about the activity restriction:

> Someone walks in and says, "Lie on the couch; now you can't get up any more." Your hair is dirty, you can't brush your teeth, that's too bad. Now, take out of your pocket your new watch, your car keys, your wallet, your credit cards, and your checkbook; you won't be needing these any more. . . . (p. 497)

The negotiation phase involved the women's confrontation of their multisituated reality, while negotiating their needs and wants that conflicted with that reality. In the final phase, the women shifted their focus from prevention of preterm delivery to preparation for parenthood. The proposed grounded theory that women manage their activity restriction through negotiations in which they attempt to balance perceived risks against their own needs represents a new perspective on preterm birth prevention.

Clinical Relevance

Prematurity is one of the most significant perinatal problems in the United States. It is associated with high morbidity and mortality rates and long-term sequelae. Prevention of preterm labor is paramount, and therefore this study addressed an issue of great clinical relevance. Durham conducted a strong study that attended to many of the aspects of Glaser and Strauss' (1967) grounded theory method.

The findings from this study can inform nurses' efforts to help women cope with activity restrictions for home management of their preterm labor. Knowledge of the three phases of preterm labor management can help nurses to provide timely and appropriate counseling. During the diagnostic phase, health care professionals can provide continuity of care by calling these women after they are discharged from the hospital. After the shock of the diagnosis wears off, the mothers-to-be have many questions about their prescriptions and their risk status. During the negotiation phase, nurses can help identify creative ways for the women to manage their activity restriction. In the final phase as women near the end of their pregnancies, nurses can play a role in providing women with the information they need to prepare for labor, delivery, and parenthood because the activity restriction prevents them from attending traditional childbirth classes.

RESEARCH EXAMPLE OF AN ANALYSIS FOR AN ETHNOGRAPHIC STUDY

Research Summary

Russell's (1996) ethnographic study focused on the care-seeking process used by elders residing in a continuing care retirement community. During 8 months of fieldwork in a retirement community, Russell collected data on the elders' process of eliciting care and engaging caregivers in care interactions. Data were collected through in-depth semistructured interviews with 12 elders, participant observation of 34 elders in the facility's adult care center, and a focus group interview with 4 elders. Each of the data collection methods yielded different perspectives about the participants' care seeking. The interviews and focus group sessions were taped and fully transcribed, and the researcher took field notes after observational sessions. Data collection and data analysis were done concurrently. The data were entered into computer files for organization and management.

The first step involved comparing and contrasting data elements from different sources to generate a categorization scheme. The result was the development of a codebook with more than 150 codes and definitions. The codes were organized and reorganized into larger units that enabled the researcher to identify patterns, features, sequences, and relationships in elders' care seeking. Field notes and memos were maintained to document new ideas about the analysis, including both theoretical and methodologic insights.

The basic unit of analysis was a specific care encounter. More than 275 such units were demarcated in the textual database. Each case was characterized in terms of certain structural elements, such as actors, contexts, and behaviors. These cases were used to develop and test an emerging conceptualization of the care-seeking process.

According to Russell's analysis, the care-seeking process comprises two phases, which she labeled "Care Eliciting" and "Care Engaging." Figure 14-4 shows Russell's diagram of the care-seeking process. The Initiating Stage, which begins when elders decide that assistance is needed, is shaped by the elders' preferences (*i.e.,* their desires and expectations relating to care) and their beliefs in terms of the appropriateness of a potential caregiver. One woman with a paid helper articulated her preferences as follows:

> It's hard for me to ask her sometimes to do things. I think they (hired people) should see what needs to be done and go ahead and do it without being asked. I don't ask her to do more. I'm afraid I'll lose her. (p. 49)

Stage 2, the Alerting Stage, involves both verbal and nonverbal strategies designed to alert others to their desire for assistance. Stage 3, the Negotiating Stage, begins when a caregiver becomes engaged in an elder's care. The negotiations between the elder and caregiver varied in terms of content, history of the relationship, and "doing"—the extent to which elders did for themselves or worked with caregivers to accomplish their care. Finally, stage 4 is the Eval-

CARE-ELICITING PHASE	CARE-ENGAGING PHASE

1. Initiating Stage
  Preferences
  Beliefs
	3. Negotiating Stage
	  Content
	  History
	  Doing

2. Alerting Stage
  Verbal
  Nonverbal
	4. Evaluating Stage
	  Care Settings
	  Caregivers
	  Care

FIGURE 14-4. Russell's (1996) diagram of sequences in the care-seeking process.

uation Stage, the periodic appraisal that the elders undertake to make further decisions regarding the caretaking. This stage was characterized by the elders' perceptions about the care settings, caregivers, and the care itself. Russell concluded that the findings support viewing elders' care seeking as an interactional and developmental process.

Clinical Relevance

Researchers have only recently begun to lay a foundation for better understanding the lives of older adults who receive care from others. Russell's use of multiple fieldwork methods helped to address this gap in knowledge.

As noted by Russell, people are often relegated to total dependence when they can no longer take care of themselves in one or more aspects of their lives. Russell's research suggests that this practice should be avoided. The elders in Russell's study desired to remain as independent as possible and to be active participants in their care when assistance was needed. Careful listening to elders can guide nurses to the appropriate amount of information and care that elders want and believe they need. By attending to each elder's needs, nurses can help avoid inducing excess dependency of their aging patients. Fostering older adults' autonomy and demonstrating sensitivity to the uniqueness of each older adult are important features of nursing care for elders.

RESEARCH EXAMPLE OF A PHENOMENOLOGICAL ANALYSIS

Research Summary

Beck (1998) conducted a descriptive phenomenological study of the experience of panic disorder in new mothers. The purposive sample consisted of six women who had experienced their initial onset of panic disorder during the postpartum period. Data collection lasted 11 months. Each mother participated in an in-depth interview in which she described her experiences living with panic after delivery. All interviews, which lasted from 50 minutes to 2 hours, were audiotaped and transcribed.

Colaizzi's (1978) method was used to analyze the verbatim transcripts. After reading the transcripts, significant statements were extracted, their meanings were formulated, and the statements were categorized into theme clusters. The findings were then integrated into an exhaustive description of the phenomenon of postpartum panic and validated by two of the mothers who had participated in the study.

Data analysis yielded 214 significant statements describing mothers' experiences of panic. These significant statements were organized into the following six themes:

1. The terrifying physical and emotional components of panic paralyzed women, leaving them feeling totally out of control.
2. During panic attacks, women's cognitive functioning abruptly diminished, whereas between these attacks, women experienced a more insidious decrease in their cognitive functioning.
3. During the panic attacks, women feverishly struggled to maintain their composure, leading to exhaustion.
4. Because of the terrifying nature of panic, preventing further panic attacks was paramount in the lives of the women.
5. As a result of recurring panic attacks, negative changes in women's lifestyles ensued, lowering their self-esteem and leaving them to bear the burden of disappointing not only themselves but also their families.
6. Mothers were haunted by the prospect that their panic could have residual effects on themselves and their families.

Clinical Relevance

Implications for nursing practice with mothers suffering from postpartum onset of panic disorder can be derived from each of these six themes. For example, based on theme 1, education would be a crucial nursing intervention to help decrease the terrifying effects of panic. Anticipatory guidance can be provided regarding the possibility of panic attacks after delivery.

As another example, a nursing intervention that could be derived from theme 3 could focus on the overwhelming exhaustion that mothers experience as they try to hide their panic attacks from others. Nurses can foster a trusting, supportive environment that would allow mothers to reveal that they were having these unexpected, frightening panic attacks. Another example of a nursing intervention that can be based on the findings of this study comes from theme 4. To help mothers prevent further panic attacks, nurses can suggest the women keep diaries in which they make notes to try to identify their panic triggers.

SUMMARY POINTS

- Qualitative analysis is a challenging, labor-intensive activity—and one that is guided by few standardized rules.
- Although there are no universal strategies for qualitative analysis, four prototypical styles have been identified: (1) a **quasi-statistical style** that begins with preestablished themes and that lends itself to basic descriptive statistical analysis; (2) a **template analysis style** that involves the development of an analysis guide (**template**) to sort the data; (3) an **editing analysis style** that involves an interpretation of the data on which a **categorization scheme** is based; and (4) an **immersion/crystallization style** that is characterized by the analyst's total immersion in and reflection of text materials.
- Qualitative analysis typically involves four types of intellectual processes: comprehending, synthesizing, theorizing, and **recontextualizing** (exploration of the developed theory in terms of its applicability to other settings or groups).
- The first major step in analyzing qualitative data is to organize and index the materials for easy retrieval, typically by coding the content of the data according to a categorization scheme.
- Traditionally, researchers have organized their data by developing **conceptual files**, which are physical files in which coded excerpts of data relevant to specific categories are placed. However, there are now computer programs that perform basic indexing functions and also offer various enhancements that facilitate data analysis.
- The actual analysis of data begins with a search for **themes**, which involves the discovery of commonalities across subjects as well as natural variation in the data.
- The next analytic step generally involves a validation of the thematic analysis. Some researchers use **quasi-statistics**, which involves a tabulation of the frequency with which certain themes or relations are supported by the data.
- In a final analytic step, the analyst tries to weave the thematic strands together into an integrated picture of the phenomenon under investigation.
- Grounded theory uses the constant comparative method of data analysis.
- There are two broad types of codes in grounded theory: **substantive codes** (in which the empirical substance of the topic is conceptualized) and **theoretical codes** (in which the relationships among the substantive codes are conceptualized).
- Substantive coding involves **open coding** to capture what is going on in the data, and then **selective coding**, in which only variables relating to a core variable are coded. The **core variable**, a behavior pattern that has relevance for participants, is sometimes a **basic social process** (BSP) that involves an evolutionary process of coping or adaptation.

- There are numerous different approaches to phenomenological analysis, including the descriptive methods of Colaizzi, Giorgi, and Van Kaam, in which the goal is to find common patterns of experiences shared by particular instances.
- In Van Manen's approach, which involves efforts to grasp the essential meaning of the experience being studied, the researcher searches for themes, using either a **holistic approach** (viewing text as a whole); **selective approach** (pulling out key statements and phrases); or **detailed approach** (analyzing every sentence).
- Some researchers identify neither a specific approach nor a specific research tradition; rather, they might say that they used **qualitative content analysis** as their analytic method.

➤ ➤ ➤ ➤ *CRITICAL THINKING ACTIVITIES*

Chapter 14 of the accompanying *Study Guide to Accompany Essentials of Nursing Research,* 5th edition offers various exercises and study suggestions for reinforcing the concepts presented in this chapter. In addition, you can address the following:

1. Read the method section from the qualitative research study in the Appendix of this book, and then answer the questions in Box 14-1.

2. What is the basic social process that was identified in Sayre's study of psychiatric inpatients (the research example described in Chapter 9)? The citation is: Sayre, J. (2000). The patient's diagnosis: Explanatory models of mental illness. *Qualitative Health Research, 10,* 71–83.

*For additional review, see questions 198–205 on the study CD provided with Polit: Study Guide to Accompany Essentials of Nursing Research.

SUGGESTED READINGS

Methodologic References

Beck, C. T. (1994). Reliability and validity issues in phenomenology. *Western Journal of Nursing Research, 16,* 254–267.

Beck, C. T. (1999). Grounded theory. In J. Fain (ed.). *Reading, understanding, and applying nursing research.* Philadelphia: F. A. Davis.

Becker, H. S. (1970). *Sociological work.* Chicago: Aldine.

Colaizzi, P. (1978). Psychological research as the phenomenologist views it. In: R. Valle & M. King (Eds.). *Existential phenomenological alternatives for psychology.* New York: Oxford University Press.

Crabtree, B. F., & Miller, W. L., Eds. (1992). *Doing qualitative research.* Newbury Park, CA: Sage.

Diekelmann, N., Allen, D., & Tanner, C. (1989). *The NLN criteria for appraisal of baccalaureate programs: A critical hermeneutic analysis.* New York: NLN Press.

Giorgi, A. (1985). *Phenomenology and psychological research.* Pittsburgh, PA: Duquesne University Press.

Glaser, B. G. (1978). *Theoretical sensitivity: Advances in the Methodology of grounded theory*. Mill Valley, CA: Sociology Press.

Glaser, B. G., & Strauss, A. L. (1967). *The discovery of grounded theory: Strategies for qualitative research*. Chicago: Aldine.

Miles, M. B., & Huberman, A. M. (1994). *Qualitative data analysis* (2nd ed.). Beverly Hills, CA: Sage.

Morse, J. M., & Field, P. A. (1995). *Qualitative research methods for health professionals* (2nd ed.). Thousand Oaks, CA: Sage.

Strauss, A., & Corbin, J. (1990). *Basics of qualitative research*. Newbury Park, CA: Sage.

Van Kaam, A. (1966). *Existential foundations of psychology*. Pittsburgh, PA: Duquesne University Press.

Van Manen, M. (1990). *Researching lived experience*. New York: State University of New York.

Substantive References

Barroso (1999). Long-term nonprogressors with HIV disease. *Nursing Research, 48,* 242–249.

Beck, C. T. (1998). Postpartum onset of panic disorder. *Image—The Journal of Nursing Scholarship, 30,* 131–135.

Caliandro, G., & Hughes, C. (1998). The experience of being a grandmother who is the primary caregiver for her HIV-positive grandchild. *Nursing Research, 47,* 107–113.

Durham, R. F. (1999). Negotiating activity restriction: A grounded theory of home management of preterm labor. *Qualitative Health Research, 9,* 493–503.

King, K. M., & Jensen, L. (1994). Preserving the self: Women having cardiac surgery. *Heart & Lung, 23,* 99–105.

Polit, D. F., London, A., & Martinez (2000). *Food security and hunger in poor, mother-headed families in four U.S. cities*. New York: MDRC, Inc.

Russell, C. K. (1996). Elder care recipients' care-seeking process. *Western Journal of Nursing Research, 18,* 43–62.

PART VI

CRITICAL APPRAISAL AND UTILIZATION OF NURSING RESEARCH

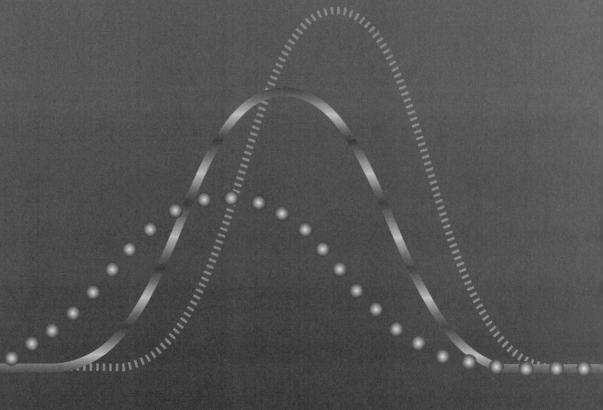

Critiquing Research Reports

● ●

Student Objectives

On completion of this chapter, the student will be able to:

○ describe aspects of a study's findings important to consider in developing an interpretation of quantitative and qualitative studies
○ describe strategies for interpreting hypothesized, unhypothesized, or mixed results in quantitative studies
○ distinguish practical and statistical significance
○ describe the purpose, features, and dimensions of a research critique
○ evaluate the substantive, methodologic, and ethical dimensions of a study
○ evaluate a researcher's interpretation of his or her results
○ define new terms in the chapter

● ●

New Terms

Critique	Results
Interpretation	Unhypothesized results
Methodologic decisions	
Mixed results	

Throughout this book, we have provided guidelines for critiquing various aspects of nursing research projects reported in the nursing literature. This chapter describes the purposes of a research critique and offers some further tips on how to evaluate research reports. One important aspect of a research critique involves the reviewer's interpretation of the study findings. Therefore, we begin this chapter by offering some suggestions on interpreting research results.

INTERPRETING STUDY RESULTS

The analysis of research data provides the **results** of the study. These results need to be evaluated and interpreted, which is often a challenging task. **Interpretation** should take into consideration the study's aims, its theoretical underpinnings, the existing body of related research knowledge, and the limitations of the adopted research methods. The interpretive task involves a consideration of the following aspects of the study findings:

• The credibility and accuracy of the results
• The meaning of the results

- The importance of the results
- The extent to which the results can be generalized or have potential for use in other contexts
- The implications for practice, theory, or research

In this section, we review issues relating to these interpretive aspects for quantitative and qualitative research reports.

Interpreting Quantitative Results

Quantitative research results often offer the consumer more interpretive opportunities than qualitative ones—in large part, because a quantitative report can summarize much of the study data, whereas qualitative reports contain only illustrative examples of the data. Readers of quantitative reports need to give careful thought to the possible meaning behind the numbers.

The Credibility of Quantitative Results

One of the first tasks you will face in interpreting quantitative results is assessing how accurate and believable they are. A thorough assessment of the accuracy of the results relies on your critical thinking skills and on your understanding of research methods. The evaluation should be based on an analysis of evidence, not on personal opinions and "gut feelings." Both external and internal evidence can be brought to bear. External evidence comes primarily from the body of prior research. If the results are consistent, the credibility of the findings is enhanced. If the results are inconsistent with prior research, possible reasons for the discrepancy should be sought. What was different about the way the data were collected, the sample was selected, key variables were operationalized, extraneous variables were controlled, and so on?

Internal evidence for the accuracy of the findings comes from an evaluation of the methods used. You will need to evaluate carefully all the major methodologic decisions made in planning and executing the study to determine whether alternative decisions might have yielded different results. This issue is discussed in greater detail later in this chapter.

A critical analysis of the research methods and conceptualization, and an examination of various types of external and internal evidence, almost inevitably indicates some limitations. These limitations must be taken into account in interpreting the results.

The Meaning of Quantitative Results

In quantitative studies, the results are usually in the form of test statistic values and probability levels, which do not in and of themselves confer meaning. The statistical results must be translated conceptually and interpreted. In this section, we discuss the interpretation of various types of research outcomes within a statistical hypothesis testing context.

CONSUMER TIP:

Many research reports do not formally specify the hypotheses that are being tested, but rather present research questions or a statement of purpose (see Chap. 5). However, every time researchers use an inferential statistic such as a *t*-test, ANOVA, chi-squared test, and so on, they are using statistics to test a hypothesis. The hypothesis being tested is that, in the population, the groups being compared are different, or that there are true, reliable relationships between variables. When hypotheses are not stated but statistical tests are performed, you may have to infer the hypotheses, which are likely to be nondirectional. ■

Interpreting Hypothesized Significant Results. When statistical tests support the researcher's hypotheses, the task of interpreting the results may be straightforward because the rationale for the hypotheses presumably offers an explanation of what the findings mean. However, hypotheses can be correct even when the researcher's explanation of what is going on is not. As a reviewer, you will need to be sure that the researcher does not go beyond the data in interpreting the results. For example, suppose a nurse researcher hypothesized that a relationship exists between a pregnant woman's level of anxiety about the labor and delivery experience and the number of children she has already borne. The data reveal that a negative relationship between anxiety levels and parity does exist ($r = -.40$; $p < .05$). The researcher concludes that childbirth experience reduces anxiety. Is this conclusion supported by the data? The conclusion seems logical, but, in fact, there is nothing within the data that leads to this interpretation. An important, indeed critical, research precept is: correlation does not prove causation. The finding that two variables are related offers no evidence about which of the two variables—if either—caused the other. Alternative explanations for the findings should always be considered. If competing interpretations can be excluded on the basis of the data or previous research findings, so much the better, but interpretations should always be given adequate competition. Throughout the interpretation process, you should bear in mind that the support of research hypotheses through statistical testing never constitutes proof of their veracity. Hypothesis testing is probabilistic, and it is always possible that obtained relationships were due to chance. Also, if there are reasons to question the study's credibility, there may also be reasons to challenge the findings.

Example of corroboration of a hypothesis:

Hayes (1998) used an experimental design to test the hypothesis that the delivery of well-structured medication instructions specifically designed for older adults discharged from the emergency department would increase knowledge of discharge regimens. The hypothesis was fully supported.

Interpreting Nonsignificant Results.   Nonsignificant results pose interpretive problems. Standard statistical procedures are geared toward disconfirmation of the null hypothesis. Failure to reject a null hypothesis (*i.e.*, obtaining results indicating no relationship between the independent and dependent variables) could occur for either of two reasons: (1) because the null hypothesis is true (i.e., there really is no relationship among research variables), or (2) because the null hypothesis is false (*i.e.*, a true relationship exists but the data failed to reveal it). Neither you nor the researcher knows which of these situations prevails. In the first situation, the problem is likely to be in the logical reasoning or the conceptualization that led the researcher to the stated hypotheses. The second situation (a false null hypothesis), by contrast, generally reflects methodologic limitations, such as internal validity problems, a small or atypical sample, or a weak statistical procedure. These limitations should previously have been identified in assessing the credibility of the results. Thus, the interpretation must consider both substantive and methodologic reasons for nonsignificant results. Whatever the underlying cause, there is never justification for interpreting a retained null hypothesis as proof of a lack of relationship among variables. The safest interpretation is that nonsignificant findings represent a lack of evidence for either truth or falsity of the hypothesis.

Note, however, that there is a decided bias against publishing the results of studies in which the results are nonsignificant. This may reflect reviewers' beliefs that nonsignificant results are likely to reflect methodologic limitations.

Example of nonsignificant results:

Schultz, Bridgham, Smith, and Higgins (1998) hypothesized that antepartum and postpartum patients would have different perceptions about the caring behavior of hospital nurses. Based on self-reported perceptions of 42 patients, there were no significant differences between the two patient groups.

Interpreting Unhypothesized Significant Results.   Although this does not happen frequently, there are situations in which the researcher obtains significant results that are the opposite of the research hypothesis; these are referred to as **unhypothesized results.** For example, a researcher might predict a negative relationship between patient satisfaction with nursing care and the length of stay in the hospital, but a significant positive relationship might be found. In such cases, it is less likely that the methods are flawed than that the reasoning or theory is incorrect. In attempting to explain such findings, you should pay particular attention to the results of previous research and alternative theories. It is also useful, however, to consider whether there is anything unusual about the sample that might lead its members to behave or respond atypically.

Example of unhypothesized significant results:

Pellino (1997) tested the Theory of Planned Behavior to predict postoperative analgesic use following elective orthopedic surgery. The theory predicted that patients with high levels of perceived control would be more likely to intend to use analgesics than those with low levels of perceived control. However, just the opposite was found to be true, leading Pellino to conclude that the findings "raise issues for research in the use of medications." (p. 104)

Interpreting Mixed Results. The interpretive process is often confounded by **mixed results:** some hypotheses are supported by the data, whereas others are not. Or a hypothesis may be accepted when one measure of the dependent variable is used but rejected with a different measure. When only some results run counter to a theoretical position or conceptual scheme, the research methods are the first aspect of the study deserving critical scrutiny. Differences in the validity and reliability of the various measures may account for such discrepancies, for example. On the other hand, mixed results may suggest that a theory needs to be qualified, or that certain constructs within the theory need to be reconceptualized.

Example of mixed results:

Neitzel, Miller, Shephard, and Belgrade (1999) tested the effects of implementing evidence-based postoperative pain management strategies on patient, provider, and fiscal outcomes. As hypothesized, there were significant effects on provider behavior (*e.g.,* decreased use of meperidine) and nurses' knowledge as well as on costs. However, patient outcomes (*e.g.,* decreased pain intensity, increased satisfaction) were not affected by the intervention.

The Importance of Quantitative Results

In quantitative studies, results supporting the hypotheses are described as being significant. A careful analysis of study results involves an evaluation of whether, in addition to being statistically significant, they are important.

The fact that statistical significance was attained in testing the hypothesis does not necessarily mean the results were of value. Statistical significance indicates that the results were unlikely to be a function of chance. This means that the observed group differences or observed relationships were probably real—but not necessarily important. With large samples, even modest relationships are statistically significant. For instance, with a sample of 500 subjects, a correlation coefficient of .10 is significant at the .05 level, but a relationship of this magnitude might have little practical value. As a reviewer, therefore, you should pay attention to the numeric values obtained in an analysis in addition to the significance level when assessing the implications of the findings.

Conversely, the absence of statistically significant results does not mean that the results are unimportant—although, because of problems in interpreting nonsignificant results, the case is more complex. Suppose a study compared two alternatives for making a clinical assessment (*e.g.*, body temperature). Suppose that a researcher retained the null hypothesis (*i.e.*, found no statistically significant differences between the two methods). If the study involved a small sample, the nonsignificant results would be difficult to interpret. If a very large sample was used, however, there would be a low probability of a Type II error. In such a situation, it might reasonably be concluded that the two procedures yield equally accurate assessments. If one of these procedures were more efficient, less painful, or less costly than the other, the nonsignificant findings could, indeed, be clinically important.

Another criterion for assessing the importance of quantitative research results concerns whether the findings are trivial or obvious. If the findings do little more than confirm common sense, their contribution to knowledge is marginal.

The Generalizability of Quantitative Results

Another aspect of quantitative results that you should assess is their generalizability. Researchers are rarely interested in discovering relationships among variables for a specific group of people at a specific point in time. The aim of nursing research is to gain insights for the improvement of nursing practice. Therefore, an important interpretive question is whether the intervention will work or whether the relationships will hold in other settings, with other people. Part of the interpretive process involves asking the question: To what groups, environments, and conditions can the results of the study be applied?

The Implications of Quantitative Results

After you have formed conclusions about the accuracy, meaning, importance, and generalizability of the results, you are ready to draw inferences about their implications. You might consider the implications of the findings with respect to future research (What should other researchers working in this area do?) or theory development (What are the implications for nursing theory?). However, you are most likely to consider the implications for nursing practice (How, if at all, should the results be used by other nurses in their practice—or by me in my own role as a nurse?). Of course, if you have reached the conclusion that the results have limited credibility or importance, they may be of little utility to your practice.

Interpreting Qualitative Results

It is usually difficult for a reviewer to interpret qualitative findings thoroughly because the researcher is selective in the amount and types of data included in the report for a reviewer's perusal. Nevertheless, you should strive to consider the same five interpretive dimensions for a qualitative study as for a quantitative one.

The Credibility of Qualitative Results

As with the case of quantitative reports, you should question whether the results of a qualitative inquiry are believable. It is reasonable to expect authors of qualitative reports to provide evidence of the credibility of the findings, as described in Chapter 12—although this does not always happen. Because readers of qualitative reports are exposed to only a portion of the data, they must rely on the researcher's efforts to corroborate the findings through such mechanisms as peer debriefings, member checks, audits, and triangulation.

CONSUMER TIP:

Even when peer debriefings or member checks have been undertaken, you should realize that they do not unequivocally establish proof that the results are believable. For example, member checks may not always be effective in illuminating flaws. Perhaps some participants are too polite to disagree with the researcher's interpretations. Or perhaps they become intrigued with a conceptualization they themselves would never have developed on their own—a conceptualization that is not necessarily accurate. ■

In thinking about the believability of qualitative results—as with quantitative results—it is advisable to adopt the posture of a person who needs to be persuaded and to expect the researcher to marshal solid evidence with which to persuade you.

The Meaning of Qualitative Results

In qualitative studies, explication and analysis of the data often occur simultaneously. That is, the researchers make sense of the data as they are coding it, developing a thematic analysis and integrating the themes into a unified whole. Efforts to validate the qualitative analysis are necessarily efforts to validate the thematic or interpretive development as well. Thus, in a qualitative study, the meaning of the data flows from the analysis, and it is seldom necessary to puzzle through the findings in search of a deeper meaning. Moreover, the qualitative researcher rarely establishes *a priori* hypotheses, and thus the task of gleaning meaning does not involve elucidating unhypothesized or mixed results.

The Importance of Qualitative Results

Qualitative research is especially productive when it is used to describe and explain poorly understood phenomena. But the amount of prior research on a topic is not a sufficient barometer for deciding whether the findings can make a contribution to nursing knowledge. The phenomenon must be one that merits rigorous scrutiny. For example, some people prefer the color green and others like red. Color preference may not, however, be a sufficiently important topic for an in-depth inquiry. Thus, you must judge whether the topic under study is important or trivial.

In a critical evaluation of a study's importance, you should also consider whether the findings themselves are trivial. Perhaps the topic is worthwhile, but you may feel after reading the report that nothing new has been learned—which can result when the data are too "thin" or when the conceptualization is shallow. Qualitative researchers often attach catchy labels to their themes and processes, but you should ask yourself whether the labels have really captured an insightful construct that goes beyond common knowledge.

The Transferability of Qualitative Results

Although qualitative researchers do not strive for generalizability, the application of the results to other settings and contexts must be considered. If the findings are only relevant to the study participants, they cannot be useful to nursing practice. Thus, in interpreting qualitative results, you should consider how transferable the findings are. In what other types of settings and contexts would you expect the phenomena under study to be manifested in a similar fashion? Of course, to make such an assessment, the author of the report must have described in sufficient detail the context in which the data were collected. Because qualitative studies are context bound, it is only through a careful analysis of the key parameters of the study context that the transferability of results can be assessed.

The Implications of Qualitative Results

If the findings are judged to be believable and important, and if you are satisfied with your interpretation of the meaning of the results, you can begin to consider what the implications of the findings might be. As with quantitative studies, the implications can be multidimensional. First, you can consider the implications for further research: Should the similar study be undertaken in a new settings? Can the study be expanded (or circumscribed) in meaningful or productive ways? Do the results suggest that an important construct has been identified that merits the development of a formal measuring instrument? Does the emerging theory suggest hypotheses that could be tested through controlled quantitative research? Second, do the findings have implications for nursing practice? For example, could the health-care needs of a subculture (*e.g.*, the homeless) be identified and addressed more effectively as a result of the study? Finally, do the findings shed light on fundamental processes that are incorporated into nursing theory?

RESEARCH CRITIQUE

If nursing practice is to be based on scientific knowledge, the worth of studies appearing in the nursing literature must be critically appraised. Sometimes, consumers mistakenly believe that if a research report was accepted for publication, the study must be sound. Unfortunately, this is not necessarily the case. Indeed, most research has limitations and weaknesses, and, for this reason, no single study can provide unchallengeable answers to research questions. Nevertheless, the methods of disciplined inquiry continue to provide us with the best possible means of answering certain questions. Knowledge is accumulated not by an individual researcher conducting a single, isolated study but rather through the conduct of several studies addressing the same or similar research questions and through the subsequent critical appraisal of these studies by others. Thus, consumers who can thoughtfully critique research reports also play a role in the advancement of nursing knowledge.

Critiquing Research Decisions

The quality of a study depends on the decisions the researcher made in conceptualizing, designing, and executing the study and in interpreting and communicating the study results. Each study tends to have its own peculiar flaws because each researcher, in addressing the same or a similar research question, makes different decisions about how the study should be done. It is not uncommon for researchers who have made different **methodologic decisions** to arrive at different answers to the same research question. It is precisely for this reason that consumers must be knowledgeable about research methods. You must be able to evaluate research decisions so that you can determine how much faith should be put in the conclusions. You must ask: What other approaches could have been used to study this research problem? and, If another approach had been used, would the results have been more reliable, credible, or replicable? In other words, you need to evaluate the impact of the researcher's decisions on the study's ability to reveal the truth.

Much of this book has been designed to acquaint you with a range of methodologic options for the conduct of research—options on how to design a study, measure variables, select a sample, analyze data, and so on. We hope a familiarity with these options will provide you with the tools to challenge a researcher's decisions when it is appropriate to do so.

Purposes of a Research Critique

A research **critique** is not just a summary of a study but rather a careful appraisal of its merits and flaws. A critique can vary in scope and length, depending on its intended purpose. As a student, you may be asked to prepare a thorough and comprehensive critique of a research report. The purpose of such a critique is to cultivate critical thinking, to induce you to use newly acquired skills in research methods, and to obtain documentation of those skills. Comprehensive critiques are also sometimes prepared by researchers writing commentaries for publication or by discussants at research conferences.

Critiques are often prepared by scholars and researchers to help journal editors in making publication decisions and to offer guidance to researchers on how their research reports could be effectively revised. These critiques typically are not long and generally focus primarily on key substantive and methodologic issues. These critiques may be written in narrative, essay form or may take the form of a bulleted list of the study's strengths and weaknesses.

Practicing nurses also critique research reports—sometimes in writing, and sometimes orally in discussion groups or journal clubs. These critiques, which are especially important in relation to the utilization of research results (see Chap. 16), tend to focus on the scientific merit of the study and on its implications for nursing practice. Their purpose is to help practicing nurses think about how study findings can be used and, sometimes, actually to plan a utilization project.

Regardless of the scope of a critique, its function is not to hunt dogmatically for and expose mistakes. A good critique objectively identifies areas of adequacy and inadequacy, virtues as well as faults. Sometimes, the need for this balance is obscured by the terms *critique* and *critical appraisal*, which connote unfavorable observations. The merits of a study are as important as its limitations in coming to conclusions about the worth of its findings. Therefore, the research critique should reflect a thoughtful, objective, and balanced consideration of the study's validity and significance.

Each chapter in this text has offered guidelines for evaluating various research decisions as well as various aspects of written research reports. In preparing a written critique, these guidelines should be reviewed. Box 15-1

BOX 15-1

GUIDELINES FOR THE CONDUCT OF A WRITTEN RESEARCH CRITIQUE

1. Be sure to comment on the study's strengths as well as its limitations. The critique should be a balanced consideration of the worth of the research. Each research report has *some* positive features. Be sure to find them and note them.

2. Give specific examples of the study's strengths and limitations. Avoid vague generalizations of praise and fault finding.

3. Try to justify your criticisms. Offer a rationale for how a different approach would have solved a problem that the researcher failed to address.

4. Be as objective as possible. Try to avoid being overly critical of a study because you are not particularly interested in a topic or because you have a world view that is inconsistent with the underlying paradigm.

5. Be sensitive in handling negative comments. Try to put yourself in the shoes of the researcher receiving the critical appraisal. Do not be condescending or sarcastic.

6. Suggest realistic alternatives that the researcher (or future researchers) might want to consider. Don't just identify problems—offer some recommended solutions, making sure that the recommendations are practical ones.

7. Evaluate all aspects of the study—its substantive, theoretical, methodologic, ethical, interpretive, and presentational dimensions.

presents some further, more general tips for those preparing a formal research critique.

ELEMENTS OF A RESEARCH CRITIQUE

Each research report has several important dimensions that should be considered in a comprehensive critical evaluation of the study's worth (although some dimensions may be given limited consideration in targeted critiques). The aspects we review here include the substantive and theoretical; methodologic; ethical; interpretive; and presentation and stylistic aspects.

Substantive and Theoretical Dimensions

In preparing a critique, you need to determine whether the study was important in terms of the significance of the problem, the soundness of the conceptualizations, the appropriateness of the theoretical framework, and the insightfulness of the analysis and interpretation. The research problem should have obvious relevance to some aspect of nursing. It is not enough that a problem be interesting if it offers no possibility of contributing to nursing knowledge or improving nursing practice.

Many problems that are relevant to nursing are still not necessarily worthwhile substantively. You may need to ask a question such as, Given what we know about this topic, is this research the right next step? Knowledge tends to be incremental. Researchers must consider how to advance knowledge on a topic in the most beneficial way. They should avoid unnecessary replications of a study once a body of research clearly points to an answer, but they also should not leap several steps ahead when there is an insecure foundation. Sometimes, replication is exactly what is needed to enhance the credibility or generalizability of earlier findings. Thus, the study problem must be considered in terms of the existing body of research.

Another issue that has both substantive and methodologic implications is the congruence between the study question and the methods used to address it. There must be a good fit between the research problem on the one hand and the overall study design, data collection methods, and analytic approach on the other. Questions that deal with poorly understood phenomena, with processes, with the dynamics of a situation, or with in-depth description, for example, are usually best addressed with flexible designs, unstructured methods of data collection, and qualitative analysis. Questions that involve the measurement of well-defined variables, cause-and-effect relationships, or the effectiveness of some specific intervention, however, are usually better suited to more structured, quantitative approaches using designs that maximize research control.

A final issue to consider is whether the researcher has appropriately placed the research problem into a larger theoretical context. As we stressed in Chapter 7, a researcher does little to enhance the value of the study if the connection between the research problem and a conceptual framework is contrived. But a research problem that is genuinely framed as a part of a larger intellectual problem usually can go farther in advancing knowledge than a problem that ignores its theoretical underpinnings.

Methodologic Dimensions

Researchers make a number of important decisions regarding how best to answer their research questions or test their research hypotheses. It is your job as consumer to evaluate critically the consequences of those decisions. In fact, the heart of the research critique lies in the appraisal of the researcher's methodologic decisions.

Although the researcher makes hundreds of decisions about the methods for conducting a study, some are more consequential than others. In a quantitative study, you should focus critical attention on the following four major decisions:

- *Decision 1, Research Design:* What design will yield the most unambiguous and meaningful (internally valid) results about the relationship between the independent and dependent variables, or the most valid descriptions of the concepts under study?
- *Decision 2, Research Sample:* Who should participate in the study? What are the characteristics of the population to which the findings should be generalized? How large should the sample be, from where should participants be recruited, and what sampling approach should be used to select the sample?
- *Decision 3, Data Collection:* How should the research data be gathered? How can the variables be operationalized and reliably and validly measured?
- *Decision 4, Data Analysis:* What statistical analyses will provide the most appropriate tests of the research hypotheses or answers to the research questions?

In a quantitative study, these methodologic decisions are typically made up-front, and the researcher then executes the prespecified plan. In a qualitative study, by contrast, the researcher makes ongoing methodologic decisions while in the process of collecting and analyzing data—after the very important decisions about the research setting and research tradition have been made. In a qualitative study, the major methodologic decisions you should consider in your critique are as follows:

- *Decision 1, Setting:* Where should the study take place? What setting will yield the richest information about the phenomenon under study?
- *Decision 2, Data Collection:* What should the data sources be, and how should the data be gathered? Should multiple sources of data (*e.g.,* unstructured interviews and observations) be used to achieve method triangulation?

- *Decision 3, Sample:* Who should participate in the study? How can participants be selected to enhance the theoretical richness of the study? How many participants will be needed to achieve data saturation? How much time should be spent in the field to achieve "prolonged engagement"?
- *Decision 4, Data Quality:* What types of evidence can be obtained to support the credibility, transferability, dependability, and confirmability of the data, the analysis, and the interpretation?

Because of practical constraints, research studies almost always involve making compromises between what is ideal and what is feasible. For example, a quantitative researcher might ideally like to work with a sample of 500 subjects, but because of limited resources, may have to be content with a sample of 200 subjects. A qualitative researcher might realize that 3 years of field work would yield an especially rich and deep understanding of the culture or group under study, but cannot afford to devote this much time to the effort. The person doing a research critique cannot realistically demand that researchers attain these methodologic ideals but must be prepared to evaluate how much damage has been done by failure to achieve them.

Ethical Dimensions

In performing a comprehensive critique, you should consider whether there is evidence of ethical violations. If there are any potential ethical problems, you will need to consider the impact of those problems on the scientific merit of the study as well as on the subjects' well-being.

There are two main types of ethical transgressions in research studies. The first class consists of inadvertent actions or activities that the researcher did not foresee as creating an ethical dilemma. For example, in one study that examined married couples' experiences with sexually transmitted diseases, the researcher asked the husband and wife each to complete, privately, a self-administered questionnaire. The researcher offered to mail back copies of the questionnaires to couples who wanted an opportunity to discuss their responses. This offer was intended as a means of enhancing couple communication. However, some subjects may have felt compelled to say, under spousal pressure, that they wanted to have a copy of their responses returned in the mail, when, in fact, they did not. The use of the mail to return these sensitive completed questionnaires was also questionable. In this case, the ethical problem was inadvertent and could easily be resolved (*e.g.*, the researcher could give out blank copies of the questionnaire for the couples to go over together).

In other cases, the researcher is aware of potential ethical problems, but consciously decides that the violation is minor in relation to the knowledge gain. For example, the researcher may decide not to obtain informed consent from the parents of minor children attending a family planning clinic because such consent might discourage participation in the study and lead to a biased sample of clinic users; it could also violate the minors' right to confidential treatment at the clinic. When the researcher knowingly elects not to follow the ethical principles outlined in Chapter 4, both the decision and the researcher's rationale should be evaluated.

Interpretive Dimensions

Research reports almost always conclude with a discussion, conclusions, or implications section. In this final section, the researcher offers an interpretation of the findings, considers whether the findings support a theoretical framework, and discusses what the findings might imply for nursing.

As a reviewer, you should be somewhat wary if the discussion section fails to point out any limitations. The researcher is in the best position to detect and assess the impact of sampling deficiencies, practical constraints, data quality problems, and so on, and it is a professional responsibility to alert readers to these difficulties. Moreover, when a researcher notes methodologic shortcomings, readers know that these limitations were taken into account in the interpretation of results. As an example, Carty, Bradley, and Winslow (1996) conducted a study of women's perceptions of fatigue during pregnancy and postpartum. Women who were discharged within 3 days of delivery were compared with women who were discharged after 3 days with respect to fatigue levels. The researchers found few differences between the two groups with regard to hours slept, perceptions of tiredness, and impact of tiredness on daily life. However, the researchers included a word of caution in their discussion section:

> The following limitations should be considered when interpreting the findings: The women in this study chose their discharge time, those who went home early had significant follow-up by nurses, and the questionnaire developed for this study does not have established reliability (p. 77).

Of course, researchers are unlikely to note all relevant shortcomings of their own work. For instance, in the above example, the authors failed to point out that the absence of significant group differences could have resulted from the use of a relatively small sample. Thus, the inclusion of comments about study limitations in the discussion section, although important, does not relieve you of the responsibility of appraising methodologic decisions.

Your task as reviewer is to contrast your own interpretation with that of the researcher and to challenge conclusions that do not appear to be warranted by the results. If your objective evaluation of the research methods and findings leads to an interpretation notably different from that of the researcher, the interpretive dimension of the study merits critical commentary.

In addition to contrasting your interpretation with that of the researchers, your critique should also draw conclusions about the stated implications of the study. Some researchers make grandiose claims or offer unfounded recommendations on the basis of modest results. Some guidelines for evaluating the researcher's interpretation and implications are offered in Box 15-2.

> **BOX 15-2**
>
> ## GUIDELINES FOR CRITIQUING THE INTERPRETATIVE DIMENSIONS OF A RESEARCH REPORT
>
> 1. Does the discussion section offer conclusions or interpretations for all the important results?
>
> 2. Are the interpretations consistent with the results? Do the interpretations give due consideration to the limitations of the research methods?
>
> 3. What types of evidence in support of the interpretation does the researcher offer? Is that evidence persuasive? Are the results interpreted in light of findings from other studies?
>
> 4. Are alternative explanations for the findings mentioned, and is the rationale for their rejection presented?
>
> 5. In quantitative studies, does the interpretation distinguish between practical and statistical significance?
>
> 6. Are generalizations made that are not warranted on the basis of the sample used?
>
> 7. Does the researcher offer implications of the research for nursing practice, nursing theory, or nursing research? Are the implications appropriate, given the study's limitations?
>
> 8. Are specific recommendations for practice or future studies made? Are the recommendations consistent with the findings and consistent with the body of knowledge on the topic?

Presentation and Stylistic Dimensions

Although the worth of the study is primarily reflected in the dimensions discussed thus far, the manner in which the information is communicated in the research report is also fair game in a comprehensive critical appraisal. Box 15-3 summarizes the major points that should be considered in evaluating the presentation of a research report.

An important consideration is whether the research report has provided sufficient information for a thoughtful critique of the other dimensions. For example, if the report does not describe how participants were selected, the reviewer cannot comment on the adequacy of the sample, but he or she can criticize the researcher's failure to include information on sampling. When vital pieces of information are missing, the researcher leaves the reader little choice but to assume the worst because this would lead to the most cautious interpretation of the results.

The writing in a research report, as in any published document, should be clear, grammatical, concise, and well organized. Unnecessary jargon should be minimized, but colloquialisms generally should be avoided. Inadequate organization is another presentation flaw in some research reports.

BOX 15-3

GUIDELINES FOR CRITIQUING THE PRESENTATION OF A RESEARCH REPORT

1. Does the report include a sufficient amount of detail to permit a thorough critique of the study's purpose, conceptual framework, design and methods, handling of critical ethical issues, analysis of data, and interpretation?

2. Is the report well written and grammatical? Are pretentious words or jargon used when a simpler wording would have been possible?

3. Is the report well organized, or is the presentation confusing? Is there an orderly, logical presentation of ideas? Are transitions smooth, and is the report characterized by continuity of thought and expression?

4. Is the report sufficiently concise, or does the author include a lot of irrelevant detail? Are important details omitted?

5. Does the report suggest overt biases?

6. Is the report written using tentative language as befits the nature of disciplined inquiry, or does the author talk about what the study did or did not "prove"?

7. Is sexist language avoided?

8. Does the title of the report adequately capture the key concepts and the population under investigation? Does the abstract (if any) adequately summarize the research problem, study methods, and important findings?

Continuity and logical thematic development are critical to good communication of scientific information, but these qualities are often difficult to attain.

Styles of writing do differ for qualitative and quantitative reports, and it is unreasonable to apply the standards considered appropriate for one paradigm to the other. Quantitative research reports are typically written in a more formal, impersonal fashion, using either the third person or passive voice to connote objectivity. Qualitative studies are likely to be written in a more literary style, using the first or second person and active voice to connote proximity and intimacy with the data and the phenomenon under study. Regardless of style, however, you should, as a reviewer, be alert to indications of overt biases, unwarranted exaggerations, emotionally laden comments, or melodramatic language.

In summary, the research report is meant to be an account of how and why a problem was studied and what results were obtained. The report should be accurate, clearly written, cogent, and concise. It should reflect scholarship, but not pedantry, and it should be written in a manner that piques the reader's interest and curiosity.

RESEARCH EXAMPLES

The appendix offers two research reports—one qualitative and the other quantitative—in their entirety. The guidelines in this chapter and throughout the book can be used to conduct a critical appraisal of these studies. (In addition, there are two complete research reports in the accompanying *Study Guide for Essentials of Nursing Research*, 5th edition, as well as a fictitious research report with a complete critique.)

In this section, we describe two studies by nurse researchers and present excerpts from published written critiques. Note that these comments are not comprehensive—they do not cover all the dimensions of a research critique as described in this chapter. However, the excerpts should provide a flavor for the kinds of things that are noted in a critique. Additionally, we present excerpts from the researchers' responses to the critique.

Research Example of a Quantitative Report and Critical Comments

Levesque, Ducharme, and Lachance (1999) used the Lazarus and Folkman Stress and Coping Model to study whether there were differences in family caregiving for institutionalized elders with and without dementia. Their published report was accompanied by commentaries by two reviewers.

Research Summary

According to the Lazarus and Folkman model, it is not only the presence of stressors that affects the well-being of caregivers but also the caregivers' cognitive appraisal of the stressors and the resources available in the situations. Based on the model and consistent with literature on home caregiving, it was expected that there would be more stress among caregivers of an institutionalized demented than nondemented relative.

Lévesque and her colleagues collected their data from a sample of primary caregivers of demented (N = 220) and nondemented (N = 88) relatives, who were recruited through more than 100 public nursing homes in and near Montreal. The in-home interviews lasted about 90 minutes and included measures of stressors (*e.g.,* the relative's functional impairment), appraisal of stressors, social support, coping strategies, and caregiver well-being (*e.g.,* psychological distress).

The findings revealed that the caregivers of a demented relative were exposed to more stressors than caregivers of a nondemented relative, and functional impairment and depressive behaviors were appraised as more disturbing. However, caregivers of a demented relative had more formal and informal social support. There were no significant differences in the level of psychological distress between the two groups of caregivers, although differences were significant when the amount of social support was statistically controlled. Caregivers seemed to use the same coping strategies whether or not their relative suffered from dementia.

Critical Comments and Response

Gerdner (1999) commented that the study made an important contribution to the literature on the caregiving experience, and also noted that the findings were consistent with other research on caregivers. She pointed out that the study "provides a basis to examine the effects of additional variables on caregiver stress" (p. 492), such as the caregivers' perception of the quality of care their loved one is receiving. Gerdner encouraged further research, noting that "a design that incorporates quantitative and qualitative data would add to the depth of findings" (p. 493).

In another review, Jirovec (1999) also praised the study. However, she had some critical comments as well:

> Comparing the stressors associated with caregiving for the two types of institutionalized elders found differences in functional impairment, disruptive behaviors, and caregiving tasks. More light might have been shed on this caregiving experience if analysis of covariance was used and functional ability used as the control variable. We would then see the significant differences in functional impairment between the groups and other differences not due to functional impairment. (p. 494)

Jirovec also questioned the particular scale the researchers used to measure depression:

> The depression scale was not validated with demented patients, and a more valid depression scale would need to be used to draw conclusions about depression in institutionalized demented elders versus non-demented elders (p. 494).

In their response to Jirovec's comment, Lévesque and her colleagues noted that there was no theoretical basis (in the Lazarus and Folkman model) for using functional impairment as a covariate. However, when they performed the requested analysis, they found that the significant group differences persisted even with functional impairment controlled. They also provided evidence that the depression scale they used was valid for use with demented people.

Clinical Relevance

As Jirovec (1999) noted in her critical commentary, Lévesque and colleagues' study addressed an often neglected area of research. Caregiving does not end when a loved one is institutionalized, and these caregivers may be at risk in terms of their psychological well-being. The reviewer noted that the study "makes an important contribution to our understanding of the caregiving experience when an elder has been institutionalized" (p. 494).

Gerdner (1999) pointed out that the researchers' findings regarding additional caregiver stress factors will facilitate the design of nursing strategies to enhance both formal and informal support of these caregivers. Examples of these potential stressors on primary caregivers include (1) factors surrounding the decision for placement in an institution, (2) caregivers' perception of the quality of care their loved one is receiving, and (3) length of time the family member has been in the primary caregiver role. Nurses can explore with care-givers how these variables have affected their response to their loved one's institutionalization. Also important to clinical practice is the acknowledg-ment by nurses of the family caregivers' expertise and knowledge in caring for their loved ones. By drawing on their extensive experience, nurses can help establish positive family–staff relationships.

RESEARCH EXAMPLE OF A QUALITATIVE REPORT AND CRITICAL COMMENTS

Butler, Banfield, Sveinson, and Allen (1998) conducted a qualitative study to describe women's experiences with changes in sexual function following treatment for gynecological cancer. Their research report, which appeared in *Western Journal of Nursing Research,* was followed by commentaries by two reviewers.

Research Summary

Butler and her colleagues conducted a multimethod study that explored issues of sexual health for women with cervical and endometrial cancer. The qualitative portion of their study involved in-depth interviews with a sample of 17 women, using a semistructured interview guide. The questions were designed to stimulate discussion about the effects of cancer and its treatment on how the participants viewed themselves as women, as partners, and as mothers. The interviews, which were taped and transcribed, lasted about 90 minutes. Content analysis was used for data analysis. Three of the investiga-tors independently coded the data; intercoder agreement was high.

Although the study's purpose was to pursue issues relating to sexual func-tioning, the women described a broader concept of sexual health in which functioning was only one aspect contributing to the view of self as a sexual being. The analysis revealed multiple components that need to be considered in developing a conceptual model of sexual health.

One of the central categories the women discussed was the effect of rela-tionships—with health care personnel, family, friends, and partners—on their sexual well-being. The absence of discussions about sexual health by nurses and physicians suggested to the women that their sexuality was not really a medical concern. This interpretation was shared with their partners, resulting in couples making efforts to adjust with little information or support. The authors concluded that health care professionals should examine their own values and beliefs about sexuality and assess their knowledge and comfort level about these topics.

Critical Commentary and Response

Downe-Wamboldt (1998) praised Butler and her colleagues for undertak-ing an interesting study on an important topic and encouraged them to con-tinue with research in this area: "The important topic of sexual health in the context of cancer care has received little attention from researchers, and this article makes a valuable contribution to the nursing literature" (p. 700).

Downe-Wamboldt did not offer any criticism of the actual study, except to note its limited generalizability, but made some suggestions about improving the report itself:

> To more meaningfully interpret the findings, it would have been helpful to have a description of the specific questions that were asked that provided the data for the study. Were there any questions that the women found too sensitive or were not comfortable to answer? The identified themes and relevant quotations generally provided a clear picture of how the themes emerged from the data. One notable exception is the theme of sexual health influenced by the environment. It is difficult to assess the validity of this theme based on the quality and quantity of quotations provided. (pp. 700–701)

Alteneder (1998), who wrote a second commentary, also expressed a desire for more information than was provided in the report:

> The authors said that nurses rarely discussed sexual functioning; however, it would be of interest to the reader what the nurses did cover when they spoke on this topic. . . . Because 6 of the participants had no longer continued to be sexually active post-treatment, information about why they were no longer active would have added to the description of the women. (p. 702)

This second commentator further suggested that the researchers could have improved the study by interviewing the women's partners; she also expressed some misgivings about the data collection:

> I have some concern about the use of the semistructured interview guide, which was reviewed for content and face validity by three oncology nurses and one physician. I feel that this type of study should be open to learn from the participants, and the restricting structure might inhibit the type of information received by the investigator. (p. 702)

In their response, Butler and her colleagues provided the commentators with some of the information they were seeking (e.g., the six women's reasons for not being sexually active). They acknowledged the need for replication of the study and also commented on data quality issues:

> The purpose statement may not have adequately reflected the depth of exploration provided by the semistructured interview guide. . . . The study participants did not appear to have any difficulty with questions asked during the interview and openly described how the cancer affected their well-being. (p. 704)

Clinical Relevance

In her critical commentary, Downe-Wamboldt (1998) noted that Butler and colleagues' study addressed an important gap in nursing knowledge and makes a valuable contribution to the nursing literature. Minimal research has been conducted on sexual health in cancer care. After treatment for gynecological cancer, many women try to cope with changes in their sexual health with insufficient help from clinicians.

Some methodologic concerns raised by the two reviewers have implications for the credibility of this study's findings, such as the restrictive nature of the semi-structured interview. This type of interview may have hindered the emergence of flow of rich data. Another limitation was the limited data supporting the theme of sexual health influenced by the environment.

Despite these limitations, the study has made a valuable contribution to health professionals' understanding of key issues for women who have undergone treatment for gynecological cancer. Alteneder (1998) noted that sexuality has not been a concern of health professionals when they are establishing priorities for treating cancer. The findings suggest that nurses should examine their beliefs, knowledge, and attitudes regarding sexuality to facilitate their comfort in discussing sensitive sexual health issues with their female patients and partners. Open discussions with women who have had gynecological cancer treatment are critical to help foster their sexual expression, communication, and intimacy.

• • • • • SUMMARY POINTS

- The **interpretation** of research findings is a search for the broader meaning and implications of the results of an investigation.
- Interpretation of both qualitative and quantitative results typically involves five steps: (1) analyzing the credibility of the results; (2) determining their meaning; (3) considering their importance; (4) determining the generalizability or transferability of the findings; and (5) assessing the implications in regard to theory, nursing practice, and future research.
- A research **critique** is a careful, critical appraisal of the strengths and limitations of a study.
- A reviewer preparing a comprehensive review should consider five major dimensions of the study: the substantive and theoretical, methodologic, ethical, interpretive, and presentation and stylistic dimensions. Many critiques focus primarily on the methodologic dimension.
- Researchers designing a study must make a number of important **methodologic decisions** that affect the quality and integrity of the research. Consumers preparing a critique must evaluate the decisions the researchers made to determine how much faith can be placed in the results.

➤ ➤ ➤ ➤ CRITICAL THINKING ACTIVITIES

Chapter 15 of the accompanying *Study Guide to Accompany Essentials of Nursing Research*, 5th edition offers various exercises and study suggestions for reinforcing the concepts presented in this chapter. In addition, you can address the following:

1. Prepare a written critique of one of the two studies that appear in the Appendix.

2. Read one or both of the studies that appear as research examples in this chapter, together with the two commentaries. To what degree to you agree with the commentaries? What additional comments would you have to offer the researchers? To what extent did the researchers' responses address the concerns of the commentators?

For additional review, see questions 206–215 on the study CD provided with Polit: Study Guide to Accompany Essentials of Nursing Research.

SUGGESTED READINGS

Methodologic References

Beck, C. T. (1990). The research critique: General criteria for evaluating a research report. *Journal of Obstetric, Gynecologic, and Neonatal Nursing, 19,* 18–22.

Beck, C. T. (1993). Qualitative research: The evaluation of its credibility, fittingness, and auditability. *Western Journal of Nursing Research, 15,* 263–266.

Burns, N. (1989). Standards for qualitative research. *Nursing Science Quarterly, 2,* 254–260.

Rasmussen, L., O'Conner, M., Shinkle, S., & Thomas, M. K. (2000). The basic research review checklist. *Journal of Continuing Education in Nursing, 31*(1), 13–18.

Ryan-Wenger, N. M. (1992). Guidelines for critique of a research report. *Heart & Lung, 21,* 394–401.

Substantive References

Alteneder, R. A. (1998). Commentary. *Western Journal of Nursing Research, 20,* 701–703.

Butler, L., Banfield, V., Sveinson, T., & Allen, K. (1998). Conceptualizing sexual health in cancer care. *Western Journal of Nursing Research, 20,* 683–699.

Carty, E. M., Bradley, C., & Winslow, W. (1996). Women's perceptions of fatigue during pregnancy and postpartum. *Clinical Nursing Research, 5,* 67–80.

Schultz, A. A., Bridgham, C., Smith, M. E., & Higgins, D. (1998). Perceptions of caring: Comparison of antepartum and postpartum patients. *Clinical Nursing Research, 7,* 363–378.

Downe-Wamboldt, B. (1998). Commentary. *Western Journal of Nursing Research, 20,* 700–701.

Gerdner, L. A. (1999). Commentary. *Western Journal of Nursing Research, 21,* 491–493.

Hayes, K. S. (1998). Randomized trial of geragogy-based medication instruction in the emergency department. *Nursing Research, 47,* 211–218.

Jirovec, M. M. (1999). Commentary. *Western Journal of Nursing Research, 21,* 493–494.

Lévesque, L., Ducharme, F., & Lachance, L. (1999). Is there a difference between family caregiving of institutionalized elders with or without dementia? *Western Journal of Nursing Research, 21,* 472–491.

Neitzel, J. J., Miller, E. H., Shepherd, M. F., & Belgrade, M. (1999). Improving pain management after total joint replacement surgery. *Orthopaedic Nursing, 18,* 37–45.

Pellino, T. A. (1997), Relationships between patient attitudes, subjective norms, perceived control, and analgesic use following elective orthopedic surgery. *Research in Nursing & Health, 20,* 97–105.

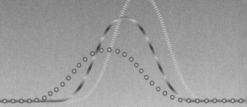

Using Research Findings in Nursing Practice

● ●

Student Objectives

On completion of this chapter, the student will be able to:

○ describe a continuum along which research utilization can occur
○ give examples of how research can be used in the five phases of the nursing process
○ discuss the current status of research utilization within nursing
○ identify barriers to utilizing nursing research and strategies for improving utilization
○ describe the general steps in an individual and organizational utilization project
○ evaluate the extent to which a nurse researcher adequately addresses the issue of utilization in the discussion section of a research report
○ define new terms in the chapter

● ●

New Terms

Clinical relevance
Collaborative research
Conceptual utilization
Cost–benefit assessment
CURN project
Decision accretion
Implementation potential
Instrumental utilization
Iowa Model of Research in Practice
Knowledge creep

Knowledge-focused triggers
Problem-focused triggers
Research-based nursing protocol
Research utilization
Rogers' Diffusion of Innovations Model
Scientific merit
Stetler Model
WICHE project

Most nurse researchers would like to have their findings incorporated into nursing protocols, decisions, and curricula. In addition, most nurses working in clinical settings are aware of the benefits of research-based practice. That is, there is a growing interest in developing a practice in which there is solid evidence from disciplined research that specific nursing actions are clinically appropriate and cost-effective and result in positive outcomes for clients.

A number of changes in nursing education and research have been prompted by the desire to develop a better knowledge base for nursing practice. In education, most nursing schools now include courses to instill some degree of research competence in their students. In the research arena, there has been a dramatic shift toward a focus on clinical nursing problems. These two changes alone, however, have not been enough to lead to widespread integration of research findings into the delivery of nursing care. There was an assumption—or at least a hope—that the production of clinically relevant studies would lead to improved nursing practice, if there was an audience of practicing nurses who could critically evaluate these studies. Research utilization, as the nursing community has come to recognize, is a complex and nonlinear phenomenon. In this chapter, we discuss various aspects of research utilization and provide information on how you can use research findings to improve your practice.

WHAT IS RESEARCH UTILIZATION?

Broadly speaking, **research utilization** refers to the use of some aspect of a study in an application unrelated to the original research. Current conceptions of research utilization recognize a continuum in terms of the specificity or diffuseness of the use to which knowledge is put. At one end of the continuum are discrete, clearly identifiable attempts to base a specific action on research findings. For example, a series of studies demonstrated that the optimal placement time of a glass thermometer for accurate oral temperature determination is 9 minutes (Nichols & Verhonick, 1968). When nurses specifically altered their behavior from shorter placement times to the empirically based recommendation of 9 minutes, this constituted research utilization at this end of the continuum, which has been referred to as **instrumental utilization** (Caplan & Rich, 1975).

Research also can be used more diffusely in a manner that promotes awareness or enlightenment. Caplan and Rich (1975) refer to this end of the utilization continuum as **conceptual utilization.** Thus, practicing nurses may read a research report indicating that nonnutritive sucking among preterm infants had a beneficial effect on the number of days to the infant's first bottle feeding. Nurses may be reluctant to alter their own behavior or to suggest an intervention based on a single study, but their reading of the report may make them more observant in their own work with preterm infants and may lead them to watch for the effects of nonnutritive sucking in their own setting. Conceptual utilization, then, refers to situations in which users are influenced in their thinking about an issue based on one or more studies but do not put this knowledge to any specific, documentable use. Qualitative research, because it has the potential to offer rich insights into human needs, behaviors, and experiences, is especially likely to have implications for conceptual utilization.

The middle ground of this continuum involves the partial impact of research findings on nursing activities. This middle ground frequently is the result of a slow evolutionary process that does not reflect a conscious decision to use an innovative procedure but rather reflects what Weiss (1980) has termed knowledge creep and decision accretion. **Knowledge creep** refers to an evolving "percolation" of research ideas and findings. **Decision accretion** refers to the manner in which momentum for a decision builds over a period of time based on accumulated information gained through readings, informal discussions, meetings, and so on.

Research utilization at all points along this continuum is an appropriate goal for nurses.

RESEARCH UTILIZATION IN NURSING

Numerous commentators have noted that progress in using nursing research results has proceeded slowly—too slowly for many who are anxious to establish a scientific base for nursing actions. In this section, we consider the possibilities for research utilization and evidence of the extent to which utilization has occurred.

Incorporating Research Into Practice: The Potential

The nursing process is complex and requires nurses to make many decisions. In the course of delivering patient care, nurses collect information, make assessments and diagnoses, develop plans for appropriate nursing actions, initiate interventions, and evaluate the effects of nursing interventions. These activities correspond to the five phases of nursing outlined in the Standards of Clinical Nursing Practice established by the American Nurses Association (1991). Within each phase, research findings can assist nurses in making more informed decisions and in taking actions that have a solid, scientifically based rationale.

- *Assessment phase.* Nurses collect information to assess patient needs from a variety of sources. The information may come from interviews with clients, family members, and other health professionals as well as from records, charts, and observations. Research can focus on how best to collect accurate information, what types of information to collect, how to integrate assessment data, and how to interpret the data.
- *Diagnosis phase.* Based on an analysis of assessment information, nurses are expected to develop nursing diagnoses. Research can play an important role in helping nurses to make more accurate nursing diagnoses by validating the etiology of a diagnosis against recorded assessment information. In addition, research can help to determine the frequency of occurrence for defining characteristics associated with a diagnosis. Continued efforts in this area will promote the clustering of nursing diagnostic groups and the refinement of nursing diagnoses.
- *Planning phase.* The planning phase of the nursing process involves decisions concerning what nursing actions or interventions are needed; when the actions are most appropriately instituted; who the recipients of the interventions should be; and under what conditions the interventions are to be implemented. Research findings can fruitfully be used in planning care by indicating the nursing interventions that are especially effective for particular cultural groups, settings, types of problem, and client characteristics.

- *Intervention phase.* Ideally, professionally accountable nurses would base as many of their nursing interventions as possible on research findings. Consider, for example, the many decisions made by nurses working the night shift in a nursing home. At what point do they decide that the nursing interventions are no longer producing the desired results for a resident in the process of dying? What alterations in nursing interventions are available that facilitate the transition from a state of life to a state of death? What response might be expected from other residents of the home, and how might their stresses be alleviated? The systematic documentation of successful nursing interventions can benefit other nurses facing similar situations.
- *Evaluation phase.* The last stage of the nursing process involves the evaluation of the degree to which goals developed at the planning stage have been met. Research can help document success or failure in achieving desired outcomes. Successful outcomes enhance nurses' confidence in implementing the plan in other similar situations. When outcomes are not successful, nurses need to reexamine the assessment, diagnoses, plan, and interventions. Such information, collected systematically, can lead to improvements in nursing care.

Incorporating Research Into Practice: The Record

As we have just seen, there is ample potential for utilizing research throughout the nursing process. However, there is considerable concern that nurses have thus far failed to realize fully this potential. This concern is based on some evidence suggesting that nurses are not always aware of research results and do not effectively incorporate these results into their practice.

One of the first pieces of evidence about the gap between research and practice came from a study by Ketefian (1975), who reported on the oral temperature determination practices of 87 registered nurses (RNs). The results of a series of studies had clearly demonstrated that the optimal placement time for oral temperature determination using glass thermometers is 9 minutes. In Ketefian's study, only 1 of the 87 nurses reported the correct placement time, suggesting that few nurses were aware of the research findings.

In another study of research utilization, Kirchhoff (1982) investigated the discontinuance of coronary precautions in a national sample of 524 intensive care nurses. Several studies had failed to demonstrate that the practices of restricting ice water and rectal temperature measurement were necessary, yet Kirchhoff's results indicated that these coronary precautions were still widely practiced.

Coyle and Sokop (1990), replicating a study by Brett (1987), investigated practicing nurses' adoption of 14 nursing innovations reported in the nursing literature. The criteria used to select the 14 studies included scientific merit; significance and usefulness of the research findings to the practice setting; and the suitability of the findings for application to practice. A sample of 113 nurses practicing in 10 hospitals (randomly selected from the medium-sized hospitals in North Carolina) completed questionnaires that measured the nurses' awareness and use of the study findings. Coyle and Sokop used Brett's original scheme to categorize each study according to its stage of adoption: awareness (indicating knowledge of the innovation); persuasion (indicating the nurses' belief that nurses should use the innovation in practice); occasional use in practice; and regular use in practice. Only 1 of the 14 innovations was at the regular-use stage of adoption. Six of the innovations were in the persuasion stage, indicating that the nurses knew of the innovation and thought it should be incorporated into nursing practice but were not basing their own nursing decisions on it. Table 16-1 describes 4 of the 14 nursing innovations, one for each of the four stages of adoption, according to Coyle and Sokop's results.

TABLE 16-1. Extent of Adoption of Four Nursing Practices*					
STAGE	**NURSING INNOVATION**	**AWARE** (%)	**PERSUADED** (%)	**USE SOMETIMES** (%)	**USE ALWAYS** (%)
Awareness	Elimination of lactose from the formulas of tube-feeding diets for adult patients minimizes diarrhea, distention, flatulence, and fullness and reduces patient rejection of feedings (Horsley, Crane, & Haller, 1981)	38	36	13	19
Persuasion	Accurate monitoring of oral temperatures can be achieved in patients receiving oxygen therapy by using an electronic thermometer placed in the sublingual pocket (Lim-Levy, 1982)	68	55	35	29
Occasional use	A formally planned and structured preoperative education program preceding elective surgery results in improved patient outcomes (King & Tarsitano, 1982)	83	81	48	23
Regular use	A closed sterile system of urinary drainage is effective in maintaining the sterility of urine in patients who are catheterized for less than 2 weeks; continuity of the closed drainage system should be maintained during irrigations, sampling procedures, and patient transport (Horsley, Crane, Haller, & Bingle, 1981)	94	91	84	6

*Based on findings reported in Coyle, L. A. & Sokop, A. G. (1990). Innovation adoption behavior among nurses. *Nursing Research, 39,* 176–180. The sample consisted of 113 practicing nurses.

More recently, Rutledge and colleagues (1996) studied the extent to which oncology staff nurses adopted eight research-based practices. More than 1,000 nurses were surveyed. The researchers found that awareness levels were high, with between 53% and 96% of the oncology nurses reporting awareness of the eight practices. Awareness and use were strongly linked: almost 90% of aware nurses used seven of the practices at least some of the time.

The results of the recent studies are more encouraging than the studies by Ketefian and Kirchhoff because they suggest that, on average, the practicing nurses are aware of many innovations based on research results, are persuaded that the innovations should be used, and are beginning to use them on occasion. Although it is clear that a gap exists between knowledge production and knowledge utilization in nursing (as well as in other disciplines) it is also clear that nurses are becoming enlightened by a growing body of research that is challenging traditional ways of practicing nursing.

Efforts to Improve Utilization of Nursing Research

There has been considerable discussion about the need to reduce the gap between nursing research and nursing practice, and several formal efforts to achieve that goal have been undertaken. In this section, we briefly describe a few of these projects.

The WICHE Project

One of the earliest research utilization projects was the Western Interstate Commission for Higher Education (WICHE) Regional Program for Nursing Research Development. The 6-year **WICHE project** investigated the feasibility of increasing nursing research activities through regional collaborative activities. The three major project activities were: (1) collaborative, nontargeted research (bringing together nurses from different settings to address mutually identified nursing problems); (2) collaborative, targeted research (multiple studies in different settings all designed to investigate the concept of quality of care); and (3) research utilization (Krueger, Nelson, & Wolanin, 1978).

Nurses who participated in the WICHE project were given the opportunity to identify problems that needed research-based solutions and were then provided with opportunities to develop skills in reading and evaluating research for use in practice. They also developed detailed plans for introducing research innovations into their clinical practice settings. The final report indicated that the project was successful in increasing research utilization, but it also identified a stumbling block. The problem that posed the greatest difficulty was finding scientifically sound, reliable nursing studies with clearly identified implications for nursing care.

The CURN Project

One of the best-known nursing research utilization projects is the Conduct and Utilization of Research in Nursing (CURN) project, a 5-year project awarded to the Michigan Nurses Association by the Division of Nursing in the 1970s. The major objective of the **CURN project** was to increase the use of research findings in the daily practice of RNs by (1) disseminating current findings; (2) facilitating organizational changes needed for implementing innovations; and (3) encouraging the conduct of **collaborative research** that has relevance to nursing practice.

One of the activities of the CURN project was to stimulate the conduct of research in clinical settings. The project resulted in a set of nine volumes on various clinical problems. The titles of these volumes (*e.g., Pain; Preventing Decubitus Ulcers; Structured Preoperative Teaching;* and *Reducing Diarrhea in Tube-Fed Patients*) indicate that a wide range of clinical issues were studied.

The CURN project also focused on helping nurses to use research findings in their practice. CURN project staff saw research utilization primarily as an organizational process (Horsley, Crane, & Bingle, 1978). According to their view, the commitment of organizations that employ practicing nurses to the research utilization process is essential for research to have any impact on nursing practice. The CURN project team concluded that research utilization by practicing nurses is feasible—but only if the research is relevant to practice and if results are broadly disseminated.

Other Utilization Projects

In the past decade, utilization projects have been undertaken by growing numbers of nurses, and descriptions of those projects are appearing with greater regularity in the nursing literature. Two examples of broadly focused projects are cited here to illustrate approaches that have been used to close the research–practice gap.

Bostrom and Wise (1994) described a project implemented at a western hospital. The Retrieval and Application of Research in Nursing (RARIN) project was designed to facilitate the transfer of clinically relevant nursing information to nursing practice. A major component of the project involved training nurses to retrieve scientific information electronically.

A project in California focused on building organizational capacity as a tool for increasing research utilization (Rutledge & Donaldson, 1995). The Orange County Research Utilization in Nursing (OCRUN) project developed a regional network of 20 nursing service organizations and six academic institutions. During a 3-year period, nearly 400 nurses participated in continuing education courses that focused on the development of research utilization competency. The project influenced nurse executives' perceptions of organizational readiness for change and ultimately influenced participating organizations' utilization processes.

Hundreds of more focused utilization projects are being implemented to address specific clinical issues. A few of these are described in the Research Example section of this chapter.

BARRIERS TO UTILIZING NURSING RESEARCH

Typically, several years elapse between the design of a study and it's completion. Several more years may elapse between the time results are reported and the time practicing nurses learn about them and attempt to incorporate them into practice. Thus, it is not unusual for there to be an interim of 5 to 10 years between the identification of a research problem and the implementation of a solution—if, in fact, there is ever an effort to implement. In the next section of this chapter, we discuss some strategies for bridging the gap between nursing research and nursing practice. First, however, we review some barriers to research utilization in nursing. These barriers can be broadly grouped into four categories relating to the source of the barrier—the research itself, practicing nurses, organizational settings, and the nursing profession.

Research Characteristics

For many nursing problems, the state of the art of research knowledge is at a fairly rudimentary level. Results reported in the literature often do not warrant their incorporation into practice. Methodologic flaws often raise questions about the soundness or generalizability of study findings. Thus, a major impediment to research utilization by practicing nurses is that, for many problems, an extensive base of valid and trustworthy study results has not been developed.

As we have repeatedly stressed, most studies have flaws of one type or another. If nurses were to wait for the perfect study before basing clinical decisions on research findings, they would have a very long wait indeed. It is precisely because of the limits of research methods that replication is essential. When repeated efforts to address a research question in different settings yield similar results, there can be greater confidence in the findings. Single studies rarely provide an adequate basis for making changes in nursing practice. Therefore, another utilization constraint is the dearth of published replications.

Nurses' Characteristics

Practicing nurses have characteristics that constrain research utilization. Perhaps the most obvious is the educational preparation of nurses. Most practicing nurses—graduates of diploma or associate degree programs—have not received any formal instruction in research and may lack the skills to judge the merits of a study. Courses on research methodology are now typically offered in baccalaureate nursing programs but, generally, insufficient attention is paid to research utilization. The ability to critique a research report is a necessary, but not sufficient, condition for effectively incorporating research results into daily decision making.

Another characteristic is one that is common to most humans: people are often resistant to change. Change requires effort, retraining, and restructuring one's work habits. Change may also be perceived as threatening (*e.g.,* changes may be perceived as affecting job security). Thus, there is likely to be some opposition to introducing innovations in the practice setting. However, there is evidence from a survey of more than 1,200 nurses that nurses value nursing research and want to be involved in research-related activities (Rizzuto, Bostrom, Suter, & Chenitz, 1994); hence, the time may be ripe for innovation.

Organizational Characteristics

Some of the impediments to research utilization, as the CURN project staff so astutely noted, stem from the organizations that train and employ nurses. Organizations, to an even greater degree than individuals, resist change unless there is a strong organizational perception that there is something fundamentally wrong with the status quo. In many settings, the organizational climate is simply not conducive to research utilization. To challenge tradition and accepted practices, a spirit of intellectual curiosity and openness must prevail.

Few practice settings have established a reward system for utilizing research in practice or for discussing research findings appropriate to clients. Research review and utilization are often considered appropriate activities only when time is available, but available time is generally limited. In a national survey of nearly 1,000 clinical nurses, one of the greatest reported barriers to research utilization was "insufficient time on the job to implement new ideas," which was reported as a moderate or great barrier by about 75% of the sample (Funk, Champagne, Wiese, & Tornquist, 1991).

Organizations may be reluctant to expend the necessary resources for utilization projects or for implementing changes to organizational policy. (Resources may be required for staff release time, for administrative review, for evaluating the effects of an innovation, and so on.) With the push toward cost containment in health care settings, resource constraints may pose a barrier to research utilization.

Characteristics of the Nursing Profession

Some of the impediments that contribute to the gap between research and practice are more global, reflecting the state of the nursing profession or, even more broadly, the state of western society.

One issue is that it has sometimes been difficult to encourage clinicians and researchers to interact and collaborate. They generally work in different settings and have different professional concerns. Relatively few systematic attempts have been made to form collaborative arrangements, and even fewer of these arrangements have been institutionalized as permanent entities. Moreover, attempts to develop such collaboration will not necessarily be welcomed by either group. Lack of trust sometimes undermines collaboration between nurse researchers and nurse clinicians.

A related issue concerns communication between practitioners and researchers. Most practicing nurses do not read nursing research journals, and they may be too overwhelmed by technical jargon or statistical analysis to understand fully such reports when they do read them. Furthermore, nurse researchers too infrequently attend to the needs of clinical nurses. For research utilization to happen, there must be two-way communication between practicing nurses and nurse researchers. The recent emergence of two journals—*Applied Nursing Research* and *Clinical Nursing Research*—represents an important step in this direction.

Phillips (1986) noted another barrier to bridging the research–practice gap: the historical "baggage" that has defined nursing in such a way that practicing nurses may not perceive themselves as independent professionals capable of recommending changes based on research results. If nurses believe that their role is to wait for direction from the medical community, and if they believe they have no power to be self-directed, they will have difficulty initiating research-based innovations. In the previously mentioned national survey, the barrier perceived by the largest percentage of nurses was their feeling that they did not have "enough authority to change patient care procedures" (Funk et al., 1991).

SCOPE OF RESPONSIBILITY FOR RESEARCH UTILIZATION

Where does the responsibility for bridging the gap between research and practice lie? Should practicing nurses pursue research-based innovations? Should organizations and their administrative staffs take the lead? Or should the direction come from researchers themselves? In our view, the entire nursing community must be involved in the process of putting research into practice.

Strategies for Researchers

There are a number of strategies that researchers can implement to foster better adoption of their research results, including the following:

- *Do high-quality research.* A major impediment to utilizing nursing research results is that there is often an inadequate scientific basis for introducing innovations or for making changes.
- *Replicate.* Researchers must make a commitment to replicating studies and publishing the results of those efforts.
- *Collaborate with practitioners.* Researchers will never succeed in influencing nursing practice unless they become better attuned to the needs of practicing nurses and the problems they face in delivering care. Researchers should seek opportunities to exchange ideas for research problems with nurse clinicians, to involve them in the conduct of research, and to seek their input in interpreting study results.

- *Disseminate aggressively.* It is a researcher's responsibility to find a means of communicating research results to practicing nurses. It is especially important from a utilization standpoint for researchers to report their results in specialty journals and at conferences, colloquia, and workshops that nurse clinicians attend.
- *Communicate clearly.* It is not always possible to present study results in a way that is readily comprehensible to nonresearchers. Researchers need to be encouraged, however, to avoid unnecessary jargon, to construct tables carefully so that a nonresearcher can get a sense of the findings, and to compose the abstract so that virtually any intelligent reader can understand the research problem, general approach, and salient results.
- *Suggest clinical implications.* Researchers should suggest how the results of their research can be utilized by practicing nurses, while at the same time pointing out study limitations. If an implications section became a standard feature of research reports, the burden of utilization would be much lighter for the nurse clinician.

As a consumer, you can and should evaluate the extent to which researchers have adopted these strategies to enhance research utilization.

Strategies for Practicing Nurses

Practicing nurses cannot by themselves launch institution-wide utilization projects, but their behaviors and attitudes are, nevertheless, critical to the success of any efforts to implement research-based procedures. Furthermore, individual nurses can engage in and benefit from conceptual utilization. Therefore, every nurse has an important role to play in utilizing nursing research. The following are some strategies for nurses:

- *Read widely and critically.* Professionally accountable nurses continue their nursing education by keeping abreast of important developments. Nurses should read regularly journals relating to their specialty, including the research reports in them. Research newsletters and columns with research briefs are alternative sources of information on research developments in a field.
- *Attend professional conferences.* Many nursing conferences include presentations of studies that have clinical relevance. Conference participants usually hear of an innovation sooner than those who learn of it in a journal. Furthermore, those attending a conference get an opportunity to meet the researcher and to ask questions about practice implications.
- *Learn to expect evidence that a procedure is effective.* Every time nurses or nursing students are told about a standard nursing procedure, they have a right to ask the question: Why? Nurses need to develop expectations that the decisions they make in their clinical practice are based on sound rationales.

- *Seek environments that support research utilization.* Organizations differ in their openness to research utilization; therefore, nurses interested in basing their practice on research have some control through their employment decisions.
- *Become involved in a journal club.* Many organizations that employ nurses sponsor journal clubs that meet to review research articles that have potential relevance to practice. Generally, members take turns critically appraising a study and presenting the critique to the club's members. If there is no such club in existence, nurses can consider initiating one (see, for example, Tibbles & Sanford, 1994).
- *Collaborate with a nurse researcher.* Collaboration is a two-way street. Practicing nurses who have identified a clinical problem in need of a solution and who lack strong research skills should consider initiating a collaborative relationship with a local nurse researcher. Collaboration could also be a useful approach for undertaking institutional utilization projects.
- *Pursue and participate in institutional utilization projects.* Sometimes, ideas for utilization projects come from staff nurses. Although large-scale utilization projects require organizational support, individual nurses or groups of nurses can propose such a project to the nursing department. For example, an idea for such a project may emerge within a journal club. If the idea for a research utilization effort originates from within the administration, nurses are still likely to play an important role in carrying out the project. Several studies have found that nurses who are involved in research-related activities (*e.g.*, a utilization project or data collection activities) develop more positive attitudes toward research and better research skills (*e.g.*, Dufault, Bielecki, Collins, & Willey, 1995; Bostrom & Suter, 1993).
- *Pursue appropriate personal utilization projects.* Not all findings from research studies require organizational commitment or policy directives. For example, an ethnographic study might reveal that the health beliefs of an immigrant group are distinctive, and this may lead a nurse to ask informally several additional questions of clients of that immigrant group during assessment. If the nurse discovers that important new information is gleaned, it may then be appropriate to recommend a more formal utilization project involving changes to the standard assessment protocols. Of course, not all research findings are amenable to such informal personal utilization projects. If the results of a study suggest an action or decision that is contrary to organizational policy or that has potential risk for clients, nurses should not pursue such projects without supervisory approval.

Strategies for Administrators

Organizations that employ nurses play a fundamental role in supporting or undermining nurses' efforts to develop a scientific base of practice. In the national survey of clinical nurses, respondents viewed "enhancing administrative support and encouragement" as the single most effective means of facilitating research utilization (Funk et al., 1991). Although you are likely not an administrator, some strategies are described to alert you to the kinds of issues they face. To promote research utilization, administrators should engage in the following strategies:

- *Foster a climate of intellectual curiosity.* If there is administrative opposition to change, the staff's interest in research utilization is not likely to become ignited. Open communication is important in persuading staff nurses that their experiences and problems are important and that the administration is willing to consider innovative solutions.
- *Offer emotional or moral support.* Administrators need to make their support visible by informing staff and prospective staff of such support, by establishing research utilization committees, by helping to develop journal clubs, and by serving as role models for staff nurses.
- *Offer financial or resource support for utilization.* Utilization projects typically require some resources. If the administration expects nurses to engage in utilization activities on their own time and at their own expense, the message is that research utilization is unimportant to those managing the organization.
- *Reward efforts for utilization.* Administrators use various criteria to evaluate nursing performance. Although research utilization should not be a primary criterion for evaluating nurses' performance, its inclusion as one of several important criteria is likely to have an impact on their behavior.

THE UTILIZATION PROCESS

A number of different models of research utilization have been developed during the past few decades. These models offer guidelines for designing and implementing a utilization project in a practice setting. Some models focus on the use of research from the perspective of an individual clinician, whereas others focus on utilization from an organizational perspective. This section discusses mechanisms for applying research findings to nursing practice.

Individual Utilization

Individual nurses can read research reports and put the information to use in practice. One especially prominent utilization model for individual clinicians is the **Stetler Model** of research utilization. This model involves six sequential phases that are designed to "facilitate critical thinking about the pragmatic application of research findings" (Stetler, 1994, p. 20):

1. *Preparation.* In this phase, you would specify your underlying purpose and identify a relevant study that could provide insight and direction relevant to that purpose.

2. *Validation.* This phase involves an evaluation of the selected study, focusing in particular on whether it is sufficiently sound for potential application in practice. (The utilization process stops at this point if the study is rejected.) The end product of the validation phase is a summary that translates the findings of an acceptable study in day-to-day terms and that indicates application constraints and qualifiers.

3. *Comparative evaluation.* This phase has four criteria that, taken together, are used to determine the desirability and feasibility of applying findings from a validated study to your practice. These criteria are summarized in Table 16-2.

4. *Decision making.* The end result of the comparative evaluation is to make a decision about utilizing the study findings. In the decision-making phase, there are four possible outcomes:
   - Use now to change practice, without waiting for additional information
   - Consider use, but wait for additional information (*e.g.,* through discussions with others)
   - Delay use until further research has been conducted
   - Reject use (no further steps necessary)

5. *Translation and application.* This phase is intended to make you think through the exact details and extent of the application, by specifying how the findings will be used (*e.g.,* as background information, as part of a routine nursing practice) and by identifying any caveats or special circumstances of its use.

6. *Evaluation.* In the final phase, the application would be evaluated, either informally (*e.g.,* through discussions with peers) or more formally through an assessment of measurable outcomes.

TABLE 16-2.   Criteria for Comparative Evaluation Phase of the Stetler Model of Research Utilization*

1. Fit of setting
   Similarity of characteristics of sample to your client population
   Similarity of study's environment to the one in which you work

2. Feasibility
   Potential risks of implementation to patients, staff, and the organization
   Readiness for change among those who would be involved in a change in practice
   Resource requirements and availability

3. Current Practice
   Congruency of the study with your theoretical basis for current practice behavior

4. Substantiating Evidence
   Availability of confirming evidence from other studies
   Availability of confirming evidence from a meta-analysis or integrative review

*Adapted from Stetler, C. B. (1994). Refinement of the Stetler/Marram model for application of research findings to practice. *Nursing Outlook, 42,* 15–25.

Although the Stetler Model was designed as a tool for individual practitioners, it has also been used by small groups of nurses.

Example of an application of the Stetler Model:

The application of the six phases of the Stetler Model to the problem of bereavement care by a group of nurses has been carefully described in an article by Hanson and Ashley (1994).

Organizational Utilization

Research utilization—especially instrumental utilization—is often addressed by groups of individuals interested in the same practice issue. Formal utilization projects follow systematic procedures that have been described in a number of research utilization models. One such model is the **Iowa Model of Research in Practice** (Titler et al., 1994), which involves a series of activities with two critical decision points: (1) deciding whether there is a sufficient research base for utilization and (2) deciding whether the change is appropriate for adoption in practice. Some utilization projects have used as a framework **Rogers' Diffusion of Innovations Model**, which describes a process involving five stages: knowledge, persuasion, decision, implementation, and confirmation (Rogers, 1995). In this section, we discuss how a research utilization project can be planned and executed, using a model that we have adapted from several existing utilization models.

Selection of a Utilization Topic

Nurses interested in utilizing research findings in their nursing practice generally set about the task in one of two ways. One approach to utilization, shown schematically as path A in Figure 16-1, begins with the identification of a clinical problem that needs solution (in the Iowa Model of Research in Practice, this corresponds to what is called **problem-focused triggers**). Such a problem identification may arise in the normal course of clinical practice or in the context of a quality assessment or quality improvement effort. This problem identification approach is likely to have staff support if the selected problem is one that numerous nurses have encountered. This approach to utilization is likely to have considerable clinical relevance because a specific clinical situation generated interest in the problem in the first place.

The second major approach to conducting a utilization project, shown schematically as path B in Figure 16-1, begins with the research literature—corresponding to the **knowledge-focused triggers** identified in the Iowa model. This approach could occur if, for example, a utilization project emerged as a result of discussions within a journal club. In this approach, a preliminary assessment would need to be made of the **clinical relevance** of the research. The central issue here is whether a problem of significance to nurses will be solved by making some change or introducing a new interven-

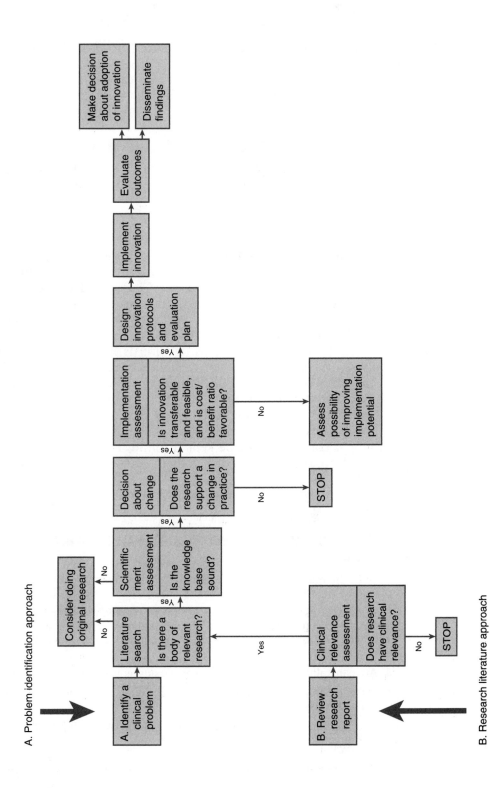

A. Problem identification approach

B. Research literature approach

FIGURE 16-1. A model for research utilization.

tion. Five questions relating to clinical relevance (shown in Box 16-1) can be applied to a research report or set of related reports. If the answer is yes to any of these questions, the next step in the process can be pursued, but if it is determined that the research base is not clinically relevant, it would be necessary to start all over.

 CONSUMER TIP:

The method of selecting a topic does not appear to have any bearing on the success of a utilization project. However, what is important is that the nursing staff who will implement an innovation are involved in the topic selection. ■

Literature Retrieval and Evaluation of Scientific Merit

The next step is a literature search to determine the extent to which nurse researchers have addressed the problem (see Chap. 6). If the research base related to the identified problem is limited, there are two choices: to abandon the original problem and perhaps select an alternative one, or to consider initiating an original research project on the topic (*i.e.,* to initiate steps to create or enhance the knowledge base). This decision is likely to depend on the research skills of the staff and on the availability of research consultants.

Next, the knowledge base must be critically evaluated. We have discussed the criteria for **scientific merit** throughout this text, and, in each chapter, we presented guidelines for assessing whether the findings and conclusions of a study are trustworthy and believable. When it comes to utilization, however, some additional concerns must be kept in mind. First and foremost is the issue of replication, the repeating of a study in a new setting with a new sam-

BOX 16-1

CRITERIA FOR EVALUATING THE CLINICAL RELEVANCE OF A BODY OF RESEARCH

1. Does the research have the potential to help solve a problem faced by practicing nurses?

2. Does the research have the potential to help with clinical decision making with regard to (1) making appropriate observations, (2) identifying client risks or complications, or (3) selecting an appropriate intervention?

3. Are clinically relevant theoretical propositions tested by the research?

4. If the research involves an intervention, does the intervention have potential for use in clinical settings?

5. Can the data collection measures used in the research be applied to clinical practice?

ple of subjects. It is unwise to base a utilization project on a single study, even if the study is extremely rigorous. Ideally, there would be several replications—each providing similar evidence of the effectiveness of the innovation being considered. Another issue in a utilization-focused assessment is whether any of the studies were conducted in a clinical setting, with real clients.

The end product of this step in the process is likely to be a written integrative review, or an overall summary statement accompanied by a table that synthesizes major features of research on the topic. Although written documentation synthesizing the literature may not be needed in all utilization projects, it is highly desirable—and may be needed to secure funding or approval for the project.

 CONSUMER TIP:

In some cases, it may be possible to base a utilization project on an existing published integrated review (or meta-analysis). However, it is always wise to make sure that the review is as up-to-date as possible and that new findings published after the review are taken into consideration. ■

If the existing knowledge base inspires little confidence that the research results could effectively be utilized by nurses, there are the two alternatives suggested previously: to go back to the drawing board and select a new problem, or to investigate the possibility of doing original research to improve the knowledge base. If the knowledge base is sound, the synthesis will suggest one of two things: (1) that current practices are sound and supported by research evidence—in which case the process would end; or (2) that a research-based innovation should be tested. In the latter case, the subsequent step is to conduct an implementation assessment.

Implementation Assessment

Even when there is a sound knowledge base about a clinically significant problem, it is not necessarily true that a utilization project can be planned and implemented. A number of other issues must be considered to determine the **implementation potential** of an innovation in a particular setting. These issues include the transferability of the knowledge, the feasibility of implementation, and the cost–benefit ratio of the innovation. Box 16-2 presents some assessment questions for these categories.

* *Transferability.* The main issue in the transferability of findings question is whether it makes good sense to implement the innovation in the new practice setting. If there is some aspect of the practice setting that is fundamentally incongruent with the innovation in terms of its philosophy, types of client it serves, its personnel, or its financial or administrative structure, it makes little sense to try to adopt the innovation, even if a clinically significant innovation has been shown to be effective in other contexts.

BOX 16-2

CRITERIA FOR EVALUATING THE IMPLEMENTATION POTENTIAL OF AN INNOVATION

Transferability of the Findings

1. Will the innovation "fit" in the proposed new setting?

2. How similar are the target populations in the research and in the new setting?

3. Is the philosophy of care underlying the innovation compatible with the philosophy prevailing in the new setting?

4. Is there a sufficiently large number of clients in the new setting who could benefit from the innovation?

Feasibility

1. Will nurses have the authority to carry out the innovation and to terminate it if it is considered undesirable?

2. Is there reasonable consensus among staff, administrators, and medical personnel that the innovation should be tested? Are there major pockets of resistance that could undermine efforts to implement and evaluate the innovation fairly?

3. Are the skills needed to carry out the utilization project—both the implementation and the clinical evaluation—available within the nursing staff? If not, are there avenues to collaborate with others with the necessary skills?

4. Does the organization have the equipment and facilities necessary for the innovation? If not, is there a way to obtain needed resources?

5. If nursing staff need to be released from other practice activities to learn about and implement the innovation, what is the likelihood that this could happen?

Cost–Benefit Ratio

1. What are the risks to which clients would be exposed during the implementation of the innovation? What are the potential benefits?

2. What are the risks of maintaining current practices (*i.e.,* the cost of *not* trying the innovation)? What are the benefits?

3. What are the short-term and long-term material costs of implementing the innovation?

4. What are the material costs of *not* implementing the innovation (*i.e.,* could the new procedure result in some efficiencies that could lower the cost of providing care)?

5. What are the potential nonmaterial costs of implementing the innovation to the organization (*e.g.,* lower staff morale, staff turnover, absenteeism)?

6. What are the potential nonmaterial benefits of implementing the innovation (*e.g.,* improved staff morale, improved staff recruitment, positive community publicity)?

- *Feasibility.* The feasibility questions address a number of practical concerns about the availability of staff and resources, the organizational climate, the need for and availability of external assistance, and the potential for clinical evaluation. An important issue here is whether nurses will have control over the innovation. When nurses do not have full control over the new procedure, it is important to recognize the interdependent nature of the utilization project and to proceed as early as possible to establish necessary cooperative arrangements.
- *Cost–Benefit Ratio.* A critical part of any decision to proceed with a utilization project is a careful assessment of the costs and benefits of the innovation. The **cost–benefit assessment** should encompass likely costs and benefits to various groups, including clients, staff, and the overall organization. Clearly, the most important factor is the client. If the degree of risk in introducing a new procedure is high, then the potential benefits must be great. Moreover, if there are risks to client well-being, it is essential to have evidence from several methodologically rigorous studies confirming that the new practice is effective. A cost–benefit assessment should consider the opposite side of the coin as well: the costs and benefits of *not* implementing the innovation. It is sometimes easy to forget that the *status quo* bears its own risks and that failure to change, especially when such change is based on a firm knowledge base, is costly to clients, to organizations, and to the entire nursing community.

If the implementation assessment suggests that there might be problems in testing the innovation within that particular practice setting, the team can either identify a new problem and begin the process anew or consider adopting a plan to improve the implementation potential (*e.g.,* seeking external resources if cost considerations were the inhibiting factor).

 CONSUMER TIP:

Documentation of the implementation potential of an innovation is highly recommended. Committing ideas to writing is useful because it can help to resolve ambiguities, can serve as a problem-solving tool if there are barriers to implementation, and can also be used to persuade others of the value of the project. ∎

Implementing and Evaluating the Innovation

If all the implementation criteria are met, the team can then proceed to design the protocol for the innovation. The protocol should clearly indicate the research basis for the new practice and stipulate the exact procedures to be followed. Ideally, the protocol would stipulate the desired outcomes of the innovation in measurable terms.

Implementation of the innovation in the practice setting may be straightforward but is more likely to require advance preparation to make sure that relevant staff understand the reason for the change, have a positive attitude toward it, and are willing to cooperate in its implementation. In some cases, formal staff training may be needed.

A utilization project should always include an evaluation component to assess (1) whether the innovation was, in fact, implemented; (2) what problems were encountered during its implementation; (3) what the outcomes were for patients and staff; and (4) whether the innovation is cost-effective. A variety of research designs can be used for the latter two criteria—the most rigorous being an experimental design. However, in most cases, a less formal evaluation will be more feasible, comparing, for example, hospital records before and after the innovation, and collecting fairly simple data about patient and staff satisfaction. Evaluation data should be gathered over a sufficiently long period (typically 6 to 12 months) to allow for a true test of a "mature" innovation. The end result of this process is a decision about whether to adopt the innovation.

CONSUMER TIP:

A final optional step, but one that is highly advisable, is the dissemination of the results of the utilization project so that other practicing nurses can benefit. ∎

Other Utilization Approaches

Research can be incorporated into nursing practice even without undertaking a formal utilization project. Increasingly, **research-based nursing protocols** are being published in the literature and are essentially ready for adoption—although it is wise to undertake an implementation assessment to determine whether the adoption of a new protocol is sensible. If the publication of the protocol is not recent, it is also prudent to ensure that current research and theory on the topic remain consistent with the protocol.

Examples of research-based nursing protocols:

Two examples of published reports with full research-based protocols include Medoff-Cooper (1994), who developed a protocol for transitioning preterm infants to an open crib, and Beyea and Nicoll (1995), who presented procedures for the administration of intramuscular injections.

Additionally, in 1992, the Agency for Health Care Policy and Research (AHCPR) within the U.S. Department of Health and Human Services (recently renamed the Agency for Healthcare Research and Quality, or AHRQ) began to convene panels of experts to summarize the state-of-the-art research on certain topics and to develop clinical practice guidelines. The guidelines summarize research on a topic, offer mechanisms for assessing and managing the clinical problem, and suggest methods to evaluate outcomes. Among the existing guidelines that are likely to be relevant to your practice include the guidelines on pain management in infants and children; prediction and prevention of pressure sores in adults; and identification and treatment of urinary incontinence. The next section presents a description of a utilization project that was based on AHCPR guidelines on continence for women.

⊞ WORLD WIDE WEB SITES

AHCPR/AHRQ clinical practice guidelines can be downloaded from the Internet. Relevant addresses are:
http://www.ahrq.gov and http://www.guidelines.gov.

RESEARCH EXAMPLES

Many utilization projects are being undertaken by nurses in practice settings, and during the 1990s, many of these projects were described in the nursing literature. Table 16-3 provides examples of several research utilization projects. Another project, described in greater detail below, illustrates the potential of such projects to result in improved nursing care.

Research Summary

The Association of Women's Health, Obstetric, and Neonatal Nurses (AWHONN) has conducted three major research utilization projects. The most recently reported is a project that focused on urinary incontinence in women (Samselle et al., 2000a, 2000b). Using the AHCPR guidelines as a starting point, AWHONN initiated a project with the aim of developing an evidence-based protocol for urinary incontinence in women and designing procedures to facilitate the protocol's implementation into clinical practice.

TABLE 16-3. Examples of Research Utilization Projects

INNOVATION	RESULT OF UTILIZATION PROJECT	CITATION
Use of a standardized protocol to identify delirium in elderly hospital patients	Continued use of assessment protocol on all newly admitted patients aged 75 years and older	Lacko, Bryan, Dellasega, & Salerno, 1999
Structured support for breastfeeding mothers	Adoption as part of quality improvement efforts; change in awareness of and attitude toward research utilization	Janken, Blythe, Campbell, & Carter, 1999
Use of saline flushes in lieu of heparinized flushes for adult patients	Change fully implemented on all units in three hospitals that previously used heparin locks	Shively et al., 1997
Alternatives to use of restraints	Reduced use of restraints for patients in two nursing homes and two extended care units	Stratmann, Vinson, Magee, & Hardin, 1997

The project consisted of three 1-year phases that began in 1995. Phase I (Planning) involved the development of the evidence-based protocol by a team of nurses. The end product was a protocol that provided step-by-step procedures for (1) assessing all women for urinary incontinence; (2) conducting a baseline evaluation of symptomatic women; (3) giving behavioral instruction for bladder training and pelvic floor muscle training; and (4) when indicated, referring women for specialized care. During the planning phase, the project's advisory team also developed data management forms.

The second phase involved the implementation of the protocols. Clinical sites (general ambulatory women's health care settings) were recruited through mailings to AWHONN membership. Of those responding, 36 sites from across the United States were selected to participate (21 ultimately did participate). Coordinators from each site were brought together for a training session on the use of and rationale for the protocol. Each site was asked to administer screening questions to the first 100 nonpregnant female clients seen at the site and to follow the protocol's procedures.

Phase III of the project, Evaluation, involved an assessment of the outcomes. The evaluation addressed two broad questions:

1. Did change occur in clinical practice after clinicians were trained to identify urinary incontinence and to intervene using an evidence-based protocol?
2. Were patient outcomes positively affected after the protocol was instituted in the clinical setting?

The protocol was implemented in the 21 sites, and the process had a number of positive aspects. Participating nurses reported increased respect for the importance of evidence-based practice as well as greater professional satisfaction. A negative outcome concerned the increased demands on the clinicians' time and the problems arising from billing practices that made it difficult to justify the time required.

Nevertheless, the findings indicated that a substantially higher percentage of women screened positive for urinary incontinence using the protocol (57%) than has been reported in the literature (38% to 41%), suggesting that the screening was successful in identifying women in need of intervention. It was discovered that women who had had a hysterectomy were at significantly higher risk of incontinence than other women, indicating the need for heightened vigilance when assessing this group.

Patient outcomes were studied using a one-group before–after design. Women who were exposed to the protocol's treatment (pelvic floor muscle and bladder training) and who provided feedback at a 4-month follow-up had significant improvements in the frequency of incontinent episodes, volume of leakage per episode, perceptions of "bother," and avoidance of activities due to incontinence.

The project team concluded that the results "demonstrate the effectiveness of the evidence-based protocol in actual clinical settings. The participating sites represented a wide range of practice settings, and the overall sample was reasonably diverse. . . . This supports an acceptable level of generalizability and warrants the implementation of the protocol in general ambulatory women's health care settings" (Samselle et al., 2000b, pp. 24–25.)

Clinical Relevance

As this project discovered, many women experience urinary incontinence, a problem that affects women's health and well-being. AWHONN selected an important topic that has a sound base of scientific knowledge.

A few barriers to implementing the protocol were identified, including cooperation by office staff in a few sites and billing practices. The team recommended examining the presence of financial disincentives for sites desiring to implement the protocol.

Despite some implementation problems, the findings suggest that there are clear benefits to incorporating the protocol into standard ambulatory practice. More women with incontinence were identified than has typically been reported, and women who provided feedback reported decreases in the frequency, volume, and life impact of incontinence after treatment.

However, as noted by the team, a high percentage of women identified as having an incontinence problem did not persist with treatment and provide follow-up information. Women who were least likely to continue treatment were younger, were black or Latina, and had lower severity of incontinence. Thus, further utilization research is needed to determine (1) what steps can be taken to prevent high attrition among these groups, and (2) whether the innovation is equally effective for these women. Additionally, information on net financial costs or savings would be extremely useful.

• • • • • SUMMARY POINTS

- **Research utilization** refers to the use of some aspect of a study in a clinical application unrelated to the original research.
- Research utilization exists on a continuum, with direct utilization of some specific innovation at one end (**instrumental utilization**) and more diffuse situations in which users are influenced in their thinking about an issue based on some research (**conceptual utilization**) at the other end.
- Despite the potential for research utilization at all points along this continuum throughout the nursing process, widespread utilization has not occurred.
- Several major utilization projects have been implemented (*e.g.,* the **WICHE** and **CURN projects**), which have demonstrated that research utilization can be increased but have also shed light on barriers to utilization.
- Utilization barriers include: inadequate scientific base, nurses' limited training in research and utilization, resistance to change, unfavorable organizational climates, resource constraints, and limited communication and collaboration between practitioners and researchers.

- Responsibility for research utilization should be borne by the entire nursing community.
- Many models of research utilization have been developed, including models for individual clinicians (*e.g.,* the **Stetler Model**) and models for organizations or groups of clinicians (*e.g.,* the **Iowa Model of Research-Based Practice**).
- Most models of utilization involve the following steps: selection of a topic; retrieval and critique of relevant literature; assessment of the **implementation potential** of an innovation; development of innovation protocols; implementation of the protocols; evaluation of the outcomes; and decision making regarding the adoption of the innovation.
- The assessment of the implementation potential of an innovation includes the dimensions of transferability of findings, feasibility of utilization in the particular setting, and the cost–benefit ratio of the innovation.

➤ ➤ ➤ ➤ *CRITICAL THINKING ACTIVITIES*

Chapter 16 of the accompanying *Study Guide to Accompany Essentials of Nursing Research,* 5th edition offers various exercises and study suggestions for reinforcing the concepts presented in this chapter. In addition, you can consider the following:

1. Apply Stetler's model (insofar as feasible) to one of the studies in the Appendix of this book.

2. Consider your personal situation. What are the barriers that might inhibit your use of research findings?

For additional review, see questions 216–225 on the study CD provided with Polit: Study Guide to Accompany Essentials of Nursing Research.

SUGGESTED READINGS

Methodologic References

American Nurses Association. (1991). *Standards of clinical nursing practice.* Kansas City, MO: ANA.

Bostrom, J., & Suter, W. N. (1993). Research utilization: Making the link to practice. *Journal of Nursing Staff Development, 9,* 28–34.

Bostrom, J., & Wise, L. (1994). Closing the gap between research and practice. *Journal of Nursing Administration, 24,* 22–27.

Caplan, N., & Rich, R. F. (1975). *The use of social science knowledge in policy decisions at the national level.* Ann Arbor, MI: Institute for Social Research, University of Michigan.

Dufault, M. A., Bielecki, C., Collins, E., & Willey, C. (1995). Changing nurses' pain assessment practice: A collaborative research utilization approach. *Journal of Advanced Nursing, 21,* 634–645.

Funk, S. G., Champagne, M. T., Wiese, R. A., & Tornquist, E. M. (1991). Barriers to using research findings in practice: The clinician's perspective. *Applied Nursing Research, 4,* 90–95.

Haller, D., Reynolds, M., & Horsley, J. (1979). Developing research-based innovation protocols: Process, criteria, and issues. *Research in Nursing and Health, 2,* 45–51.

Horsley, J. A., Crane, J., & Bingle, J. D. (1978). Research utilization as an organizational process. *Journal of Nursing Administration, 8,* 4–6.

Horsley, J., Crane, J., Crabtree, M., & Wood, D. (1983). *Using research to improve nursing practice: A guide.* New York: Grune & Stratton.

Krueger, J. C., Nelson, A. H., & Wolanin, M. O. (1978). *Nursing research: Development, collaboration, and utilization.* Germantown, MD: Aspen Systems Corporation.

Phillips, L. R. F. (1986). *A clinician's guide to the critique and utilization of nursing research.* Norwalk, CT: Appleton-Century-Crofts.

Rizzuto, C., Bostrom, J., Suter, W. N., & Chenitz, W. C. (1994). Predictors of nurses' involvement in research activities. *Western Journal of Nursing Research, 16,* 193–204.

Rogers, E. M. (1995). *Diffusion of innovations* (4th ed.). New York: Free Press.

Rutledge, D. N., & Donaldson, N. E. (1995). Building organization capacity to engage in research utilization. *Journal of Nursing Administration, 25,* 12–16.

Rutledge, D. N., Greene, P., Mooney, K., Nail, L. M., & Ropka, M. (1996). Use of research-based practices by oncology staff nurses. *Oncology Nursing Forum, 23,* 1235–1244.

Sandelowski, M. (1997). "To be of use": Enhancing the utility of qualitative research. *Nursing Outlook, 45,* 125–132.

Stetler, C. B. (1994). Refinement of the Stetler/Marram model for application of research findings to practice. *Nursing Outlook, 42,* 15–25.

Stetler, C. B., Morsi, D., Rucki, S., Broughton, S., Corrigan, B., Fitzgerald, J., Giuliano, K., Havener, P., & Sheridan, E. A. (1998). Utilization-focused integrative reviews in a nursing service. *Applied Nursing Research, 11,* 195–206.

Tibbles, L., & Sanford, R., (1994). The research journal club: A mechanism for research utilization. *Clinical Nurse Specialist, 8,* 23–26.

Titler, M. G., Kleiber, C., Steelman, V., Goode, C., Rakel, B., Barry-Walker, J., & Small, S. (1994). Infusing research into practice to promote quality care. *Nursing Research, 43,* 307–313.

Weiss, C. (1980). Knowledge creep and decision accretion. *Knowledge: Creation, Diffusion, Utilization, 1,* 381–404.

Substantive References

Beyea, S. C., & Nicoll, L. H. (1995). Administration of medication via the intramuscular route: An integrative review of the literature and research-based protocol for the procedure. *Applied Nursing Research, 8,* 28–29.

Brett, J. L. L. (1987). Use of nursing practice research findings. *Nursing Research, 36,* 344–349.

Coyle, L. A., & Sokop, A. G. (1990). Innovation adoption behavior among nurses. *Nursing Research, 39,* 176–180.

Hanson, J. L., & Ashley, B. (1994). Advanced practice nurses' application of the Stetler model for research utilization: Improving bereavement care. *Oncology Nursing Forum, 21,* 720–724.

Ketefian, S. (1975). Application of selected nursing research findings into nursing practice. *Nursing Research, 24,* 89–92.

Kirchhoff, K. T. (1982). A diffusion survey of coronary precautions. *Nursing Research, 31,* 196–201.

Janken, J. K., Blythe, G., Campbell, P. T., & Carter, R. H. (1999). Changing nursing practice through research utilization: Consistent support for breastfeeding mothers. *Applied Nursing Research, 12,* 22–29.

Lacko, L., Bryan, Y., Dellasega, C., & Salerno, F. (1999). Changing clinical practice through research: The case of delirium. *Clinical Nursing Research, 8,* 235–250.

McFarlane, J., & Parker, B. (1994). Preventing abuse during pregnancy: An assessment and intervention protocol. *Maternal & Child Nursing, 19,* 321–324.

Medoff-Cooper, B. (1994). Transition of the preterm infant to an open crib. *Journal of Obstetric, Gynecologic, and Neonatal Nursing, 23,* 329–335.

Nichols, G. A., & Verhonick, P. J. (1968). Placement times for oral temperatures: A nursing study replication. *Nursing Research, 17,* 159–161.

Samselle, C. M., Wyman, J. F., Thomas, K. K., Newman, D. K., Gray, M., Dougherty, M., & Burns, P. A. (2000a). Continence for women: Evaluation of AWHONN's third research utilization project. *Journal of Obstetric, Gynecologic, and Neonatal Nursing, 29,* 9–17.

Samselle, C. M., Wyman, J. F., Thomas, K. K., Newman, D. K., Gray, M., Dougherty, M., & Burns, P. A. (2000b). Continence for women: A test of AWHONN's evidence-based practice protocol in clinical practice. *Journal of Obstetric, Gynecologic, and Neonatal Nursing, 29,* 18–26.

Shively, M., Riegel, B., Waterhouse, D., Burns, D., Templin, K., & Thomason, T. (1997). Testing a community level research utilization intervention. *Applied Nursing Research, 10,* 121– 127.

Stratmann, S., Vinson, M. H., Magee, R., & Hardin, S. B. (1997). The effects of research on clinical practice: The use of restraints. *Applied Nursing Research, 10,* 39–43.

Glossary

abstract A brief description of a completed or proposed study; in research journals, usually located at the beginning of the journal article.

accessible population The population of people available for a particular study; often a nonrandom subset of the target population.

accidental sampling Selection of the most readily available persons (or units) as participants in a study; also known as *convenience sampling.*

acquiescence response set A bias in self-report instruments, especially in social psychological scales, created when study participants characteristically agree with statements ("yea-say") independent of their content.

after-only design An experimental design in which data are collected from subjects only after the experimental intervention has been introduced.

alpha (α) (1) In tests of statistical significance, the level designating the probability of committing a Type I error; (2) in estimates of internal consistency, a reliability coefficient, as in Cronbach's alpha.

analysis A process of organizing and synthesizing data in such a way that research questions can be answered and hypotheses can be tested.

analysis of covariance (ANCOVA) A statistical procedure used to test mean differences among groups on a dependent variable, while controlling for one or more extraneous variables (covariates).

analysis of variance (ANOVA) A statistical procedure for testing mean differences among three or more groups by comparing the variability between the groups to the variability within them.

anonymity Protection of participants in a study such that even the researcher cannot link individuals with the information provided.

applied research Research that concentrates on finding a solution to a practical problem.

assumptions Basic principles that are accepted as being true on the basis of logic or reason, without proof or verification.

attrition The loss of participants during the course of a study, usually a longitudinal study.

audit trail The systematic collection and documentation of materials that allow an independent auditor in an inquiry audit of qualitative data to draw conclusions about the data.

baseline measure A measure of the dependent variable prior to the introduction of an experimental intervention.

basic research Research designed to extend the base of knowledge in a discipline for the sake of knowledge or theory construction, rather than for solving an immediate problem.

basic social process (BSP) The central social process emerging through an analysis of grounded theory data.

before–after design An experimental design in which data are collected from research subjects both before and after the introduction of the experimental intervention.

beneficence A fundamental ethical principle that seeks to prevent harm and exploitation of, and maximize benefits for, study participants.

between-subjects design A research design in which there are separate groups of people being compared (e.g., smokers and non-smokers).

bias Any influence that produces a distortion in the results of a study.

bimodal distribution A distribution of data values with two peaks (high frequencies).

bivariate statistics Statistics derived from the analysis of two variables simultaneously, for the purpose of assessing the empirical relationship between them.

"blind" review The review of a manuscript or proposal such that neither the author nor the reviewer is identified to the other party.

borrowed theory A theory borrowed from another discipline or field to guide nursing practice or research.

bracketing In phenomenological inquiries, the process of identifying and holding in abeyance any preconceived beliefs and opinions about the phenomena under study.

bricolage The tendency in qualitative research to derive a complex array of data from a variety of sources, using a variety of methods.

case-control study A research design, typically found in retrospective ex post facto research, that involves the comparison of a "case" (i.e., a person with the condition under scrutiny, such as lung cancer) and a matched control (a similar person without the condition).

categorical variable A variable with discrete values rather than values incrementally placed along a continuum (e.g., a person's marital status).

category system In observational studies, the pre-specified plan for organizing and recording the behaviors and events under observation.

causal modeling The development and statistical testing of an explanatory model of hypothesized causal relationships among phenomena.

causal relationship A relationship between two variables such that the presence of one variable (the "cause") determines the presence or value of the other (the "effect").

cell (1) The intersection of a row and column in a table with two or more dimensions; (2) in an experimental design, a cell is the representation of an experimental condition in a schematic diagram.

central tendency A statistical index of the "typicalness" of a set of scores that comes from the center of the distribution of scores; the three most common indices of central tendency are the mode, the median, and the mean.

chi-squared test A nonparametric test of statistical significance used to assess whether a relationship exists between two categorical variables; symbolized as χ^2.

clinical relevance The degree to which a study addresses a problem of significance to the practice of nursing.

clinical research Research designed to generate knowledge to guide nursing practice.

clinical trial An experiment involving a test of the effectiveness of a clinical treatment, generally involving a large and heterogeneous sample of subjects.

closed-ended question A question that offers respondents a set of mutually exclusive and jointly exhaustive alternative replies, from which the best or most accurate answer must be chosen.

cluster sampling A form of sampling in which large groupings ("clusters") are selected first (e.g., nursing schools), with successive subsampling of smaller units (e.g., nursing students).

code of ethics The fundamental ethical principles that are established by a discipline or institution to guide researchers' conduct in research with human (or animal) subjects.

coding The process of transforming raw data into standardized form for data processing and analysis; in quantitative research, the process of attaching numbers to categories; in qualitative research, the process of identifying recurring words, themes, or concepts within the data.

coefficient alpha (Cronbach's alpha) A reliability index that estimates the internal consistency or homogeneity of a measure composed of several items or subparts.

coercion In a research context, the explicit or implicit use of threats (or excessive rewards) to get people to agree to participate in a study.

comparison group A group of subjects whose scores on a dependent variable are used as a basis for evaluating the scores of the group of primary interest (e.g., nonsmokers as compared to smokers); term used in lieu of control group in studies not using a true experimental design.

concealment A tactic involving the unobtrusive collection of research data without the participants' knowledge or consent, used as a means of obtaining an accurate view of naturalistic behavior when the known presence of an observer would distort the behavior of interest.

concept An abstraction based on observations of certain behaviors or characteristics (e.g., stress, pain).

conceptual model Interrelated concepts or abstractions that are assembled together in a rational scheme by virtue of their relevance to a common theme; sometimes referred to as *conceptual framework*.

conceptual utilization The use of research findings in a general, conceptual way to broaden one's thinking about an issue, although the knowledge is not put to any specific use.

concurrent validity The degree to which scores on an instrument are correlated with an external criterion, measured at the same time.

confidentiality Protection of participants in a study such that their individual identities will not be linked to the information they provide and will never be publicly divulged.

confirmability The objectivity or neutrality of qualitative data once they are obtained; a criterion for evaluating data quality.

consent form A written agreement signed by a study participant and a researcher concerning the terms and conditions of a participant's voluntary participation in a study.

constant comparison A procedure often used in a grounded theory analysis wherein newly collected data are compared in an ongoing fashion with data obtained earlier, to refine theoretically relevant categories.

construct An abstraction or concept that is deliberately invented (constructed) by researchers for a scientific purpose.

construct validity The degree to which an instrument measures the construct under investigation.

consumer An individual who reads, reviews, and critiques research findings and who attempts to use and apply the findings in practice.

content analysis The process of organizing and integrating narrative, qualitative information according to emerging themes and concepts; classically, a procedure for analyzing written or verbal communications in a systematic fashion, typically with the goal of quantitatively measuring variables.

content validity The degree to which the items in an instrument adequately represent the universe of content.

contingency table A two-dimensional table that permits a crosstabulation of the frequencies of two categorical variables.

continuous variable A variable that can take on an infinite range of values along a specified continuum (e.g., height).

control The process of holding constant possible influences on the dependent variable under investigation.

control group Subjects in an experiment who do not receive the experimental treatment and whose performance provides a baseline against which the effects of the treatment can be measured (see also *comparison group*).

convenience sampling Selection of the most readily available people as participants in a study; also known as *accidental sampling*.

core variable In a grounded theory study, a central phenomenon or pattern of behavior relevant to study participants, and used to integrate all categories of the data.

correlation A tendency for variation in one variable to be related to variation in another variable.

correlation coefficient An index that summarizes the degree of relationship between two variables. Correlation coefficients typically range from +1.00 (for a perfect positive relationship) through 0.0 (for no relationship) to -1.00 (for a perfect negative relationship).

correlation matrix A two-dimensional display showing the correlation coefficients between all combinations of variables.

correlational research Research that explores the interrelationships among variables of interest without any active intervention on the part of the researcher.

cost-benefit analysis An evaluation of the financial costs of a program or intervention relative to the financial gains attributable to it.

cost-benefit assessment The assessment of relative costs and benefits, to individuals, organizations, and society, of implementing an innovation.

covariate A variable that is statistically controlled (held constant) in analysis of covariance. The covariate is typically an extraneous, confounding influence on the dependent variable or a baseline measure of the dependent variable.

covert data collection The collection of information in a study without the participant's knowledge.

credibility Referring to confidence in the truth value of the qualitative data; a criterion for evaluating data quality.

criterion-related validity The degree to which scores on an instrument are correlated with an external criterion.

critique An objective, critical, and balanced appraisal of a research report.

Cronbach's alpha A widely-used reliability index that estimates the internal consistency or homogeneity of a measure composed of several subparts; also referred to as *coefficient alpha*.

crossover design See *repeated measures design*.

cross-sectional study A study based on observations of different age or developmental groups at a single point in time for the purpose of inferring trends over time.

crosstabulation A determination of the number of cases occurring when two variables are considered simultaneously (e.g., gender—male/female—crosstabulated with smoking status—smoker/nonsmoker). The results are typically presented in a table with rows and columns divided according to the values of the variables.

data The pieces of information obtained in the course of a study (singular is *datum*).

data analysis The systematic organization and synthesis of research data, and the testing of research hypotheses using those data.

data collection The gathering of information needed to address a research problem.

data saturation See *saturation*.

debriefing Communication with study participants, generally after their participation has been completed, regarding various aspects of the study.

deductive reasoning The process of developing specific predictions from general principles (see also *inductive reasoning*).

degrees of freedom (*df*) A concept used in conjunction with statistical tests, referring to the number of sample values that are free to vary (e.g., with a given sample mean, all but one value would be free to vary); degrees of freedom is often $N - 1$, but different formulas are relevant for different tests.

dependability A criterion for evaluating data quality in qualitative data, referring to the stability of data over time and over conditions.

dependent variable The outcome variable of interest; the variable that is hypothesized to depend on or be caused by the *independent variable*.

descriptive correlational study A study in which the researcher is primarily interested in describing relationships among variables, without seeking to establish a causal connection.

descriptive research Research studies that have as their main objective the accurate portrayal of the characteristics of persons, situations, or groups, and/or the frequency with which certain phenomena occur.

descriptive statistics Statistics that describe and summarize data (e.g., mean, standard deviation).

descriptive theory A broad characterization that thoroughly accounts for a single phenomenon.

determinism The belief that phenomena are not haphazard or random, but rather have antecedent causes; an assumption in the positivist paradigm.

directional hypothesis A hypothesis that makes a specific prediction about the direction and nature of the relationship between two variables.

discriminant function analysis A statistical procedure used to predict group membership— or status on a categorical (nominal level) variable— on the basis of two or more independent variables.

disproportionate sample A sample that results when the researcher samples differing proportions of study participants from different strata in the population to ensure adequate representation of strata that are comparatively smaller.

double-blind experiment An experiment in which neither the subjects nor those who administer the treatment know who is in the experimental or control group.

electronic database Bibliographic files that can be accessed by computer for the purpose of conducting a literature review.

element The most basic unit of a population, from which a sample will be drawn; in nursing research, the element is typically humans.

eligibility criteria The criteria used by a researcher to designate the specific attributes of the target population, and by which participants are selected for participation in a study.

emergent design A design that unfolds in the course of a qualitative study as the researcher makes ongoing design decisions reflecting what has already been learned.

emic perspective A term used by ethnographers to refer to the way members of a culture themselves view their world; the "insider's view."

empirical evidence Evidence that is rooted in objective reality, based on the collection of data using one's senses.

equivalence The degree of similarity between alternate forms of a measuring instrument.

error of measurement The deviation between true scores and obtained scores of a measured characteristic.

ethics A system of moral values that is concerned with the degree to which research procedures adhere to professional, legal, and social obligations to the study participants.

ethnography A branch of human inquiry, associated with the field of anthropology, that focuses on the culture of a group of people, with an effort to understand the world view of those under study.

ethnomethodology A branch of human inquiry, associated with sociology, that focuses on the way in which people make sense of their everyday activities and come to behave in socially acceptable ways.

ethnonursing research The study of human cultures, with a focus on a group's beliefs and practices relating to nursing care and related health behaviors.

etic perspective A term used by ethnographers to refer to the "outsider's" view of the experiences of a cultural group.

evaluation A type of research designed to determine the effectiveness of a program, treatment, practice, or policy works.

event sampling In observational studies, a sampling plan that involved the selection of integral behaviors or events.

evidence-based practice Nursing practice that uses research findings as a basis for nurses' decisions, actions, and interactions with clients.

***ex post facto* research** Research conducted after the variations in the independent variable have occurred in the natural course of events; a form of nonexperimental research in which causal explanations are inferred "after the fact."

experiment A research study in which the investigator controls (manipulates) the independent variable and randomly assigns subjects to different conditions.

experimental group The subjects who receive the experimental treatment or intervention.

experimental intervention (experimental treatment) See *intervention*; *treatment*.

external validity The degree to which the results of a study can be generalized to settings or samples other than the ones studied.

extraneous variable A variable that confounds the relationship between the independent and dependent variables and that needs to be controlled either in the research design or through statistical procedures.

extreme case sampling A sampling approach used by qualitative researchers that involves the purposeful selection of the most extreme or unusual cases.

extreme response set A bias in self-report instruments, especially in social psychological scales, created when participants express their opinions in terms of extreme response alternatives (e.g., "strongly agree") independent of the question's content.

***F*-ratio** The statistic obtained in several statistical tests (e.g., ANOVA) in which variation attributable to different sources (e.g., between groups and within groups) is compared.

face validity The extent to which a measuring instrument looks as though it is measuring what it purports to measure.

factor analysis a statistical procedure for reducing a large set of variables into a smaller set of variables by identifying underlying dimensions.

factorial design An experimental design in which two or more independent variables are simultaneously manipulated; this design permits analysis of the main effects of the independent variables, plus interaction effects.

field notes The notes taken by researchers describing the unstructured observations they have made in the field, and their interpretation of those observations.

field research Research in which the data are collected "in the field" from individuals in their normal roles, with the aim of understanding the practices, behaviors, and beliefs of individuals or groups as they normally function in real life.

findings The results of the analyses of the research data that address the research questions or hypothesis.

fixed alternative question A question that offers respondents a set of prespecified responses, from which the respondent must choose the alternative that is the most appropriate or accurate response.

focus group interview An interview with a group of individuals assembled to answer and discuss questions on a given topic.

focused interview A loosely structured interview in which the interviewer guides the respondent through a set of questions using a topic guide.

follow-up study A study undertaken to determine the outcomes of people with a specified condition or who have received a specified treatment.

framework The conceptual underpinnings of a study; often referred to as a *theoretical framework* in studies based on a theory, or as a *conceptual framework* in studies that have roots in a specific conceptual model.

frequency distribution A systematic array of numerical values from the lowest to the highest, together with a count of the number of times each value was obtained.

frequency polygon Graphic display of a frequency distribution depicting the number of times a score value occurs in a set of data.

full disclosure The communication of complete information to potential study participants regarding the nature of the research, the person's right to refuse participation, and the likely risks and benefits that would be incurred.

functional relationship An association between two variables wherein it cannot be assumed that one variable caused the other, but values for variable X change as a function of changes in variable Y.

gaining entrée The process of gaining access to study participants in qualitative field studies through the cooperation of key actors in the selected site.

generalizability The degree to which it can be inferred that the findings can be generalized from a sample to a population.

grand theory A theory aimed at describing large segments of the physical, social, or behavioral world; also referred to as a *macrotheory*.

grand tour question A broad question asked in an unstructured interview to gain a general overview of a phenomenon, on the basis of which more focused questions are subsequently asked.

grounded theory An approach to collecting and analyzing qualitative data with the aim of developing theories and theoretical propositions grounded in real-world observations.

Hawthorne effect The effect on the dependent variable resulting from subjects' awareness that they are participants under study.

hermeneutics A qualitative research tradition, drawing on interpretive phenomenology, that focuses on the lived experiences of humans, and on how they interpret those experiences.

heterogeneity The degree to which objects are dissimilar (i.e., characterized by high variability) with respect to some attribute.

histogram A graphic presentation of frequency distribution data.

historical research Systematic studies designed to establish facts and relationships about past events.

history threat A threat to the internal validity of a study; refers to the occurrence of events external to the intervention, but concurrent with it, that can affect the dependent variable of interest.

homogeneity (1) In terms of the reliability of an instrument, the degree to which the subparts are internally consistent (i.e., are measuring the same critical attribute). (2) More generally, the degree to which objects are similar (i.e., characterized by low variability).

hypothesis A prediction about relationships between variables.

impact analysis An evaluation of the effects of an intervention on outcomes of interest, net of other factors influencing those outcomes.

implementation analysis An evaluation that describes the process by which a program or intervention was implemented in practice.

implementation potential The extent to which an innovation is amenable to implementation in a new setting, an assessment of which is made in a research utilization project.

independent variable The variable that is believed to cause or influence the dependent variable; in experimental research, the manipulated (treatment) variable.

inductive reasoning The process of reasoning from specific observations to more general conceptualizations (see also *deductive reasoning*).

inferential statistics Statistics that permit inferences on whether relationships observed in a sample are likely to occur in a population.

informant A term used to refer to those individuals who provide information to researchers about a phenomenon under study, often used in qualitative studies.

informed consent An ethical principle that requires researchers to obtain the voluntary participation of subjects, after informing them of possible risks and benefits.

inquiry audit An independent scrutiny of qualitative data and relevant supporting documents by an external reviewer, a method used to determine the dependability and confirmability of qualitative data.

Institutional Review Board (IRB) A group of individuals from an institution who convene to review proposed and ongoing studies with respect to ethical considerations.

instrument The device that a researcher uses to collect data (e.g., questionnaires, scales, observation schedules, etc.).

instrumental utilization Clearly identifiable attempts to base a specific action or intervention on research findings.

integrated research design A research design that integrates qualitative and quantitative methodologies and data.

interaction effect The effect of two or more independent variables acting in combination (interactively) on a dependent variable rather than as unconnected factors.

internal consistency The degree to which the subparts of an instrument are all measuring the same attribute or dimension, as an index of the instrument's reliability.

internal validity The degree to which it can be inferred that the independent variable, rather than uncontrolled, extraneous factors, is responsible for observed effects on the dependent variable.

interrater (interobserver) reliability The degree to which two raters or observers, operating independently, assign the same values for an attribute being measured or observed.

interval measure A level of measurement in which an attribute of a variable is rank-ordered on a scale that has equal distances between points on that scale (e.g., Fahrenheit degrees).

intervention In experimental research, the experimental treatment or manipulation.

interview schedule The formal instrument, used in structured self-report studies, that specifies the wording of all questions to be asked of respondents.

inverse relationship A negative correlation between two variables; i.e., a relationship characterized by the tendency of high values on one variable to be associated with low values on the second variable.

item A single question on a test or questionnaire, or a single statement on a scale (e.g., a final examination might consist of 100 items).

journal article A report that summarizes an investigation in a professional journal.

journal club A group that meets regularly (often in clinical settings) to discuss and critique research reports appearing in research journals, often with the goal of assessing the utilization potential of the findings.

judgmental sampling A nonprobability sampling method in which the researcher selects study participants on the basis of personal judgment about which ones will be most representative or productive; also referred to as *purposive sampling.*

known-groups technique A technique for estimating the construct validity of an instrument through an analysis of the degree to which the instrument separates groups that are predicted to differ on the basis of known characteristics or a theory.

level of measurement A system of classifying measurements according to the nature of the measurement and the type of mathematical operations to which they are amenable; the four levels are nominal, ordinal, interval, and ratio.

level of significance The risk of making a Type I error, established by the researcher before statistical analysis (e.g., the .05 level).

life history A narrative self-report about a person's life experiences vis-à-vis a theme of interest to the researcher.

Likert scale A composite measure of attitudes that involves summation of scores on a set of items (statements) to which respondents are asked to indicate their degree of agreement or disagreement.

LISREL The widely-used acronym for linear structural relation analysis, typically used for testing causal models.

literature review A critical summary of research on a topic of interest, often prepared to put a research problem in context or as the basis for a utilization project.

log In participant observation studies, the observer's daily record of events and conversations.

logical positivism The philosophy underlying the traditional scientific approach; see also *positivist paradigm.*

logistic regression A multivariate regression procedure that analyzes relationships between multiple independent variables and categorical dependent variables; also referred to as *logit analysis.*

longitudinal study A study designed to collect data at more than one point in time, in contrast to a cross-sectional study.

macro-theory A theory aimed at describing large segments of the physical, social, or behavioral world; also referred to as a *grand theory.*

main effects In a study with multiple independent variables, the effects of a single independent variable on the dependent variable.

manipulation An intervention or treatment introduced by the researcher in an experimental or quasi-experimental study; the researcher manipulates the independent variable to assess its impact on the dependent variable.

matching The pairing of subjects in one group with those in another group based on their similarity on one or more dimension, done to enhance the comparability of groups.

maturation threat A threat to the internal validity of a study that occurs when changes to the outcome measure (dependent variable) result from the passage of time.

maximum variation sampling A sampling approach used by qualitative researchers that involves the purposeful selection of cases with a wide range of variation.

mean A descriptive statistic that is a measure of central tendency, computed by summing all scores and dividing by the number of subjects.

measurement The assignment of numbers to objects according to specified rules to characterize quantities of an attribute.

median A descriptive statistic that is a measure of central tendency, representing the exact middle score in a distribution of scores; the median is the value above and below which 50 percent of the scores lie.

mediating variable A variable that mediates or acts like a "go-between" in a chain linking two other variables (e.g., coping skills mediate the relationship between stressful events and anxiety).

member check A method of validating the credibility of qualitative data through debriefings and discussions with informants.

meta-analysis A technique for quantitatively combining and thus integrating the results of multiple studies on a given topic.

methodologic notes In observational field studies, the notes kept by the researcher regarding the methods used in collecting the data.

methods (research) The steps, procedures, and strategies for gathering and analyzing the data in a research investigation.

middle-range theory A theory that focuses on only a piece of reality or human experience, involving a selected number of concepts (e.g., theories of stress).

modality A characteristic of a frequency distribution describing the number of peaks; that is, values with high frequencies.

mode A descriptive statistic that is a measure of central tendency; the score or value that occurs most frequently in a distribution of scores.

model A symbolic representation of concepts or variables, and interrelationships among them.

mortality threat A threat to the internal validity of a study, referring to the differential loss of participants (attrition) from different groups.

multimethod research Generally, research in which multiple approaches are used to address a research problem; often used to designate research in which both qualitative and quantitative data are collected and analyzed.

multimodal distribution A distribution of values with more than one peak (high frequency).

multiple comparison procedures Statistical tests, normally applied after an ANOVA indicates statistically significant group differences, that compare different pairs of groups; also referred to as *post hoc tests*.

multiple correlation coefficient An index that summarizes the degree of relationship between two or more independent variables and a dependent variable; symbolized as *R*.

multiple regression analysis A statistical procedure for understanding the simultaneous effects of two or more independent (predictor) variables on a dependent variable.

multi-stage sampling A sampling strategy that proceeds through a set of stages from larger to smaller sampling units (e.g., from states, to nursing schools, to faculty members).

multivariate analysis of variance (MANOVA) A statistical procedure used to test the significance of differences between the means of two or more groups on two or more dependent variables, considered simultaneously.

multivariate statistics Statistical procedures designed to analyze the relationships among three or more variables; commonly used multivariate statistics include multiple regression, analysis of covariance, and factor analysis.

N Often used to designate the total number of study participants (e.g., "the total *N* was 500").

n Often used to designate the number of participants in a subgroup or in a cell of a study (e.g., "each of the four groups had an *n* of 125, for a total *N* of 500").

naturalistic paradigm An alternative paradigm to the traditional positivist paradigm that holds that there are multiple interpretations of reality, and that the goal of research is to understand how individuals construct reality within their context; often associated with qualitative research.

naturalistic setting A setting for the collection of research data that is natural to those being studied (e.g., homes, places of work, and so on).

negative case analysis A method used in a qualitative study to extend the understanding of the findings by searching for exceptions that will increase variation in the data.

negative relationship A relationship between two variables in which there is a tendency for higher values on one variable to be associated with lower values on the other (e.g., as temperature increases, people's productivity may decrease); also referred to as an *inverse relationship.*

negative results Research results that fail to support the researcher's hypotheses.

negatively skewed distribution An asymmetric distribution of data values, with a disproportionately high number of cases having high values—i.e., falling at the upper end of the distribution; when displayed graphically, the tail points to the left.

net effects The impacts of an intervention, over and above what would have occurred in its absence.

network sampling The sampling of participants based on referrals from others already in the sample, sometimes referred to as *snowball sampling.*

nominal measure The lowest level of measurement that involves the assignment of characteristics into categories (e.g., males, category 1; females, category 2).

nondirectional hypothesis A research hypothesis that does not stipulate in advance the expected direction of the relationship between variables.

nonequivalent control group design A quasi-experimental design involving a comparison group that was not developed on the basis of random assignment, but from whom preintervention data are obtained to assess the initial equivalence of the groups.

nonexperimental research Studies in which the researcher collects data without introducing any treatment.

nonparametric statistics A general class of inferential statistics that does not involve rigorous assumptions about the distribution of the critical variables; most often used when the data are measured on the nominal or ordinal scales.

nonprobability sampling The selection of participants or sampling units from a population using nonrandom procedures; examples include convenience, purposive, and quota sampling.

nonresponse bias A bias that can result when a nonrandom subset of people invited to participate in a study fail to do so.

nonsignificant result The result of a statistical test indicating that a relationship between variables could have occurred as a result of chance, at a given level of significance; sometimes abbreviated as *NS* in research journals.

normal distribution A distribution that is bell-shaped and symmetrical; also referred to as a *normal curve.*

null hypothesis The hypothesis that states there is no relationship between the variables under study; used with tests of statistical significance as the hypothesis to be rejected.

objectivity The extent to which two independent researchers would arrive at similar judgments or conclusions (i.e., judgments not biased by personal values or beliefs).

observational methods Techniques for acquiring data through the direct observation of phenomena.

observational notes In field studies, the observer's descriptions of observed events and conversations.

observational research Studies in which the data are collected by observing and recording behaviors or activities of interest.

obtained (observed) score The actual score or numerical value assigned to a person on a measure.

open-ended question A question in an interview or questionnaire that does not restrict the respondents' answers to preestablished alternatives.

open coding The first level of coding in a grounded theory study, used to capture what is going on in the data.

operational definition The definition of a concept or variable in terms of the operations or procedures by which it is to be measured.

ordinal measure A level of measurement that yields rank orders of a variable along some dimension.

outcome analysis An evaluation of what happens with respect to outcomes of interest after implementing a program, without use of an experimental design to assess net effects; see also *impact analysis.*

outcome variable A term sometimes used to refer to the dependent variable in experimental research, i.e., the measure that captures the outcome of the intervention.

outcomes research Research designed to document the effectiveness of health care services and the end results of patient care.

***p* value** In statistical testing, the probability that the obtained results are due to chance alone; the probability of committing a Type I error.

panel study A type of longitudinal study in which data are collected from the same people at two or more points in time.

paradigm A way of looking at natural phenomena that encompasses a set of philosophical assumptions and that guides one's approach to inquiry.

parameter A characteristic of a population (e.g., the mean age of all U.S. citizens).

parametric statistics A class of inferential statistics that involves (a) assumptions about the distribution of the variables, (b) the estimation of a parameter, and (c) the use of interval or ratio measures.

participant See *study participant.*

participant observation A method of collecting data through the observation of a group or organization in which the researcher participates as a member.

path analysis A regression-based procedure for testing causal models, typically using non-experimental data.

Pearson's *r* The most widely-used correlation coefficient, designating the magnitude of relationship between two variables measured on at least an interval scale; also referred to as the *product-moment correlation.*

peer debriefing In qualitative research, a session held with objective peers to review various aspects of the inquiry as a means of strengthening the trustworthiness of the data.

peer reviewer A person who reviews and critiques a research report, who himself/herself is a researcher (usually working on similar research problems as those under review), and who makes a recommendation about publishing the research.

perfect relationship A correlation between two variables such that the values of one variable permit perfect prediction of the values of the other; designated as 1.00 or -1.00.

personal interview A face-to-face interview between an interviewer and a respondent.

personal notes In field studies, written comments about the observer's own feelings during the research process.

phenomenon The abstract entity or concept under investigation in a study, most often used by qualitative researchers in lieu of the term "variable".

phenomenology A qualitative research tradition, with roots in philosophy, that focuses on the lived experience of humans.

pilot study A small scale version, or trial run, done in preparation for a major study.

population The entire set of individuals (or objects) having some common characteristics (e.g., all RNs in California); sometimes referred to as *universe.*

positive relationship A relationship between two variables in which there is a tendency for high values on one variable to be associated with high values on the other (e.g., as physical activity increases, pulse rate also increases).

positive results Research results that are consistent with the researcher's hypotheses.

positively skewed distribution An asymmetric distribution of values, with a disproportionately high number of cases having low values—i.e., falling at the lower end of the distribution; when displayed graphically, the tail points to the right.

positivist paradigm The traditional paradigm underlying the scientific approach, which assumes that there is a fixed, orderly reality that can be objectively studied; often associated with quantitative research.

post hoc **test** A test for comparing all possible pairs of groups following a significant test of overall group differences (e.g., in an ANOVA).

poster session A session at a professional conference in which several researchers simultaneously present visual displays summarizing their studies, while conference attendees circulate around the room perusing the displays.

posttest The collection of data after the introduction of an experimental intervention.

posttest-only design An experimental design in which data are collected from subjects only after an intervention has been introduced; also referred to as an *after-only design*.

power analysis A procedure for estimating (a) the likelihood of committing a Type II error, or (b) sample size requirements.

predictive validity The degree to which an instrument can predict a criterion observed at a future time.

pre-experimental design A research design that does not include mechanisms to compensate for the absence of either randomization or a control group.

pretest (1) The collection of data prior to the experimental intervention; sometimes referred to as *baseline data*. (2) The trial administration of a newly developed instrument to identify flaws or assess time requirements.

pretest-posttest design An experimental design in which data are collected from subjects both before and after the introduction of an intervention; also referred to as a *before-after design*.

primary source First-hand reports of facts, findings or events; in terms of research, the primary source is the original research report prepared by the investigator who conducted the study.

probability sampling The selection of participants or sampling units from a population using random procedures; examples include simple random sampling, cluster sampling, and systematic sampling.

problem statement The statement of the research problem, sometimes phrased in the form of a research question.

process analysis An evaluation focusing on the process by which a program or intervention gets implemented and used in practice.

process consent In a qualitative study, an ongoing, transactional process of negotiating consent with study participants, allowing them to play a collaborative role in the decision-making regarding their continued participation.

product moment correlation coefficient (*r*) The most widely-used correlation coefficient, designating the magnitude of relationship between two variables measured on at least an interval scale; also referred to as *Pearson's r*.

projective techniques Methods for measuring psychological attributes (values, attitudes, personality) by providing respondents with unstructured stimuli to which to respond.

prolonged engagement In qualitative research, the investment of sufficient time in the collection of data to have an in-depth understanding of the group under study; a mechanism for achieving data credibility.

proportionate sample A sample that results when the researcher samples from different strata of the population in direct proportion to their representation in the population.

prospective study A study that begins with an examination of presumed causes (e.g., cigarette smoking) and then goes forward in time to observe presumed effects (e.g., lung cancer).

psychometric evaluation An assessment of the quality of an instrument, based primarily on evidence of its reliability and validity.

purposive (purposeful) sampling A nonprobability sampling method in which the researcher selects study participants on the basis of personal judgment about which ones will be most representative or productive; also referred to as *judgmental sampling*.

Q sort A data collection method in which the participant sorts statements into a number of piles (usually 9 or 11) according to some bipolar dimension (e.g., most like me/least like me).

qualitative analysis The organization and interpretation of nonnumerical data for the purpose of discovering important underlying dimensions and patterns of relationships.

qualitative data Information collected in narrative (nonnumerical) form, such as the transcript of an unstructured interview.

qualitative research The investigation of phenomena, typically in an in-depth and holistic fashion, through the collection of rich narrative materials using a flexible research design.

quantitative analysis The manipulation of numerical data through statistical procedures for the purpose of describing phenomena or assessing the magnitude and reliability of relationships among them.

quantitative data Information collected in a numerical form.

quantitative research The study of phenomena that lend themselves to precise measurement and quantification, often involving a rigorous and controlled design.

quasi-experiment A study in which subjects are not randomly assigned to treatment conditions, but the researcher does manipulate the independent variable and exercises certain controls to enhance the internal validity of the results.

quasi-statistics An "accounting" system used to assess the validity of conclusions derived from qualitative analysis.

questionnaire A method of gathering self-report information from respondents through administration of questions in a paper-and-pencil format.

quota sampling The nonrandom selection of participants in which the researcher pre-specifies characteristics of the sample, to increase its representativeness.

r The symbol used to designate a bivariate correlation coefficient, summarizing the magnitude and direction of a relationship between two variables.

R The symbol used to designate the multiple correlation coefficient, indicating the magnitude (but not direction) of the relationship between the dependent variable and multiple independent variables, taken together.

R^2 The squared multiple correlation coefficient, indicating the proportion of variance in the dependent variable accounted for or explained by a group of independent variables.

random assignment The assignment of subjects to treatment conditions in a random manner (i.e., in a manner determined by chance alone); also known as *randomization.*

random sampling The selection of a sample such that each member of a population has an equal probability of being included.

randomization See *random assignment.*

range A measure of variability, consisting of the difference between the highest and lowest values in a distribution of scores.

ratio measure A level of measurement in which there are equal distances between score units, and that has a true meaningful zero point (e.g., weight).

raw data Data that are in the exact form in which they were collected.

reactivity A measurement distortion arising from the study participant's awareness of being observed, or, more generally, from the effect of the measurement procedure itself.

relationship A bond or association between two or more variables.

reliability The degree of consistency or accuracy with which an instrument measures the attribute it is designed to measure.

reliability coefficient A quantitative index, usually ranging in value from .00 to 1.00, that provides an estimate of how reliable an instrument is.

repeated-measures design An experimental design in which one group of subjects is exposed to more than one condition or treatment in random order; sometimes referred to as a *crossover design.*

replication The deliberate repetition of research procedures in a second investigation for the purpose of determining if earlier results can be repeated.

representative sample A sample whose characteristics are highly similar to those of the population from which it is drawn.

research Systematic inquiry that uses orderly, disciplined methods to answer questions or solve problems.

research-based practice See *evidence-based practice.*

research control See *control.*

research design The overall plan for addressing a research question, including specifications for enhancing the integrity of the study.

research problem A situation involving an enigmatic, perplexing, or conflictful condition that can be investigated through disciplined inquiry.

research question A statement of the specific query the investigator wants to answer through research.

research report A document that summarizes the main features of a study, including the research question, the methods used to address it, the findings, and the interpretation and implications of the findings.

research utilization The use of some aspect of a scientific investigation in an application unrelated to the original research.

respondent In a self-report study, the participant who responds to questions posed by the researcher.

response rate The rate of participation in a study, calculated by dividing the number of people participating by the number of people sampled.

response set bias The measurement error introduced by the tendency of some individuals to respond to items in characteristic ways (e.g., always agreeing), independently of the item's content.

results The answers to research questions, obtained through an analysis of the collected data; in a quantitative study, the information obtained through statistical tests.

retrospective study A study that begins with the occurrence of the dependent variable in the present (e.g., lung cancer) and then links this effect to some presumed cause occurring in the past (e.g., cigarette smoking).

risk–benefit ratio The relative costs and benefits, to an individual subject and to society at large, of participation in a study; also, the relative costs and benefits of implementing an innovation.

rival hypothesis An alternative explanation, competing with the researcher's hypothesis, for understanding the results of a study.

sample A subset of a population selected to participate in a study.

sample size The number of study participants in a sample.

sampling The process of selecting a portion of the population to represent the entire population.

sampling bias Distortions that arise when a sample is not representative of the population from which it was drawn.

sampling distribution A theoretical distribution of a statistic, using the values of the statistic computed from an infinite number of samples as the data points in the distribution.

sampling error The fluctuation of the value of a statistic from one sample to another drawn from the same population.

sampling frame A list of all the elements in the population, from which the sample is drawn.

sampling plan In a quantitative study, the pre-specified plan that indicates in advance what the eligibility criteria are, how the sample will be selected, and how many subjects there will be.

saturation The process of collecting data in a grounded theory study to the point where a sense of closure is attained because new data yield redundant information.

scale A composite measure of an attribute, involving the combination of several items that have a logical and empirical relationship to each other, resulting in the assignment of a score to place people on a continuum with respect to the attribute.

scientific approach A set of orderly, systematic, controlled procedures for acquiring dependable, empirical—and typically quantitative—information; the methodologic approach associated with the positivist paradigm.

scientific merit The degree to which a study is methodologically and conceptually sound.

secondary source Second-hand accounts of events or facts; in a research context, a description of a study or studies prepared by someone other than the original researcher.

selection threat (self-selection) A threat to the internal validity of the study resulting from pre-existing differences between the groups under study; the differences affect the dependent variable in ways extraneous to the effect of the independent variable.

selective coding The type of substantive coding in a grounded theory study that involves the coding of only those variables that are related to the core variable.

self-report Any procedure for collecting data that involves a direct report of information by the person who is being studied (e.g., by interview or questionnaire).

self selection A bias that can occur when the members of groups being studied are in the groups, in part, because they differentially possess traits or characteristics extraneous to the research problem, characteristics that possibly influence or are otherwise related to the research variables.

semantic differential A technique used to measure attitudes that asks respondents to rate a concept of interest on a series of bipolar rating scales.

setting The physical location and conditions in which data collection takes place in a study.

significance level The probability that an observed relationship could be caused by chance (i.e., as a result of sampling error); significance at the .05 level indicates the probability that a relationship of the observed magnitude would be found by chance only 5 times out of 100.

simple random sampling The most basic type of probability sampling, wherein a sampling frame is created by enumerating all members of a population of interest, and then selecting a sample from the sampling frame through completely random procedures.

skewed distribution The asymmetric distribution of a set of data values around a central point.

snowball sampling The selection of participants by means of referrals from earlier participants; also referred to as *network sampling*.

social desirability response set A bias in self-report instruments created when participants have a tendency to misrepresent their opinions in the direction of answers consistent with prevailing social norms.

Spearman's rank-order correlation (Spearman's rho) A correlation coefficient indicating the magnitude of a relationship between variables measured on the ordinal scale.

split-half technique A method for estimating the internal consistency reliability of an instrument by correlating scores on half of the measure with scores on the other half.

standard deviation The most frequently used statistic for measuring the degree of variability in a set of scores.

standard error The standard deviation of a sampling distribution, such as the sampling distribution of means.

statement of purpose A broad declarative statement of the goals of a research project.

statistic An estimate of a parameter, calculated from sample data.

statistical analysis The organization and analysis of quantitative data using statistical procedures, including both descriptive and inferential statistics.

statistical inference The process of inferring attributes about the population based on information from a sample, using laws of probability.

statistical significance A term indicating that the results obtained in an analysis of sample data are unlikely to have been caused by chance, at some specified level of probability.

statistical test An analytic procedure that allows a researcher to determine the probability that obtained results from a sample reflect true population results.

stipend A monetary payment to individuals participating in a study to serve as an incentive for participation and/or to compensate for time and expenses.

strata Subdivisions of the population according to some characteristic (e.g., males and females); singular is *stratum*.

stratified random sampling The random selection of study participants from two or more strata of the population independently.

structured data collection An approach to collecting information from participants, either through self-report or observations, wherein the researcher determines in advance the variables and categories of interest.

structured observation A procedure for collecting observational data in which the nature of the observations to be made are pre-specified, and a procedure for sampling observational units has been designated.

structured self-report A procedure for collecting data that involves asking a pre-specified set of questions in a pre-specified order, usually with a preponderance of closed-ended questions.

study participant An individual who participates and provides information in a research investigation.

subject An individual who participates and provides data in a study; term used primarily in quantitative research.

summated rating scale See *Likert scale*.

survey research Nonexperimental research that focusses on obtaining information regarding the activities, beliefs, preferences, and attitudes of people via direct questioning of a sample of respondents.

symmetric distribution A distribution of values that has two halves that are mirror images of the each other; a distribution that is not skewed.

systematic sampling The selection of study participants such that every kth (e.g., every tenth) person (or element) in a sampling frame or list is chosen.

target population The entire population in which the researcher is interested and to which he or she would like to generalize the results of a study.

test statistic A statistic used to test for the statistical significance of relationships between variables; the sampling distributions of test statistics are known for circumstances in which the null hypothesis is true; examples include chi-squared, F-ratio, t, and Pearson's r.

test-retest reliability Assessment of the stability of an instrument by correlating the scores obtained on repeated administrations.

theme A recurring regularity emerging from an analysis of qualitative data.

theoretical notes In field studies, notes detailing the researcher's interpretations of observed behavior.

theoretical sampling In qualitative studies (especially in grounded theory studies), the selection of sample members based on emerging findings/theory to ensure adequate representation and full variation of important themes.

theory An abstract generalization that presents a systematic explanation about the relationships among phenomena.

thick description A rich and thorough description of the research context in a qualitative study.

time sampling In observational research, the selection of time periods during which observations will take place.

time series design A quasi-experimental design that involves the collection of information over an extended time period, with multiple data collection points prior to and after the introduction of a treatment.

topic guide A list of broad question areas to be covered in a semi-structured interview or focus group interview.

transferability (1) A criterion for evaluating the quality of qualitative data, referring to the extent to which the findings from the data can be transferred to other settings or groups—analogous to generalizability; (2) also, a criterion used in an implementation assessment of a utilization project.

treatment The experimental intervention under study; the condition being manipulated.

trend study A form of longitudinal study in which different samples from a population are studied over time with respect to some phenomenon (e.g., annual Gallup polls on abortion attitudes).

triangulation The use of multiple methods or perspectives to collect and interpret data about a phenomenon, to converge on an accurate representation of reality.

true score A hypothetical score that would be obtained if a measure were infallible; the portion of the observed score not due to random error or measurement bias.

trustworthiness A term used in the evaluation of qualitative data, assessed using the criteria of credibility, transferability, dependability, and confirmability.

t-test A parametric statistical test used for analyzing the difference between two means.

Type I error An error created by rejecting the null hypothesis when it is true (i.e., the researcher concludes that a relationship exists when in fact it does not).

Type II error An error created by accepting the null hypothesis when it is false (i.e., the researcher concludes that *no* relationship exists when in fact it does).

unimodal distribution A distribution of values with one peak (high frequency).

univariate descriptive study A study that gathers information on the occurrence, frequency of occurrence, or average value of the variables of interest, one variable at a time, without focusing on interrelationships among variables.

univariate statistics Statistical procedures for analyzing a single variable for purposes of description.

unstructured interview An oral self-report in which the researcher asks questions without having a predetermined plan regarding the specific content or flow of information to be gathered.

unstructured observation The collection of descriptive information through direct observation, whereby the observer is guided by some general research questions but does not follow a prespecified plan for observing, enumerating, or recording the information.

utilization criteria The criteria used to assess whether an innovation is amenable to utilization in a practice setting; includes the criteria of clinical relevance, scientific merit, and implementation potential.

validity The degree to which an instrument measures what it is intended to measure.

validity coefficient A quantitative index, usually ranging in value from .00 to 1.00, that provides an estimate of how valid an instrument is; usually computed in conjunction with the criterion-related approach to validating an instrument.

variability The degree to which values on a set of scores are widely different or dispersed.

variable An attribute of a person or object that varies, that is, takes on different values (e.g., body temperature, age, heart rate).

variance A measure of variability or dispersion, equal to the standard deviation squared.

vignette A brief description of an event, person, or situation to which respondents are asked to react and to describe their reactions.

visual analogue scale A scaling procedure used to measure clinical symptoms (e.g., pain, fatigue) by having people indicate on a straight line the intensity of the attribute being measured.

vulnerable subjects Special groups of people whose rights in studies need special protection because of their inability to provide meaningful informed consent or because their circumstances place them at higher-than-average-risk of adverse effects; examples include young children, the mentally retarded, and unconscious patients.

weighting A correction procedure used to arrive at population values when a disproportionate sampling design has been used.

within-subjects design A research design in which a single group of subjects is compared under different conditions or at different points in time (e.g., before and after surgery).

Appendix: Research Reports

A. QUANTITATIVE STUDY

Preventing Smoking Relapse
In Postpartum Women

*Joy L. Johnson, Pamela A. Ratner, Joan L. Bottorff,
Wendy Hall, and Susan Dahinten*

- **Background:** Although many women quit smoking during pregnancy, the majority resume smoking shortly after giving birth.
- **Objectives:** To test a program to prevent smoking relapse in the postpartum period by comparing the rates of continuous smoking abstinence, daily smoking, and smoking cessation self-efficacy in treatment and control groups.
- **Methods:** In a randomized clinical trial, nurses provided face-to-face, in-hospital counseling sessions at birth, followed by telephone counseling. The target population included women who quit smoking during pregnancy and who gave birth at one of five hospitals. The 254 participating women were interviewed 6 months after delivery and assessed biochemically to determine smoking status.
- **Results:** The 6-month continuous smoking abstinence rate was 38% in the treatment group and 27% in the control group (odds ratio [OR] = 1.63, 95% confidence interval [CI] = .96 − 2.78). Significantly more control (48%) than treatment (34%) group participants reported smoking daily (OR = 1.80, 95% CI = 1.08 − 2.99). Smoking cessation self-efficacy did not vary significantly between the groups.
- **Conclusions:** Smoking cessation interventions focusing on the prenatal period have failed to achieve long-term abstinence. Interventions can be strengthened if they are extended into the postpartum period.
- **Key Words:** smoking cessation • postnatal care • telephone counseling

Since the 1960s, there has been minimal reduction in the proportion of Canadian women who smoke. Up to 15,000 Canadian women die annually from diseases attributable to smoking, and the rate of lung cancer among women is rising (Canadian Cancer Society, 1997; Ellison, Mao, & Gibbons,

Reprinted with permission from *Nursing Research* (2000;49[1]:44–52).

1995). When women smoke during pregnancy and after childbirth, they put the fetus, neonate, and growing child at risk for several health problems (Charlton, 1994; U.S. Department of Health and Human Services, 1989).

The effects of smoking during pregnancy are well known and provide a strong inducement for many women to quit. Half of women quit smoking during pregnancy and remain abstinent for 4 to 9 months (O'Campo, Faden, Brown, & Gielen, 1992; Secker-Walker et al., 1995). However, studies have revealed that approximately 70% of these women resume smoking shortly after giving birth (Fingerhut, Kleinman, & Kendrick, 1990; Mullen, Richardson, Quinn, & Ershoff, 1997; Sexton, Hebel, & Fox, 1987). Although these rates of relapse are comparable with the rates among quitters in the general population (Brandon, Tiffany, Obremski, & Baker, 1990), many pregnant women experience prolonged abstinence before relapse. These women may be unaware of the risks of smoking for their infants and themselves, or more likely they lack the support, skills, or commitment required to maintain long-term abstinence.

The purpose of this study was to test an intervention to help postpartum women to avoid or manage smoking lapses, thereby enhancing their likelihood of maintaining continuous smoking abstinence and reducing their risk of daily smoking after the birth of their babies. Three hypotheses were tested:

Hypothesis 1: The rate of continuous smoking abstinence at 6 months postpartum, based on self-report and biochemical validation, will be significantly higher in the treatment group than in the control group.

Hypothesis 2: The rate of daily smoking at 6 months postpartum will be significantly lower in the treatment group than in the control group.

Hypothesis 3: Smoking cessation self-efficacy at 6 months postpartum will be significantly higher in the treatment group than in the control group.

RELEVANT LITERATURE

It has been recognized that smoking cessation is not a binary event in which people shift from being smokers to nonsmokers (Prochaska & DiClemente, 1983; Prochaska, DiClemente, & Norcross, 1992). Accordingly, research attention has turned to understanding the factors that cause lapses and to developing interventions that prevent relapse. The work of Marlatt (1985, 1996) and Marlatt and Gordon (1985) addresses relapse after behavior change and focuses on events surrounding the initial use of the undesired substance during the postcessation period. The author conceptualizes relapse as a process influenced by cognitive and behavioral mechanisms rather than a discrete, irreversible event, and distinguishes between lapse (initial use of a substance) and complete relapse (full return to regular use of the substance). This model, widely used in relapse prevention, has been supported by empirical evidence (Baer, Holt, & Lichtenstein, 1986; Cohen & Lichtenstein, 1990; Curry et al., 1993).

The precipitants of relapse in the postpartum period include demographic and contextual variables such as contact with other smokers, parity, socio-demographic variables, amount smoked before pregnancy, and whether women quit early or late in pregnancy (Fingerhut et al., 1990; McBride, Pirie, & Curry, 1992; O'Campo et al., 1992). Greater self-efficacy and some types of coping strategies have been demonstrated to reduce the probability of post-partum relapse (McBride et al., 1992). Women require coping strategies relevant to their particular circumstances, and the coping strategies used during pregnancy may not be effective in the postpartum period (McBride et al., 1992).

Marlatt's relapse model is the cornerstone of a group of interventions referred to as "relapse prevention training" (RPT), which includes skills training to anticipate and resist lapsing in high-risk situations and cognitive restructuring to deal with self-defeating attributions after a lapse. Although not a panacea, RPT is a promising approach for the prevention of relapse. Studies in which RPT was used generally have rendered positive results, particularly with women and light smokers (Curry, Marlatt, Gordon, & Baer, 1988; Hall, Rugg, Tunstall, & Jones, 1984). Exposure to RPT has been found to be associated with long-term abstinence (Davis, Faust, & Ordentlich, 1984; Stevens & Hollis, 1989). In contrast to these positive outcomes, others have reported no effect when self-help RPT was used, perhaps because they did not incorporate tailored approaches or sufficient counseling support (Curry et al., 1988; Killen, Fortmann, Newman, & Varady, 1990; Omenn et al., 1988).

A number of studies have investigated smoking-cessation interventions with pregnant women, but few have extended their interventions to the early postpartum period (Petersen, Handel, Kotch, Podedworny, & Rosen, 1992; Secker-Walker et al., 1995). Although possibly the result of Type II error, with 175 women assigned to two study groups, Secker-Walker et al. (1995) failed to affect early postpartum relapse rates when they augmented antenatal smoking-cessation counseling with a single postpartum visit. Petersen et al. (1992) tested several interventions based on self-help materials and professional counseling during the antenatal period and the first month postpartum. The most intensive intervention, including regular counseling, significantly increased the proportion of women who remained abstinent at 8 weeks postpartum. The longer-term benefits of such interventions remain unknown.

The value of pregnancy as an intervention point for smoking cessation is being undermined by high relapse rates in the postpartum period. If abstinence during pregnancy is to result in long-term smoking cessation, more attention must be given to developing interventions to prevent and manage relapse. This experimental, pretest–posttest control group study aimed to evaluate the effectiveness of an intervention for postpartum women who quit smoking during pregnancy. Because continuous abstinence may not be a realistic goal for many individuals engaged in the smoking cessation process, the outcome measures of continuous abstinence and resumption of daily smoking were the variables of interest.

METHODS

Sample

The target population consisted of all the women who gave birth at one of five hospitals during a 7-month period and who met the following criteria: (a) identified herself as a smoker before pregnancy; (b) quit smoking once aware of pregnancy or in attempting to become pregnant; (c) ceased smoking for at least 6 weeks before delivery; (d) if smoking occurred in the 6-week period immediately before delivery, smoked on fewer than six occasions; (e) gave birth to a healthy infant not requiring hospitalization beyond discharge of the mother; (f) planned to remain in hospital for at least 24 hours; (g) was able to read and comprehend English; and (h) could be contacted by telephone.

Of the 8,837 women admitted for labor and delivery over the course of the recruitment period, 8,290 were screened. The 547 unscreened women were missed because they were discharged within a few hours of delivery (519), because they would not discuss eligibility (22), or because of another reason (6). Of 416 eligible women, 254 agreed to participate and gave their informed consent, resulting in a participation rate of 61.1%. Three of the consenting subjects were excluded from analysis: One was randomly assigned as a control participant but was inadvertently given the intervention, and two were assigned to the treatment group but did not receive any telephone contacts. The final sample was 251 women: 125 in the treatment group and 126 in the control group.

Measures

Smoking status was measured using self-report items, including those related to frequency of smoking and amount smoked. Because reports of smoking status may be unreliable (Apseloff, Ashton, Friedman, & Gerber, 1994), biochemical assessments were completed with Bedfont EC50 Smokerlyzers. Carbon monoxide (CO) readings of 10 or more parts per million (ppm) were concluded to be indicative of recent smoking. Biochemical measures such as CO readings not only validate self-reports, but also enhance the validity of self-reports, especially because the participants were uninformed about the sensitivity of the measure (Patrick et al., 1994).

When participants denied smoking but obtained CO readings of 10 ppm or more, or when they admitted to smoking but obtained CO readings of less than 10 ppm, perhaps because they smoked irregularly, they were classified as not being continuously abstinent. Self-reports were used for participants who were unable to provide a CO reading because the follow-up evaluation was conducted by telephone. Continuous abstinence referred to the complete avoidance of smoking during the entire 6-month period. Daily smoking was measured by self-reports at follow-up of one or more cigarettes typically smoked per day. Validation of participants' self-reports of daily smoking was not possible with CO monitoring because single measures of CO levels are not indicative of smoking frequency.

Smoking cessation self-efficacy was measured with the Smoking Abstinence Self-Efficacy Scale (SASE; DiClemente, 1981; Prochaska, DiClemente, Velicer, Ginpil, & Norcross, 1985), an instrument designed to assess smokers' level of confidence that they will not smoke in 20 challenging situations. The instrument consists of three subscales: (a) the negative/affective subscale measuring the degree of confidence when frustrated or facing conflict or emotional distress; (b) the habit/addictive subscale measuring the degree of confidence when the urge to smoke is felt; and (c) the positive/social subscale measuring confidence in resisting temptation in social or celebratory situations. Of the 20 items, 17 are scored with a range from 0% (not at all confident) to 100% (completely confident) (Velicer, DiClemente, Rossi, & Prochaska, 1990).

The SASE has demonstrated acceptable construct and predictive validity and acceptable internal consistency, with a Cronbach's alpha ranging from .88 to .92 (DiClemente, 1981; Prochaska et al., 1985; Velicer et al., 1990). Each subscale has demonstrated internal consistency (.92–.95), and the responses are not associated with social desirability. The data obtained in this study were subjected to factor analysis with maximum likelihood extraction and varimax rotation, which confirmed the presence of three factors. The alpha coefficients for the three subscales ranged from .80 to .88.

A number of covariates were assessed because they have been found associated with smoking and relapse. Demographic items were included to measure age, income, education, employment status, marital status, and parity. The demographic items were adapted from well-established surveys such as Canada's Health Promotion Survey (Stephens & Graham, 1993) and have undergone rigorous pretesting.

Participants were asked on a scale from 1 (not at all likely) to 10 (extremely likely) whether they expected to return to their desired weight within 6 months. Items that measured smoking history, number of cigarettes smoked daily, number of years smoked, number of prior quit attempts, and longest period of abstinence were included. Items that measured partners' smoking histories focused on smoking patterns during the pregnancy.

Social support for smoking cessation was determined by asking each woman how much encouragement from family and friends she expected to receive for her efforts to remain abstinent. The response categories were as follows: no encouragement at all, hardly any encouragement, some encouragement, and a great deal of encouragement. This item was used by Strecher, Becker, Kirscht, Eraker, and Graham-Tomasi (1985), who argued that the concept of encouragement traverses key elements of social support.

Because it has been argued that stress can interfere with the ability to make and maintain behavior changes, and that depressive moods can place people at higher risk for relapse, mental health was measured by five items taken from Canada's Health Promotion Survey (Stephens & Graham, 1993). One item measured overall happiness. The remaining items were used to create a composite scale of mental health status. The items included respondents' reported frequency of feeling "cheerful and lighthearted," "loved and wanted," "downhearted and blue," and "lonely." On factor analysis, these four items were found to measure a single factor or dimension. The smallest factor loading was .45 (59.1% of the variance was explained). The internal consistency (Cronbach's alpha) for these four items was .76. Consequently, a mental health status scale was created by taking the average of these four items (range = 1–4). Larger values were indicative of better mental health.

Physical (physiologic) dependence on nicotine or addiction was measured with the 10-item Revised Fagerstrom Tolerance Questionnaire (RTQ), which accounts for amount smoked, patterns of smoking, and ability to refrain from smoking (e.g., in banned areas and when sick) (Fagerstrom, 1978; Tate & Schmitz, 1993). Five-point Likert scales were used to score each item. Reported scores were averaged across the 10 items, with lower scores indicating relatively weaker dependence.

The RTQ has demonstrated concurrent validity with various withdrawal responses, including body temperature and heart rate elevation. Tate and Schmitz (1993) tested the RTQ with four samples of smokers and reported reliability coefficients ranging from .72 to .85. Test–retest reliability over 1 to 1.5 months duration was .88. Factor analysis identified one common factor (40% of total-item variance explained). In the current study, the questions were posed retrospectively to capture physical dependence before cessation.

Intervention

A postpartum counseling intervention was designed to prevent or interrupt the relapse process by teaching skills to deal with high-risk situations and cognitive restructuring techniques to deal with lapses. The intervention was based on the following principles derived from Marlatt's relapse model (Marlatt, 1985; Marlatt & Gordon, 1980, 1985): (a) Smoking cessation is a process, and relapse is not an irrevocable state; (b) smoking cessation is influenced by cognitive and behavioral mechanisms; (c) maintaining abstinence requires a sense of control and self-efficacy; (d) lapses are most likely to occur in high-risk situations; (e) it is possible to prevent lapses from leading to complete relapse by helping individuals cognitively to restructure lapse events; and (f) cessation efforts need to be reinforced with long-term follow-up sessions.

Nurses were hired and trained to provide the one-to-one counseling intervention. The in-hospital component consisted of sharing information and beginning skill building. The nurse began by learning about the woman's smoking experiences and the context of the smoking cessation effort. After advising about the importance of remaining a nonsmoker, the nurse reviewed potential effects of smoking on the health of the newborn, the family, and the woman herself. The skill-building component focused on teaching the woman to recognize high-risk situations in which she may be tempted to smoke, and to problem solve about how to manage those situations. The nurse reviewed cognitive strategies for dealing with lapses and modeled them using situations provided by the woman. When feasible, the woman was encouraged to role-play the strategy.

The counseling was augmented with materials developed for the study and tailored to the particular circumstances of postpartum women including (a) a pamphlet outlining the risk of smoking during the postpartum period, with strategies to deal with cravings, and a pamphlet focusing on the effects of secondhand smoke on children; (b) a two-sided "self-help" card directed toward problem solving for high-risk situations and cognitively restructuring lapses; and (c) materials to facilitate the maintenance of smoke-free environments, including signs to place on coffee tables, on doors, and in automobiles.

Eight subsequent at-home telephone counseling sessions were provided by the nurse who initially enrolled the participant. These sessions focused on efforts to maintain smoking cessation, review of high-risk situations and their management, possible lapses, guidance in problem solving, and support and encouragement. The telephone sessions were held weekly during the first month postpartum and biweekly during the second and third months. The telephone contacts ranged from 1 to 20 minutes ($M = 4.5$, $SD = 1.5$). It was noted that the average duration of the telephone contacts increased progressively over time, with the first telephone contact lasting an average of 3.7 minutes ($SD = 1.8$) and the eighth contact lasting, on the average, 5.3 minutes ($SD = 2.7$). Although the treatment group participants were expected to receive all eight telephone contacts, it was difficult to meet the study design expectations because participants often were found to be too busy or not available. Only 24.8% of the participants received eight contacts: 42.4% missed one contact; 21.6% missed two; 8% missed three; and 3.2% missed four or five.

Procedure

Group assignment was random, with identification numbers randomly assigned to two groups, in blocks of 50, via a computer software package. The intervention was provided only to the women assigned to the treatment group. The control group received "usual care," which did not include any information about the effects of smoking or prevention of smoking relapse. In the hospital, all participants were administered a baseline questionnaire, and two breath samples were collected to measure CO in expired air. At 6 months after delivery, all participants were interviewed in their homes by research assistants who had not delivered the intervention, and who were blind to group assignment. Carbon monoxide in expired air also was determined.

RESULTS

Participants ($N = 251$) ranged in age from 15 to 40 years ($M = 27.6$, $SD = 5.5$) with educational attainment ranging from some elementary school to earned postgraduate degrees (*Mdn* = completed technical/trade school). Their total annual household income, before deductions and taxes, ranged from less than $9,000 to more than $150,000 (*Mdn* = $40,000–$49,999). The majority (60.6%) usually worked for pay on a full-time basis, and 19.9% worked part-time. Most participants (60.2%) were married and living with a spouse; 23.9% lived with a common-law partner, 14.7% were single (never married), and the rest were either separated or divorced. The current birth was the first child for the majority of participants (74.1%). Three quarters of the participants (74.9%) were born in Canada, and the remainder were born in 40 different countries. Similarly, 75.3% reported that English was their first language. The demographics of the study groups differed only regarding their country of origin: The treatment group was more likely to have been born outside Canada (Table 1).

Baseline Data

Almost all of the participants (94.4%) intended to breast-feed, and expected to do so for 2 weeks to 2 years (34.1% expected to breast-feed for more than 6 months). The mean score for perceived likelihood of achieving desired weight within 6 months was 7.5 (SD = 2.3), suggesting that the majority were confident of weight loss. Two thirds of the participants (68.1%) were reportedly "very happy," 30.3% "pretty happy," and 1.6% "not too happy." The mean score on the composite mental health scale was 3.1 (SD = 0.6). The two study groups differed statistically only with respect to their mental health: The treatment group reported slightly better mental health (Table 1).

The participants reported that 4 to 52 weeks had elapsed since they quit smoking (*M* = 32.9, *SD* = 7.1). Only 10 of the participants (4%) reported smoking in the week immediately preceding the baseline interview, and all had smoked five or fewer cigarettes during that week. Seven of those 10 participants were assigned to the treatment group. As reported, 22 of the participants (8.8%) had smoked during the 6 weeks immediately before baseline data collection (5.6% of the control group and 12% of the treatment group): χ^2 (1, *N* = 251) = 2.50 with Yates' Continuity Correction; *p* = .11. The self-reports of recent smoking were consistent with the two CO breathalyzers, except for those of two participants who obtained CO readings slightly above 10 ppm while reporting complete abstinence for at least 6 weeks.

Almost all of the respondents (93.6%) reported that the primary reason why they quit smoking was concern for the health of their unborn baby. Other reasons for quitting included (a) concern for their own health (3.2%), (b) nausea too great to smoke (2.8%), and (c) recognition that it was a good opportunity to quit (.4%). Almost all (90.8%) reported that they intended to remain nonsmokers postpartum. A small percentage of the participants (15.5%) had made no other smoking cessation attempts (defined as lasting more than 24 hours). Almost one half of the participants (45.8%) had made one or two previous attempts to quit; 30.8% had made 3 to 10 previous attempts; and the remaining 8% reported 11 or more attempts.

TABLE 1. Comparisons of Control and Treatment Groups by Demographic and Personal Characteristics (at Baseline)

VARIABLES	CONTROL (*n* = 126)	TREATMENT (*n* = 125)	STATISTICS t	STATISTICS χ^2
Age (mean, years)	27.4	27.8	−0.54	
Education level (%)				
Less than high school	17.5	14.4		
High school or equivalent	23.0	28.8		
Some/completed trade/community college	33.3	40.0		
Some/completed university	26.2	16.8		4.51
Annual household income (%)[a]				
≤$29,999	29.8	24.8		
$30,000–$49,999	23.7	28.3		
$50,000–$69,999	21.1	18.6		
$70,000+	25.4	28.3		1.35
Marital status (%)				
Married and living with spouse	62.7	57.6		
Common-law/live-in relationship	22.2	25.6		
Separated/divorced/widowed/single	15.1	16.8		0.69
First child (%)				
Yes	69.8	78.4		
No	30.2	21.6		1.97[b]
Employment status (%)				
Does not work for pay	21.4	17.6		
Works part-time	20.6	19.2		
Works full-time	57.9	63.2		0.82
Born in Canada (%)				
Yes	82.5	67.2		
No	17.5	32.8		7.06[b,c]
First language spoken (%)				
English	80.2	70.4		
Other	19.8	29.6		2.71[b]
Intention to breast-feed (%)				
Yes	96.0	92.8		
No	4.0	7.2		0.71[b]
Expected duration of breast-feeding (mean, weeks)	30.6	32.7	−0.90	
Desired weight achieved within 6 months (mean)	7.4	7.6	−0.81	
Happiness (%)				
Very happy	67.5	68.8		
Not too or pretty happy	32.5	31.2		0.01[b]
Mental health (mean)	3.0	3.1	−2.0[c]	

[a]*n* = 227 (9.6% missing cases).
[b]Yates' Continuity Correction used.
[c]$p < .05$.

Before quitting, the participants reported smoking less than 1 to as many as 38 cigarettes daily ($M = 10.4$, $SD = 7.2$). Averaged scores on the 10-item RTQ ranged from 1.6 to 4.5 ($M = 2.7$, $SD = .6$), indicating low to moderate physical dependence. Participants were fairly confident that they could resist the urge to smoke in various situations. Their average SASE scores on the negative/affective, habit/addictive, and positive/social subscales were: 67.1% ($SD = 26.2\%$), 87.3% ($SD = 15\%$), and 73.1% ($SD = 21.8\%$), respectively.

Among the 234 women with partners, 47.4% of the partners were smokers at baseline; 15% quit along with the woman; 26.5% never smoked; and 11.1% had quit at some time in the past. Approximately one third of the participants (29.6%) reported that all or most of the people with whom they spent their time smoked; 30.4% reported that some of their social contacts smoked; and the remaining 40% reported that very few if any of the people with whom they had contact smoked. Most participants (72.5%) expected to receive a great deal of encouragement from their family and friends to help them remain nonsmokers. Among all the smoking-related variables, no statistically significant differences were noted between the control and treatment groups (Table 2).

Data From 6-Month Follow-Up Interview

Some participants were difficult to locate, so the follow-up interviews occurred between 24.1 and 50 weeks after baseline data collection ($M = 28.1$, $SD = 3.1$). Eleven of the interviews (4.6%) were conducted at locations other than the participants' homes (e.g., restaurants, shopping malls), and 19 (7.9%) were conducted over the telephone (as a result, the breathalyzer was not completed). Ten participants (4%) either refused to participate or could not be located (six from the control group and four from the treatment group). These women were included in the analyses, where possible, and coded as failing to maintain continuous abstinence and as daily smokers. Self-efficacy scores were not imputed for these women.

Hypothesis 1. At 6 months postpartum, the rate of continuous smoking abstinence was higher in the treatment (37.6%) than the control (27%) group, although the difference did not achieve statistical significance: χ^2 (1, $N = 251$) = 2.8, $p = .10$ with Yates' continuity correction; OR = 1.63; 95% CI = .96 − 2.78.

Hypothesis 2. Significantly more participants in the control group than in the treatment group reported smoking daily: 47.6% vs. 33.6%, χ^2 (1, $N = 251$) = 4.6, $p = .03$ with Yates' continuity correction; OR = 1.80; 95% CI = 1.08 − 2.99.

Hypothesis 3. The 6-month smoking cessation self-efficacy scores for each subscale were subjected to between-groups analysis of covariance. The independent variables were group assignment and baseline scores for the respective self-efficacy subscale. After adjustment for baseline scores, self-efficacy did not vary significantly on any of the three subscales.

TABLE 2. Comparisons of Control and Treatment Groups by Smoking-Related Factors (at Baseline)

VARIABLES	CONTROL (n = 126)	TREATMENT (n = 125)	STATISTICS t	χ^2
Time elapsed since quit date (at birth; mean, weeks)	33.0	32.8	0.31	
Reason for smoking cessation (%)				
Health of unborn	96.0	91.2		
Other	4.0	8.8		1.71[a]
Intend to remain nonsmoking postpartum (%)				
Yes	91.3	90.4		
No/don't know	8.7	9.6		0.00[a]
Number of previous quit attempts (mean)	2.8	3.2	−1.01	
Number of cigarettes/day while smoking (mean)	10.4	10.5	−0.05	
Revised Fagerstrom tolerance (RTQ; mean)	2.6	2.7	−0.91	
Smoking abstinence self-efficacy (SASE)				
Negative/affective subscale	67.3	66.9	0.12	
Habit/addictive subscale	86.9	87.7	−0.40	
Positive/social subscale	73.7	72.5	0.45	
Husband/partner's smoking status (%)[b]				
Never smoked	26.3	26.7		
Quit for the pregnancy	11.9	18.1		
Quit before pregnancy	11.9	10.3		
Current smoker	50.0	44.8		1.98
Social contacts who smoke (%)				
All or most	32.0	27.2		
Some	24.8	36.0		
Very few or none	43.2	36.8		3.71
Expected encouragement for nonsmoking from family and friends (%)				
None/hardly any	8.9	8.9		
Some	20.2	17.1		
A great deal	71.0	74.0		0.39

Note: p < .05.
[a]Yates' Continuity Correction used.
[b]n = 234 (6.8% reported no partner).

Multivariate Analysis. The rejection of Hypothesis 3 led to the question of how the intervention successfully reduced daily smoking among the treatment group. To explore possible answers to this question, a stepwise multiple logistic regression analysis was conducted to identify predictors of daily smoking, including variables that may have confounded or interacted with

TABLE 3. Mixed Effects Logistic Regression Model of Daily Smoking

VARIABLES	OR	95% CI
Group assignment		
Treatment	.56[c]	.32–.98
Control[a]	1.00	
Negative/affective self-efficacy (at baseline)[b]	.82[c]	.73–.91
Mental health (at baseline)	.44[c]	.27–.74

[a]Reference group.
[b]Variable scaled to 10% unit increments.
[c]$p < .05$.
OR = odds ratio; CI = confidence interval.

the intervention. No demographic variables were found to be significant. Only two smoking-related variables were associated with daily smoking at 6 months (Table 3). Participants having relatively strong negative/affective self-efficacy or relatively high mental health scores at baseline were less likely to smoke daily. Neither of these variables was found to confound or interact with the intervention.

DISCUSSION

Although the intervention did not prove effective in ensuring continuous smoking abstinence, the control group, as compared with the treatment group, was almost twice as likely to resume daily smoking. These findings are encouraging because they suggest that nurses can successfully intervene and help women in their commitment to achieve smoking cessation. Although continuous abstinence is the desired long-term goal, this rigid outcome measure of smoking status contradicts current thinking about the process of smoking cessation. Theorists have recommended that smoking behavior not be conceptualized as a binary event (Marlatt, 1985, 1996; Miller, 1996; Prochaska & DiClemente, 1983). Prochaska and DiClemente's (1983) model of behavior change acknowledges that those in the process of cessation may smoke at times. The question for researchers is this: "At what point is smoking a normal part of the cessation process rather than an indication of complete relapse?"

An appropriate set of outcome criteria for research purposes, sensitive to the process of change, must be identified. Donovan (1996) described five definitions of relapse in the addiction literature: (a) a gradual and insidious process, (b) a discrete event of substance use (lapse), (c) a return to original patterns of substance use (amount and frequency, relapse), (d) daily use for a specified time period, and (e) substance use that requires treatment. Collectively, these definitions point to the complex and dynamic nature of the relapse process. Miller (1996) went so far as to suggest that we should abandon the concept of relapse and preferably identify terms that describe the "normal" resolution process for addictive behaviors such as smoking.

The intervention was effective in preventing the resumption of daily smoking regardless of individual differences in self-efficacy and mental health. Apart from the group differences in resumption of daily smoking, the identified covariates suggest that those with relatively better mental health and stronger negative/affective self-efficacy (i.e., degree of confidence in resisting urges to smoke when frustrated, facing conflict, or undergoing emotional distress) at the outset are likely to avoid relapsing to daily smoking. However, the intervention did not affect self-efficacy. Participants with relatively strong baseline negative/affective self-efficacy scores were more successful in avoiding daily smoking, but overall, the self-efficacy scores were not improved in the intervention group. Indeed, the baseline self-efficacy scores were somewhat higher, on the average, than the 6-month scores, in both groups.

Why did the intervention not operate through self-efficacy, as hypothesized, and why then was it effective at all? It may be that the measure of self-efficacy used in this study, the SASE, was not appropriate for this particular population. The SASE focuses on common high-risk situations (e.g., being at a bar or cocktail lounge having a drink) and asks respondents to assess their confidence in abstaining from smoking. At baseline, many of the situations described in the SASE were not relevant to the participants' cessation experiences (e.g., while pregnant they avoided alcohol consumption). Women who have just given birth and are facing "new terrain" may be unable realistically to predict their ability to resist the temptation to smoke.

Stotts, DiClemente, Carbonari, and Mullen (1996) noted that the process of smoking cessation for pregnant women is somewhat different than for nonpregnant female smokers. Cessation during pregnancy was observed to be relatively easy, to require minimal use of coping strategies, and to result in high self-efficacy. The researchers speculated that this putative success results from specific factors that typically promote smoking cessation among pregnant women (e.g., social stigma, concern for baby's health, nausea). They therefore argue that abstinence may be better conceived as "stopping" rather than "quitting" smoking. Women who stop smoking for pregnancy may not have gone through the experiential and behavioral processes usually associated with the action phase of smoking cessation. In addition, new mothers (74.1% were primiparas in the current study) may not anticipate that the challenges in the postpartum period are different, and possibly more difficult, than those faced while pregnant.

Rather than by strengthening self-efficacy, the intervention may have been effective because of the social support provided during the initial 3-month postpartum period. Unlike other intervention studies, this study focused on the provision of sustained support, specifically targeted toward the maintenance of smoking cessation during a critical period when smoking relapse is likely.

Paradoxically, whereas the strength of the intervention may have rested on meeting the particular needs of the participants, such an approach poses a threat to research design validity. Tailoring interventions to respond to individual need may make it more difficult to ensure that the same intervention at the same dose is provided to all subjects. Fluctuations in delivery of the intervention may account for the weaker than anticipated effect. A limitation related to external validity is the 39% refusal rate among eligible women. It may have been that women with particular characteristics were attracted to receiving assistance with their smoking cessation maintenance.

Although current smoking cessation interventions for childbearing women tend to focus on the prenatal period, entry into the difficult action phase of smoking cessation may commence in the postpartum period. Smoking cessation programs designed to take advantage of the "window of opportunity" provided by pregnancy can be strengthened if interventions are extended into the postpartum period, focusing on the action phase of the smoking cessation process as well as relapse prevention.

Accepted for publication July 8, 1998.

This project was funded by the Tobacco Demand Reduction Strategy of Health Canada through a grant provided by the National Health Research and Development Program. Pilot work funding was provided by the British Columbia Medical Services Foundation. In-kind support was provided by the Nursing Consortium of the British Columbia Research Institute in Child and Family Health. Ms. Hall acknowledges the Social Sciences and Humanities Research Council provision of a doctoral fellowship and the British Commonwealth for a scholar award. Ms. Dahinten acknowledges the British Columbia Health Research Foundation's provision of a doctoral studentship. Address reprint requests to Joy L. Johnson, PhD, RN, School of Nursing, University of British Columbia, T201-2211 Wesbrook Mall, Vancouver, BC V6T 2B5 Canada; E-mail: johnson@nursing.ubc.ca.

Joy L. Johnson, PhD, RN, is Associate Professor and National Health Research and Development Program Health Research Scholar, School of Nursing, University of British Columbia, Vancouver, Canada.

Pamela A. Ratner, PhD, RN, is an Assistant Professor, School of Nursing, and Assistant Director, Institute of Health Promotion Research, University of British Columbia, Vancouver, Canada.

Joan L. Bottorff, PhD, RN, is the Associate Director of Research, an Associate Professor, and a National Health Research and Development Program Health Research Scholar, School of Nursing, University of British Columbia, Vancouver, Canada.

Wendy Hall, PhD, RN, is an Associate Professor and Doctoral Candidate, School of Nursing, University of British Columbia, Vancouver, Canada.

Susan Dahinten, MSN, RN, is a Doctoral Candidate, School of Nursing, University of British Columbia, Vancouver, Canada, and an Assistant Professor, Faculty of Nursing, University of Brunswick, Fredericton, Canada.

REFERENCES

Apseloff, G., Ashton, H. M., Friedman, H., & Gerber, N. (1994). The importance of measuring cotinine levels to identify smokers in clinical trials. *Clinical Pharmacology and Therapeutics, 56*, 460–462.

Baer, J. S., Holt, C. S., & Lichtenstein, E. (1986). Self-efficacy and smoking reexamined: Construct validity and clinical utility. *Journal of Consulting and Clinical Psychology, 54*, 846–852.

Brandon, T. H., Tiffany, S. T., Obremski, K. M., & Baker, T. B. (1990). Postcessation cigarette use: The process of relapse. *Addictive Behaviors, 15*, 105–114.

Canadian Cancer Society. (1997). *Canadian cancer statistics 1997*. Toronto: Author.

Charlton, A. (1994). Children and passive smoking: A review. *Journal of Family Practice, 38*, 267–277.

Cohen, S., & Lichtenstein, E. (1990). Perceived stress, quitting smoking, and smoking relapse. *Health Psychology, 9*, 466–478.

Curry, S. J., Marlatt, G. A., Gordon, J., & Baer, J. S. (1988). A comparison of alternative theoretical approaches to smoking cessation and relapse. *Health Psychology, 7*, 545–556.

Curry, S. J., Wagner, E. H., Cheadle, A., Diehr, P., Koepsell, T., Psaty, B., & McBride, C. (1993). Assessment of community-level influences on individuals' attitudes about cigarette smoking, alcohol use, and consumption of dietary fat. *American Journal of Preventive Medicine, 9*, 78–84.

Davis, A. L., Faust, R., & Ordentlich, M. (1984). Self-help smoking cessation and maintenance programs: A comparative study with 12-month follow-up by the American Lung Association. *American Journal of Public Health, 74*, 1212–1217.

DiClemente, C. C. (1981). Self-efficacy and smoking cessation maintenance: A preliminary report. *Cognitive Therapy and Research, 5*, 175–187.

Donovan, D. M. (1996). Assessment issues and domains in the prediction of relapse. *Addiction, 91*, S29–S36.

Ellison, L. F., Mao, Y., & Gibbons, L. (1995). Projected smoking-attributable mortality in Canada, 1991–2000. *Chronic Diseases in Canada, 16*(2), 84–89.

Fagerstrom, K. O. (1978). Measuring degree of physical dependence to tobacco smoking with reference to individualization of treatment. *Addictive Behaviors, 3*, 235–241.

Fingerhut, L. A., Kleinman, J. C., & Kendrick, J. S. (1990). Smoking before, during, and after pregnancy. *American Journal of Public Health, 80*, 541–544.

Hall, S. M., Rugg, D., Tunstall, C., & Jones, R. T. (1984). Preventing relapse to cigarette smoking by behavioral skill training. *Journal of Consulting and Clinical Psychology, 52*, 372–382.

Killen, J. D., Fortmann, S. P., Newman, B., & Varady, A. (1990). Evaluation of a treatment approach combining nicotine gum with self-guided behavioral treatments for smoking relapse prevention. *Journal of Consulting and Clinical Psychology, 58*, 85–92.

Marlatt, G. A. (1985). Relapse prevention: Theoretical rationale and overview of the model. In G. A. Marlatt & J. R. Gordon (Eds.), *Relapse prevention: Maintenance strategies in the treatment of addictive behaviors* (pp. 3–70). New York: Guilford Press.

Marlatt, G. A. (1996). Taxonomy of high-risk situations for alcohol relapse: Evolution and development of a cognitive–behavioral model. *Addiction, 91*, S37–S49.

Marlatt, G. A., & Gordon, J. R. (1980). Determinants of relapse: Implications for the maintenance of behavior change. In P. O. Davidson & S. M. Davidson (Eds.), *Behavioral medicine: Changing health lifestyles* (pp. 191–215). New York: Brunner/Mazel.

Marlatt, G. A., & Gordon, J. R. (Eds.). (1985). *Relapse prevention: Maintenance strategies in the treatment of addictive behaviors*. New York: Guilford Press.

McBride, C. M., Pirie, P. L., & Curry, S. J. (1992). Postpartum relapse to smoking: A prospective study. *Health Education Research, 7*, 381–390.

Miller, W. R. (1996). What is a relapse? Fifty ways to leave the wagon. *Addiction, 91*, S15–S27.

Mullen, P. D., Richardson, M. A., Quinn, V. P., & Ershoff, D. H. (1997). Postpartum return to smoking: Who is at risk and when. *American Journal of Health Promotion, 11*, 323–330.

O'Campo, P., Faden, R. R., Brown, H., & Gielen, A. C. (1992). The impact of pregnancy on women's prenatal and postpartum smoking behavior. *American Journal of Preventive Medicine, 8*, 8–13.

Omenn, G. S., Thompson, B., Sexton, M., Hessol, N., Breitenstein, B., Curry, S., Michnich, M., & Peterson, A. (1988). A randomized comparison of worksite-sponsored smoking cessation programs. *American Journal of Preventive Medicine, 4*, 261–267.

Patrick, D. L., Cheadle, A., Thompson, D. C., Diehr, P., Koepsell, T., & Kinne, S. (1994). The validity of self-reported smoking: A review and meta-analysis. *American Journal of Public Health, 84*, 1086–1093.

Petersen, L., Handel, J., Kotch, J., Podedworny, T., & Rosen, A. (1992). Smoking reduction during pregnancy by a program of self-help and clinical support. *Obstetrics and Gynecology, 79*, 924–930.

Prochaska, J. O., & DiClemente, C. C. (1983). Stages and processes of self-change of smoking: Toward an integrative model of change. *Journal of Consulting and Clinical Psychology, 51*, 390–395.

Prochaska, J. O., DiClemente, C. C., & Norcross, J. C. (1992). In search of how people change: Applications to addictive behaviors. *American Psychologist, 47*, 1102–1114.

Prochaska, J. O., DiClemente, C. C., Velicer, W. F., Ginpil, S., & Norcross, J. C. (1985). Predicting change in smoking status for self-changers. *Addictive Behaviors, 10*, 395–406.

Secker-Walker, R. H., Solomon, L. J., Flynn, B. S., Skelly, J. M., Lepage, S. S., Goodwin, G. D., & Mead, P. B. (1995). Smoking relapse prevention counseling during prenatal and early postnatal care. *American Journal of Preventive Medicine, 11*, 86–93.

Sexton, M., Hebel, R., & Fox, N. L. (1987). Postpartum smoking. In M. J. Rosenberg (Ed.), *Smoking and reproductive health* (pp. 222–226). Littleton, MA: PSG Publishing.

Stephens, T., & Graham, D. F. (Eds.). (1993). *Canada's health promotion survey 1990: Technical report.* Ottawa: Minister of Supply and Services.

Stevens, V. J., & Hollis, J. F. (1989). Preventing smoking relapse, using an individually tailored skills-training technique. *Journal of Consulting and Clinical Psychology, 57*, 420–424.

Stotts, A. L., DiClemente, C. C., Carbonari, J. P., & Mullen, P. D. (1996). Pregnancy smoking cessation: A case of mistaken identity. *Addictive Behaviors, 21*, 459–471.

Strecher, V. J., Becker, M. H., Kirscht, J. P., Eraker, S. A., & Graham-Tomasi, R. P. (1985). Evaluation of a minimal-contact smoking cessation program in a health care setting. *Patient Education and Counseling, 7*, 395–407.

Tate, J. C., & Schmitz, J. M. (1993). A proposed revision of the Fagerstrom Tolerance Questionnaire. *Addictive Behaviors, 18*, 135–143.

U.S. Department of Health and Human Services. (1989). *Reducing the health consequences of smoking: 25 years of progress: A report of the Surgeon General.* Superintendent of Documents (DHHS Publication No. CDC 90-8411). Washington, DC: Author.

Velicer, W. F., DiClemente, C. C., Rossi, J. S., & Prochaska, J. O. (1990). Relapse situations and self-efficacy: An integrative model. *Addictive Behaviors, 15*, 271–283.

Defensive Mothering in HIV-Positive Mothers

Deborah Ingram, Sally A. Hutchinson

The grounded theory study discussed in this article provides an explanatory schema that illuminates the mothering experiences of women living with HIV infection. Eighteen HIV-positive mothers provided 24 in-depth interviews. The grounded theory method was used for data analysis. Defensive mothering was the basic social psychological process that these HIV-positive mothers used in response to their diagnosis and the inherent stigma. Their defensive posture afforded these mothers and their children some degree of psychological protection. Defensive mothering involved much mental work and included three subprocesses: preventing the spread of HIV, preparing the children for a motherless future, and protecting themselves through thought control.

More than 70,000 cases of AIDS have been reported among women in the United States, and 1 in every 700 women in the United States is believed to be infected with HIV (Centers for Disease Control, 1995). By the year 2000, it is estimated that women will represent a full 30% of reported cases of AIDS in the United States (Guinan & Leviton, 1995). AIDS is among the top five leading causes of death among women of childbearing age in the United States (Chu, Buehler, & Berkelman, 1990). Clinical experience suggests that the "emerging epidemic" (Rose, 1996, p. 28) of HIV presents a unique challenge to women, especially mothers. HIV complicates fulfillment of the maternal role, a social expectation for women. However, little research or theory exists about the psychosocial aspects of mothering when HIV positive. The purpose of this grounded theory research was to generate a substantive theory about the experiences of HIV-positive mothers.

MOTHERING

The cultural norms and values in most Western societies encourage repro-duction and emphasize motherhood as a valued role for women. Pregnancy

QUALITATIVE HEALTH RESEARCH, Vol. 9 No. 2, March 1999 243-258 © 1999 Sage Publications, Inc.

elevates a woman's status in some communities and is often an opportunity for women to feel good about themselves. Babies represent sources of love, acceptance, and a legacy for the future, even for a woman with no sense of future for herself (Levine & Dubler, 1990; Shayne & Kaplan, 1991). Theories and research specific to mothering reflect these values. Leifer (1980) found that women regarded having children as basic to the meaning of life and essential to their view of themselves as women and adults. Rubin (1984) studied the processes involved in maternal role attainment. She found that deviations from the norm resulted in profound doubt about competence and self-worth. Successful attainment of the maternal role required supportive human feedback and a sense of connection. Mercer (1986) studied maternal role attainment and developed a theoretical framework of role theory from an interactionist approach. Her variables of interest included attachment, gratification in the maternal role, maternal behavior, social stress, and maternal self-concept. Based on 25 years of research, she formulated the maternal role attainment theory, a theory that extended Rubin's work to include many kinds of mothers: older, younger, ill, and mothers with defective children. Her theory focused on women from pregnancy through the first year after birth. Her research clearly indicated that both maternal and child health affect role attainment (Bee, Legge, & Oetting, 1994; Mercer & Ferketich, 1990).

There exists a general lack of recognition and support for the experience of women who deviate from the accepted cultural norm regarding maternal identity and experience. Such deviations include childlessness, infertility, abortion, stillbirth, and the birth of imperfect children (Layne, 1990; Miall, 1989; Whiteford & Gonzalez, 1995). Mothers using crack cocaine or other drugs deviate from our cultural norms about mothering. Despite negative views held toward drug-using mothers, researchers found that these women valued mothering highly, were motivated through mothering to change their chaotic lifestyles, and considered mothering a priority in their lives (Kearney, Murphy, Irwin, & Rosenbaum, 1995; Kearney, Murphy, & Rosenbaum, 1994; Pursley-Cotteau & Stern, 1996).

Many drug-using mothers are also HIV positive and, therefore, even further violate our beliefs about acceptable mothering. Like mothers using crack cocaine or other drugs, HIV-positive women who choose to have children are often considered cruel and uncaring. Social debates reinforce the idea of the irresponsible woman and the vulnerable fetus. The issues of coerced abortion, criminalized childbirth, and legalized sterilization surface regarding the reproduction practices of women who are HIV positive and/or drug users (Bayer, 1989, 1990; Edelman & Haverkos, 1989; King, 1991).

Even though negative attitudes are held toward HIV-positive mothers, little is actually known about the mothering practices of HIV-positive women. Concerns identified among HIV-positive mothers include fears of transmitting HIV to their children, addiction issues, and custody issues and decisions (Blanche et al., 1996; Pivnick, 1994). Andrews (1995) identified three theoretical perspectives when studying HIV-positive mothers: (a) the perspective of social stigma, (b) the perspective of individual psychologic response, and (c) the perspective of a context of poverty, isolation, and abuse. Andrews found that social support helped mitigate and buffer the stress. Other researchers described mothering among HIV-positive women not only as a source of self-esteem and identity but also as a means of survival (Andrews, Williams, & Neil, 1993; Hutchinson & Kurth, 1991; Pearlberg, 1991; Pfeiffer, 1991; Rose, 1993). Children were described as a link to life, as a reason to continue living, and as a source of emotional and psychological support. Hutchison and Kurth (1991) found that HIV-positive women viewed mothering as the source of their pride, identity, and attempts to right any wrongs from their pasts. Although important, the theories of mothering and the theoretical perspectives addressed above do not speak directly and comprehensively about the experiences of mothering among HIV-positive women. Thus, the purpose of this grounded theory research was to add to this literature by providing an explanatory schema that illuminates the experiences of mothers living with HIV infection.

METHOD

Sample

The research protocol was approved by a university institutional review board. The purposive sample of 18 HIV-positive mothers between the ages of 18 and 44 were clients at AIDS service organizations and clinics specializing in the care of HIV-positive individuals. Representatives handed out study information inviting interested HIV-positive women to call the researcher if they wished to participate in in-depth interviews about their experiences with mothering. Anonymity and confidentiality were guaranteed. Sample participants had known of their HIV-positive status for an average of 3 years, with a range of 1 month to 10 years. Eight of the participants were African American, 9 were Caucasian, and 1 was Latina. Half of the participants were married or cohabiting. The average number of children was two, with a range of one to five; 2 of the participants were grandmothers. Six mothers had histories of intravenous drug use, and 2 of them had relapsed at the time of the interviews. The other mothers related their HIV infection to unprotected heterosexual sex; 2 of the women considered the possibility of having received contaminated blood. Nine women had CD4 counts in the 200 to 499 range and had experienced HIV-related symptoms, primarily fatigue and oral/vaginal candida. Six had CD4 counts below 200 and had experienced an AIDS-defining illness, most commonly pneumocystis carinii pneumonia and toxoplasmosis.

Data Collection and Recording

Interviews focused on the experience of being an HIV-positive mother occurred at a place chosen by the mothers, and lasted from 1 to 2 hours. All but three interviews were audiotaped, and during those three interviews, detailed notes were taken. Audiotapes and notes were transcribed immediately after the interviews. Follow-up interviews to confirm and to expand the initial interviews occurred with 6 women by phone.

Data Analysis

The grounded theory method was used for data analysis. Grounded theorists seek to explain and to understand how individuals define their reality and how they act in relation to their beliefs and realities (Chenitz & Swanson, 1986). This article focuses on the basic social psychological process (defensive mothering) used by the HIV-positive mothers in this study. The process of defensive mothering was discovered by use of the constant comparative method, three levels of coding, theoretical sampling, and memoing—all hallmarks of the grounded theory process (Glaser, 1978, 1992; Glaser & Strauss, 1967).

The constant comparative method involved four stages (Glaser & Strauss, 1967): comparing incidents applicable to each category, integrating categories and their properties, delimiting the theory, and writing the theory. Incidents in the data were coded into as many categories as possible. Coding involved level-one codes, called substantive codes, that frequently are written in the language of the participants; level-two codes, called categories; and level-three codes, called theoretical codes (Hutchinson, 1993). Theoretical sampling refers to seeking data from participants in subsequent interviews that can densify a code or category. Thus, because data collection and analysis occurred simultaneously, initial interview questions were altered to focus on obtaining data based on emerging codes. Memoing or writing theoretical notes on the developing codes and categories moved the theory-generation process along and helped in the identification of properties, conditions, causes, and relationships among codes. The theory and its categories were delimited when saturation of the data occurred, and no new conceptual information was discovered.

According to Glaser (1978, 1992), a core variable or basic social process that explains much of the data is central to a grounded theory. The categories and properties of the theory are related to the core variable. In this study, the core variable and basic social psychological process is defensive mothering.

The simultaneous processes of data collection and analysis permitted ongoing verification of the developing theory. Validation with participants and peer review with colleagues also contributed to validity (Lincoln & Guba, 1985).

FINDINGS

Defensive Mothering

Defensive is defined in the *Oxford American Dictionary* (1980) as "used or done for defense; protective; in an attitude of defense; ready to defend oneself against criticism" (p. 223). This definition offers a sense of being guarded, cautious, or wary and describes defensive mothering. Mothers in this study felt different and set apart from others because of being HIV positive. "Being HIV positive, you definitely learn what it's like to be an outcast." Underlying the defensiveness was a fear of being exposed as HIV positive and consequently stigmatized. Mothers performed much mental work in their daily lives, assessing situations and potential consequences for themselves and their children if their HIV-positive status was exposed: "Everything you do in your life you have to worry about if someone is going to find out [that you are HIV positive]. It is hard. You have to watch everything you say and do." Stigma provides the context for mothering when HIV positive. Stigma sets the stage for defensive mothering.

Three subprocesses are fundamental to defensive mothering: preventing the spread of HIV and stigma, preparing the children for a motherless future, and protecting themselves through thought control. These subprocesses often occur simultaneously, although the mothers may focus more on one than another, depending on the exigencies in their lives.

Preventing the Spread of HIV and Stigma

Mothers realized that HIV had destroyed their health and hopes for the future. The recognition that they brought the devastation of HIV to their children was horrifying. The mothers assumed a defensive posture as they worked to prevent the spread of HIV and its concomitant stigma.

Assessing family members for HIV. With great anxiety, mothers assessed the damage caused by HIV in their families. Fear of having transmitted HIV prompted the mothers to take immediate action after their own diagnosis to discover if the virus was present in other family members and children. Ten of the mothers knew that they were infected during at least one pregnancy. However, even if they did not believe they were infected when pregnant, the mothers in this study had all of their children tested. They sought antigen testing for children born HIV positive at birth. All mothers informed their sexual partners personally or reported their names to county public health units.

Limiting the damage. Limiting the damage caused by HIV refers to preventing its spread to others. Mothers acted to block transmission through exposure to blood or body fluids by safety work. They spoke of not sharing toothbrushes or razors, of cleaning everything with bleach, and of using latex gloves. The deteriorating health of the mothers, or that of their partner and/or children, made both bleach and latex gloves commonplace. One mother whose husband also had AIDS spoke about her fear:

> What's worse than me having it is thinking my children could get it. I bleach my floors before I mop and wax them. Our floors are mopped every night. Our countertops, too. The kids put bleach in the dishwater. The bathroom is bleached down. You have to. It's a precaution worth taking. We bleach all of the underclothes. All of the underclothes are either light pink or light blue or white. I buy them that way on purpose because I bleach them. I put everybody's clothes in together on hot and pour the bleach to them.

Teaching was an important strategy of safety work and involved teaching the children about avoiding blood and body fluids and using gloves. This teaching was particularly problematic for the mothers whose children did not know that their mothers were HIV positive. One mother, whose younger son also had AIDS, spoke about her efforts with her older son who was HIV negative and unaware that his mother and younger brother had AIDS:

> I don't want [my older son] to get exposed. I talked to him about keeping things clean with bleach. I warned him about not touching bloody things. I told him I don't want him to help if I am hurt or the baby is hurt.

Mothers also taught their children about transmission of HIV through unprotected sexual contact. Some recognized their own ignorance regarding unprotected sex, which inspired them to want to help their children prevent similar experiences.

Mothers were concerned about limiting stigma. Goffman (1974) proposes that stigmas often extend beyond the stigmatized individual to their family and close associates. The mothers feared such a "courtesy stigma" directed at their children. In the previous example, the mother did not disclose her and her younger son's AIDS to her older son because of the fear of courtesy stigma. Mothers learned that even a normal event such as starting school could end in disaster for their children:

> I won't let my baby go to public school. I mean, if he went, they should know about his HIV to help protect him and other kids. But I can't take the risk that they would be mean to him. I remember the Ray boys. They burned their house. I won't let them be mean to him. What if he bit or scratched or kicked some kid? Kids do that naturally. I wouldn't have that kind of attention on him because of something innocent like that.

Monitoring for HIV and stigma. Monitoring involved the mothers' mental work of watching and worrying about the ever-present threat of HIV and stigma in the lives of their children. The hypervigilant mothers felt anxious about any physical illness and lived with the fear that their children might have been misdiagnosed as HIV negative:

> I still panic every time he gets sick. He's got a lot of asthma problems. He gets nose bleeds a lot, and I have never dealt with nose bleeds. If he has a regular common bout of diarrhea or something like that, then I panic. He is a small-frame child, for 2 years he stayed at 37 pounds. Wouldn't go up or down. That kind of put me into a state [fearing he was HIV positive].

Also, the mothers monitored the threat posed by the stigma of HIV. Mothers escorted their children in public to monitor the reaction of others:

> I live in the projects now. I've been there for over a year. It's a small town, and people know me. The hardest part is my children because people say nasty stuff to them about me. Every day I have to walk out of the apartment with them to watch these people.

Mothers moved their families if the threat became too great:

> I don't want people rejecting me and my kids. I worry about rejection. I'd leave town if anybody knew. I live where a lot of people with AIDS live. I'm going to move because I'll get labeled because of the HIV.

Preparing the Children for a Motherless Future

In spite of advances in the treatment of AIDS, mothers viewed HIV as a death sentence, predicting a bleak future for themselves and a motherless future for their children. A profound sense of loss permeated the data and accentuated the importance of mothering to these women. They carried the overwhelming burden of both their own losses and the losses of their children. They believed that children always needed their mothers, that there was no substitute for a mother, and that through their deaths they were personally responsible for a grievous loss to their children. At the heart of the mothers' defensive posture were their defenseless children whom they believed needed their protection and guidance for the uncertain amount of time left and for their motherless future: "No one can take care of them like me. I tell them nobody can love you like me. I want to do everything I can while I'm here." Another woman lamented,

> You know he's going to need a mother. You always have times when you need a mother, and I won't be there. I'm so sorry that I'm taking that away from him. There are still times when I need my mother, and she's been dead for several years now. No matter how old you get, there are times when you just want to be held by your mother, and no one else will do. Sometimes your mother is the only person you want to hold you or to answer something for you. There's trust with your mother like with no other person.

Mothers imagined horrible scenarios of their children's motherless future, and they responded defensively to the threat of a motherless future by attempting to position their children as best they could.

Teaching the children. Basic to the work of mothering was a perception that the value of a mother was found in what she did to make better people of her children. Toward that end, the mothers shared their values with their children:

> The best they can get from me is how to love and be kind, but be strong and responsible. That's what I'm teaching them now. I teach them about the Bible and prayer. We pray. Most of all I want to teach them about being good people, to treat everyone nice, to listen, and not to be disrespectful.

Mothers emphasized the importance of loving relationships:

> I taught him about relationships. Not just sex stuff, but more. To me that's what is important. I talked to him about women, more than just sex, about emotion, not just sweet talk. I talked to him about listening to each other, and touching, and holding each other. I told him to value his partner and never to abuse her or allow himself to be abused. I let him know that abuse is out there. And emotional abuse was just as bad as physical abuse. I told him that if it ever happened to him to get help. That he had to stop it if it ever happened to him, either way.

In addition, mothers felt responsible for giving their children the basic education necessary to meet future demands. They provided "how to" information about safety, household chores, the stock market, and other practical topics:

> I ran out and learned about the stock market to talk to him. I want him to have some basics. I won't be around when he will naturally be ready to make financial decisions. You know when he's more into a job or career. But I want him to know that it's important and something to pay attention to. I don't want anyone to take advantage of him. And I want him to have a good head on his shoulders for money.

Mothers felt the urgency of their situation and the complicating issue of stigma:

> I have to give him everything that he will need to make it in this world, and I don't have much time to do that. I don't know how much time I have, but I know it's not enough. It's like I've got so much to tell him as I am dying. And nobody knows that I am doing it. I'm having to cram a lifetime of teaching him everything into such a short time, and I can't even talk about it. That's how crazy it feels.

Straight talk between the mothers and their older children involved the forecasting of difficult future scenarios:

> It's like I told my daughter, I'm always going to be with her. I won't be sitting across the table with her, but I'll be here with her. I'll be in her heart. When she has a problem and she can't ask me what to do, she can think about what mom would do. She'll get the same answer 9 times out of 10 because she's got a good head on her shoulders.

Shortly after beginning her menstrual cycle, a young adolescent expressed her sadness: "She looked up, and she said, 'Well, mom, what's going to happen when I have a baby? You won't get to hold it.' I said, 'Well, you will have to hold it for me.' "

Mothers attempted to teach younger children by writing them letters about important issues. The mothers gave the letters to a trusted individual who promised to share them with the children when they were older:

> I have written [my preschool-age children] letters for every day in their lives that is important. The day she starts her first period. Mom will have a birds and bees talk, well it's written. The day they turn 18 and can vote. All of their mom's political beliefs. I just have stacks and stacks of letters for them. Well, certainly on all of the milestone days in their lives there is a letter. I have talked about values. I really tried to explain to them that choices they make in their lives early on affect the rest of their whole life, the rest of their days on this planet.

Negotiating custody and legal support. As they prepared their children for the future, the mothers felt there were things they should do, but they found them difficult to do because of immense psychic pain. These tasks included custody arrangements for minor children, legal preparation for the children's future, and their own death arrangements. The single most common issue for negotiation was custody for minor children in the event of the mother's death, especially if the baby was HIV positive: "The hardest decision that I've had was who will I ask to take care of my baby? Will they want to take care of an HIV baby if the baby doesn't come out clean? That's the hardest choice." The children who knew of their mother's HIV-positive status were concerned about where they would go after their mother's death:

> [My oldest child] said, "What is going to happen to us?" I said, "Well, we're going to have to find you somebody to love." He said, "I'll never love anybody like you." I said, "No, you won't, but you will find somebody that will ease the ache a little bit. Somebody to look out for you until you can be with me again." He will be with me one day.

In spite of the widespread anxiety surrounding this issue, none of the mothers had legal documentation about their wishes concerning custody of their minor children in the event of their deaths. All the mothers spoke to lawyers, counselors, or health care providers about custody issues, but none pursued the matter to completion. One mother spoke of the indecision associated with the impossible task of finding someone to mother her children:

> I said, "Well, what's going to happen to my kids?" [The social worker] said, "Well, have you made arrangements for that?" I said when the time came that I would do that because I'm not throwing my hands up and saying I'm dying. When the time comes, I'll make that decision. Nobody is going to push me into it because when I have to make that decision I am gone. I will think about it, and I will make plans in my heart because I am going to change my mind 80,000 times. In my heart there ain't nobody good enough for my kids.

Another mother said,

> If anything should happen to me, my mother's gonna have custody of him. It's arranged, but I haven't done it legally because every time I try to go to the legal center it depresses me too much to go. But I am gonna go next month because they say it's better if I do it now than to wait 'till I get sick. But to me it just means like I'm agreeing with the fact that I'm dying.

In spite of the reluctance to make a legal decision, all of the mothers negotiated with an identified individual to assume custody of their children. Ten of the mothers named their own mothers as the custodian, 3 named a sibling, and 3 named their partners. In custody negotiations, the biological fathers of the children generally did not represent a source of support for these HIV-positive mothers; rather, the mothers often expressed a sense of threat and mental anguish created by concerns about unfit biological fathers' gaining custody of their children:

> [My ex] is nothing but a thief and a cheat. I don't want my kids to learn from him. It's all he knows. He can't help it. That's what his father was and what his father taught him. Just how can I save my kids from that man?

Three of the mothers feared a custody battle between their ex-partners and their parents after their death:

> There is a concern when I die where my children are going to go, who is going to be taking care of them. I worry about it being a feud between my ex and [my parents]. Basically, [my parents] have been there to help where he hasn't. They feel like they have just as much rights to the children as he does. I think that is one of the things that I need to get down and work out. To me it scares me to even get started on it cause I feel like I am almost at the end of my life doing that. But I know it is something that needs to be done.

Fear of stigma and its repercussions inhibited mothers' from building supportive relationships for their children after their death. One mother said,

> You can't talk to just anyone. You can't talk to friends and teachers and people who might be able to help him when I'm gone because it's such a stigma. It's difficult because you can't line people up for him without telling them something that they could hold against him.

Another mother reported not even being able to tell her sisters: "My sisters don't know. My sisters don't have children. I've thought about them. They don't understand children. They don't understand my situation."

Preparing a legal will and making funeral arrangements were other negotiated issues. Although all of the mothers sought out resources to assist them with legal arrangements for their deaths, none of them had legal documentation because such negotiations were depressing and a symbol for giving up and accepting death.

Leaving a legacy. Leaving a legacy involved the mothers' efforts to impart to their children a positive sense of who their mothers were. The mothers feared they would die before their children were old enough to remember them or that they would be so disfigured their children would be horrified by them:

> You know my biggest fear is not dying, it is dying before my kids are old enough to remember who I am. It is part of the disease process that causes so much fear for me. I am terrified of getting dementia. That is the hardest part of being a mom, the fear that I might lose my mind, and my kids would see me that way. They would see some kind of monster. Let's face it, everybody's seen people with dementia, and some of them become very ugly, very violent, something that they never would have been in their life. That certainly scares me.

Although other terminally ill mothers might express similar fears related to dying and not being remembered by their children, HIV-positive mothers expressed the unique fear of their children thinking poorly of them because of stigma:

> I want them to know [about the HIV], but I also want them to understand that I just didn't go out and ask for AIDS. People got to believe that you don't have to sleep around with a thousand people to get AIDS. That's just not the case.

As a part of leaving a legacy, most of the mothers worked to leave special memories about the mother/child relationship in shared experiences, photo albums, video recordings, or written cards and letters:

We saved back enough money for 3 weeks so we could go to the beach one day with them. It may not be much to everybody else out there, but to us it is a day full of memories that they will never forget. I can't explain it, seeing my babies run up and down the sand and the smile and wind on their faces. It's heaven, but it is hell. Every hug and every kiss is heaven and hell. But I'll take all the hell just for the heaven and be glad for it.

Another mother said,

I watch my kids. I grab all the precious moments with a camcorder. I cry when I watch them grow up so fast. Now I understand my mom saying that we grew up so fast. I take those special moments and just hold on.

The mothers realized they would not be available to their children in the future. Therefore, they defensively prepared their children for a motherless future by teaching, negotiating custody and legal support, and leaving a legacy.

Protecting the Self Through Thought Control

Protecting themselves through thought control allowed the mothers to keep the negative thoughts and fears accompanying their illness from taking over their lives. Thought control by consciously choosing what topics were worthy of thought and refusing to think about the negative lessened the disruptive effects of HIV, enabling the mothers to defend themselves to some degree. The ravages of HIV weakened the mothers' ability to mother physically and emotionally. Grief and worry consumed mental energy, and the mothers lived in fear of being discredited as mothers by themselves and others because they were HIV positive. Therefore, because their well-being had a direct impact on their children, mothers worked to strengthen and maintain their mental well-being. A defensive stance helped them gain control of the negative thoughts that had the potential to take over their lives. They worked to preserve a positive attitude in spite of HIV and the resultant stigma and to create meaning from the inherent chaos.

Focusing on the children. The mothers said that their children helped them maintain their mental well-being as they dealt with the challenges of HIV. Focusing on their children helped them protect themselves. Their children were a reason to live and a focus for life:

I can't sleep without my baby. I won't let go of him, not physically, not any way. When he was in the hospital, that was the hardest time. The negative thoughts tried to creep in. Just seeing him makes my day. I have medicine to calm my nerves, but my baby can make me laugh better than any medicine.

Another mother said,

I see other people getting sick, preparing to die, getting herpes. I'm gonna control that. I got things to do. I'm not ready to die. I want to enjoy my kids. They need me. I want to show them around, show them fun times. I live for my kids.

Positive reframing. Positive reframing refers to having a positive attitude, to viewing the glass as half full instead of half empty. Maintaining a positive attitude was viewed as an integral part of controlling their response to the agonies of being HIV positive:

> I just found out by accident [that I was HIV positive] with my last baby. They did a routine test. I had not been tested with the other two. We were all shocked when it was positive. I was crying and calling everywhere trying to get information. But it made me sit up and take notice of what my life was like. Now I am better. It's a mind thing. I've educated myself. HIV made me a better mother, wife, and woman. Now I move on things I never did before. It brought out my better values. I am more responsible, more focused on the positive.

Another mother described the positive effects that being HIV positive had on her mothering:

> We live every second positively. I used to put other people down, but not now. I see folks in a different light. We are all just trying to get by the best we can. HIV helped me put things in a positive form, a forgiving way. I learned to love by having this disease. I'm still learning from it. In that way, I'm a better mom and better for my kids. Especially my older son. I can accept more, not hear just the bad. I don't spank anymore. I treasure every second. I listen. I don't make negative remarks. When I hear gossip, I don't comment. I only speak if I can do it in a positive way.

Previous researchers have pointed to the buffering effects of denial as positive and important to the preservation of psychological well-being, especially among individuals facing threatening situations (Lazarus, 1983; Lewinsohn & Mischel, 1980; Russell, 1993; Taylor & Brown, 1988). These women focused on finding meaning and significance in their lives. Embracing negative beliefs and attitudes about their situations was considered analogous to giving up, dying, and losing their children. Mothers recognized negative attitudes as detrimental to their health and spoke of witnessing such damaging negativity in other HIV-positive individuals:

> My partner died of AIDS. He was in a denial stage. He would not take his medication or nothing like that, and he would tell me that I was going to die. He said go ahead and use drugs, you know you're gonna die anyway. He was totally at that point to where he didn't care. I am not going to ever get in that state.

To avoid succumbing to anxiety and negativity, the mothers used diverse strategies to assist them in maintaining their mental health and well-being. The strategies helped them to focus on their children and with positive reframing. Mental health counseling was beneficial for most participants. One mother enrolled in stress management classes. Nine of the participants were active in private support groups, usually in their homes, sponsored by local AIDS service organizations. The mother of an HIV-positive toddler praised the support she received through an AIDS service organization:

He comes here, and everyone touches him and hugs him. He's learned so much. I can see the difference. He goes to preschool here every day. They teach him things, give his medicines, take him to social events, and test him here. Here they are okay. I trust them. He is so happy here.

Relying on their faith in God facilitated mothers' efforts to maintain a positive attitude:

I really didn't have a lot of anxiety when I was pregnant that something was wrong with the baby cause I knew that if I conceived him in the first place that everything was gonna be okay. So I just kind of had that faith because I was using birth control, and he still wound up here. The faith was that he was here for a reason, you know, and God didn't get me this far to drop me.

Some mothers identified making personal space apart from others and distant from other people's negativity as useful for thought control and for safeguarding their positive mental health:

I take some time just to myself. Just to be alone and smoke and drink coffee. I get up around four in the morning just to be alone.... I do it for me. When people get sick and they start to die for whatever reason, I distance myself as much as I can without being mean because I can't take it. I can't hurt anymore than I'm already hurting.

At some point in their interviews, most of the mothers spoke about their hopes for a cure. The belief in a cure helped these HIV-positive mothers live with HIV. The belief was especially important for women with HIV-positive children:

One day a cure may be found. I may not survive, but my child might. One day I feel confident a cure will come about, and I just hope that it is in my lifetime or in my children's lifetime.

DISCUSSION AND RECOMMENDATIONS

More and more women are being infected with HIV, and many of these women will be mothers struggling to cope with fears for themselves and their children. The grounded theory presented in this article contributes an explanatory schema that illuminates the experiences of this vulnerable and underserved group. Findings from this study reveal the work involved in mothering and the social psychological pain that these mothers experience in their day-to-day lives—pain that is surely as great as the physical pain associated with their illness. These mothers grieve multiple day-to-day losses and future losses in a context of stigma that exacerbates their grief. The literature on chronic sorrow seems relevant to this population. Chronic sorrow refers to a pervasive sadness that is permanent, periodic, and progressive (Hainesworth, 1996). Researchers have noted its presence among mothers of chronically mentally ill children (Eakes, 1995) and disabled children (Phillips, 1991) and among individuals living with life-threatening conditions such as cancer (Eakes, 1993) and Parkinson's disease (Lindgren, 1996).

Much has been written about grief symptoms, stages, time trajectories, and normal versus pathological grief (Demi & Miles, 1986; Pilkington, 1993; Rando, 1984; Sanders, 1989); less has been written about the anticipatory grieving that is most relevant to this study. The complicated work of anticipatory grief requires grieving losses and preparing for the death of oneself or others (Walker, Pomeroy, McNeil, & Franklin, 1994). HIV-positive mothers grieve not only the anticipated loss of their own lives but also the concomitant loss of their children, families, and friends. Because HIV-positive mothers grieve losing their children due to their own death or to the child's death if he or she is HIV positive, they experience the most painful kind of grief (Jacob & Scandrett-Hibdon, 1994). HIV-positive mothers also experience disenfranchised grief, which because of stigma cannot be openly acknowledged and publicly mourned (Doka, 1989).

Researchers have identified stigma as a problem for individuals living with HIV/AIDS (Alonzo & Reynolds, 1995; Demas, Schoenbaum, Wills, Doll, & Klein, 1995; Kadushin, 1996; Katz, 1996; O'Hare, Williams, & Ezoviski, 1996). Stigma often poses unique problems for HIV-positive mothers (Ingram & Hutchinson, in press; Moneyham et al., 1996; Pizzi, 1992; Smeltzer & Whipple, 1991). Stigma and the accompanying fear and anxiety of HIV isolate HIV-positive mothers. These women described not talking with their physicians about mothering issues, feeling anxious about attending support groups because of fear of being identified as having HIV, and not talking openly about mothering with friends and family. Many only had one or two people with whom they felt completely comfortable. Health care professionals can combat this isolation by providing support in the form of listening and education. The mothers need to know that their concerns are common for women in their circumstances. Scheduled time for private conversations about mothering will encourage them to raise questions and address their concerns; the necessary education and support can follow.

Based on this research, we assert that defensive mothering assists these women in combating the threats associated with being HIV positive and that mothers who practice defensive mothering are more likely to feel in charge of their lives. Health care professionals can help mothers learn how to be defensive by preventing the spread of infection, preparing for the children's motherless future, and protecting themselves through thought control to avoid the negativity that is inherent in being HIV positive. These propositions can be tested in additional quantitative and/or qualitative research.

The theory of defensive mothering can be used for assessment and as a foundation for clinical interventions. For example, are HIV-positive mothers knowledgeable about and comfortable with strategies to prevent the spread of infection to their children and family? How are they thinking about issues of disclosure with their children? With their families? Where are they with legal issues such as custody, wills, and funeral arrangements? What are they doing to leave a legacy? What kinds of positive experiences do they have with their children? What works for them in combating negativity? These issues are important to HIV-positive mothers and, therefore, are the issues that should be addressed in clinical practice and research.

This research with its heterogeneous sample provides a new way of thinking about HIV-positive mothers. Future studies should expand this research by using homogeneous samples of HIV-positive mothers who represent various ethnic/racial groups, mothers who are addicted and those who are not addicted, mothers who have HIV-positive children, and mothers whose children are not infected in order to discover differences and similarities that could inform care. In addition, research on HIV-positive mothers' decisions about whether to become pregnant or, if pregnant, whether to have an abortion is needed. Research on chronic sorrow, anticipatory grief, and disenfranchised grief in this population is also needed.

AUTHORS' NOTE: This research was partially funded by an Evelyn McKnight Award, American Nurses Foundation, to Dr. Ingram.

Deborah Ingram, ARNP, PhD, is a visiting assistant professor at the University of Florida College of Nursing and nurse practitioner, Women's Health Primary Care, Department of Veterans Affairs, Gainesville, Florida.

Sally A. Hutchinson, RN, PhD, FAAN, is a professor in the College of Nursing at the University of Florida Health Science Center-Jacksonville.

REFERENCES

Alonzo, A., & Reynolds, N. (1995). Stigma, HIV, and AIDS: An exploration and elaboration of a stigma trajectory. *Social Science & Medicine, 41*(3), 303–315.

Andrews, S. (1995). Social support as a stress buffer among human immunodeficiency virus-seropositive urban mothers. *Holistic Nursing Practice, 10*(1), 36–43.

Andrews, S., Williams, A., & Neil, K. (1993). The mother-child relationship in the HIV-positive family. *IMAGE: Journal of Nursing Scholarship, 25*(3), 193–198.

Bayer, R. (1989). The suitability of HIV-positive individuals for marriage and pregnancy. *Journal of the American Medical Association, 261*, 993.

Bayer, R. (1990). AIDS and the future of reproductive freedom. *The Milbank Quarterly, 68*(Suppl. 2), 179–204.

Bee, A., Legge, D., & Oetting, S. (1994). Ramona T. Mercer: Maternal role attainment. In A. Marriner-Tomey (Ed.), *Nursing theorists and their work* (pp. 390–405). St. Louis, MO: Mosby.

Blanche, S., Mayaux, M., Veber, F., Landreau, A., Courpotin, C., Vilmer, E., Ciraru-Vigneron, N., Flock, C., Tricoire, J., Noseda, G., Retbi, J., & Rouzious, C. (1996). Separation between HIV-positive women and their children: The French prospective study, 1986–1993. *American Journal of Public Health, 86*, 376–381.

Centers for Disease Control. (1995). The first 500,000 cases of AIDS. *Morbidity and Mortality Weekly Report, 44*, 398–403.

Chenitz, W. C., & Swanson, J. (1986). Qualitative research using grounded theory. In W. C. Chenitz & J. Swanson (Eds.), *From practice to grounded theory: Qualitative research in nursing* (pp. 3–15). Menlo Park, CA: Addison-Wesley.

Chu, S., Buehler, J., & Berkelman, R. (1990). Impact of the human immunodeficiency virus epidemic on mortality in women of reproductive age, United States. *Journal of the American Medical Association, 264*, 225–229.

Demas, P., Schoenbaum, E., Wills, T., Doll, L., & Klein, R. (1995). Stress, coping, and attitudes toward HIV treatment in injecting drug users: A qualitative study. *AIDS Education and Prevention, 7*(5), 429–442.

Demi, A., & Miles, M. (1986). Bereavement. *Annual Review of Nursing Research, 4*, 105–123.

Doka, K. (1989). Disenfranchised grief. In K. Doka (Ed.), *Disenfranchised grief: Recognizing hidden sorrow* (pp. 3–23). Lexington, MA: Lexington Books.

Eakes, G. (1993). Chronic sorrow: A response to living with cancer. *Oncology Nursing Forum, 20*, 1327–1334.

Eakes, G. (1995). Chronic sorrow: The lived experience of parents of chronically mentally ill individuals. *Archives of Psychiatric Nursing, 9*(2), 77–84.

Edelman, R., & Haverkos, H. (1989). The suitability of HIV-positive individuals for marriage and pregnancy. *Journal of the American Medical Association, 261*, 993.

Glaser, B. (1978). *Theoretical sensitivity.* Mill Valley, CA: Sociology Press.

Glaser, B. (1992). *Basics of grounded theory analysis.* Mill Valley, CA: Sociology Press.

Glaser, B., & Strauss, A. (1967). *The discovery of grounded theory.* Chicago: Aldine.

Goffman, E. (1974). *Stigma: Notes on the management of spoiled identity.* New York: Jason Aronson.

Guinan, M., & Leviton, L. (1995). Prevention of HIV infection in women: Overcoming barriers. *Journal of the American Medical Women's Association, 50*, 74–77.

Hainesworth, M. (1996). Helping spouses with chronic sorrow related to multiple sclerosis. *Journal of Psychosocial Nursing and Mental Health Services, 34*(6), 36–42.

Hutchinson, S. (1993). Grounded theory: The method. In P. Munhall & C. Oiler (Eds.), *Nursing research: A qualitative perspective* (2nd ed., pp. 180–212). New York: National League for Nursing.

Hutchison, M., & Kurth, A. (1991). I need to know that I have a choice: A study of women, HIV, and reproductive decision making. *AIDS Patient Care, 5*, 17–25.

Ingram, D., & Hutchinson, S. (in press). Stigma and HIV-positive mothers. *Health Care for Women International.*

Jacob, S., & Scandrett-Hibdon, S. (1994). Mothers grieving the death of a child. *Nurse Practitioner, 19*(7), 60–65.

Kadushin, G. (1996). Gay men with AIDS and their families of origin: An analysis of social support. *Health and Social Work, 21*(2), 141–149.

Katz, A. (1996). Gaining a new perspective on life as a consequence of uncertainty in HIV infection. *Journal of the Association of Nurses in AIDS Care, 7*(4), 51–60.

Kearney, M., Murphy, S., Irwin, K., & Rosenbaum, M. (1995). Salvaging self: A grounded theory of pregnancy on crack cocaine. *Nursing Research, 44*, 208–213.

Kearney, M., Murphy, S., & Rosenbaum, M. (1994). Mothering on crack cocaine: A grounded theory analysis. *Social Science Medicine, 38*, 351–361.

King, P. (1991). Helping women helping children: Drug policy and future generations. *Milbank Quarterly, 69*, 595–621.

Layne, L. (1990). Motherhood lost: Cultural dimensions of miscarriage and stillbirth in America. *Women and Health, 16*(3/4), 69–98.

Lazarus, R. (1983). The costs and benefits of denial. In S. Brenitz (Ed.), *The denial of stress* (pp. 1–30). New York: International University Press.

Leifer, M. (1980). *Psychological effects of motherhood: A study of first pregnancy.* New York: Praeger.

Levine, C., & Dubler, N. (1990). Uncertain risks and bitter realities: The reproductive choices of HIV-infected women. *Milbank Quarterly, 68*, 321–351.

Lewinsohn, P., & Mischel, W. (1980). Social competence and depression: The role of illusory self-perceptions. *Journal of Abnormal Psychology, 89*, 203–212.

Lincoln, Y., & Guba, E. (1985). *Naturalistic inquiry.* Beverly Hills, CA: Sage.

Lindgren, C. (1996). Chronic sorrow in persons with Parkinson's and their spouses. *Scholarly Inquiry for Nursing Practice, 10,* 351–370.

Mercer, R. (1986). *First-time motherhood: Experiences from teens to forties.* New York: Springer.

Mercer, R., & Ferketich, S. (1990). Predictors of parental attachment during early parenthood. *Journal of Advanced Nursing, 15,* 268–280.

Miall, C. (1989). Reproductive technology versus the stigma of involuntary childlessness. *Social Casework: The Journal of Contemporary Social Work, 70,* 43–50.

Moneyham, L., Seals, B., Demi, A., Sowell, R., Cohen, L., & Guillory, J. (1996). Experiences of disclosure in women infected with HIV. *Health Care for Women International, 17,* 209–221.

O'Hare, T., Williams, C., & Ezoviski, A. (1996). Fear of AIDS and homophobia: Implications for direct practice and advocacy. *Social Work, 41*(1), 51–58.

Oxford American Dictionary. (1980). New York: Avon.

Pearlberg, G. (1991). *Women, AIDS, and communities: A guide for action.* Metchen, NJ: Women's Action Alliance and the Scarecrow Press.

Pfeiffer, N. (1991). Highlights from the national conference on women and HIV infection. *AIDS Patient Care, 5,* 67–72.

Phillips, M. (1991). Chronic sorrow in mothers of chronically ill and disabled children. *Issues in Comprehensive Pediatric Nursing, 14,* 111–120.

Pilkington, F. (1993). The lived experience of grieving the loss of an important other. *Nursing Science Quarterly, 6*(3), 130–139.

Pivnick, A. (1994). Loss and regeneration: Influences on the reproductive decisions of HIV-positive drug-using women. *Medical Anthropology, 16*(1), 39–62.

Pizzi, M. (1992). Women, HIV infection, and AIDS: Tapestries of life, death, and empowerment. *American Journal of Occupational Therapy, 46*(11), 1021–1027.

Pursley-Cotteau, S., & Stern, P. (1996). Creating a new life: Dimensions of temperance in perinatal cocaine crack users. *Qualitative Health Research, 6,* 350–367.

Rando, T. (1984). Grief, dying, and death. Champaign, IL: Research Press Company.

Rose, M. (1993). Health concerns of women with HIV/AIDS. *Journal of the Association of Nurses in AIDS Care, 4*(3), 39–45.

Rose, M. (1996). Quality of life and coping styles of HIV-positive women with children. *Journal of the Association of Nurses in AIDS Care, 7*(2), 28–34.

Rubin, R. (1984). *Maternal identity and the maternal experience.* New York: Springer.

Russell, G. (1993). The role of denial in clinical practice. *Journal of Advanced Nursing, 18,* 938–940.

Sanders, C. (1989). *Grief: The mourning after.* New York: John Wiley.

Shayne, V., & Kaplan, B. (1991). Double victims: Poor women and AIDS. *Women and Health, 17,* 21–37.

Smeltzer, S., & Whipple, B. (1991). Women and HIV infection. *IMAGE: Journal of Nursing Scholarship, 23*(4), 249–256.

Taylor, S., & Brown, J. (1988). Illusion and well-being: A social psychological perspective on mental health. *American Psychologist, 103,* 193–210.

Walker, R., Pomeroy, E., McNeil, J., & Franklin, C. (1994). Anticipatory grief and Alzheimer's disease: Strategies for intervention. *Journal of Gerontological Social Work, 22*(3/4), 21–39.

Whiteford, L., & Gonzalez, L. (1995). Stigma: The hidden burden of infertility. *Social Science and Medicine, 40,* 27–36.

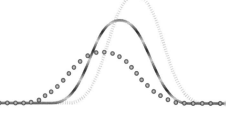

INDEX

Page numbers in bold type indicate glossary entries.

A

Absolute value, 342
Abstract, **457**
 in the research literature, 127
 in research reports, 54,55
Abstract journal, 127
Accessible population, 234, **457**
Accidental (convenience) sampling, 236-237, **457**
Acquiescence response set bias, 274, **457**
Active reading, 62
Adaptation Model (Roy), 151, 152
Administrators, research utilization strategies for, 441
Advances in Nursing Science, 8
After-only (posttest-only) design, 171, **457**
Agency for Health Care Policy and Research (AHCPR), 111, **450**
AIDSLINE database, 123
Aim, research, 97
Alpha (α), **457**
 reliability (Cronbach's alpha), 307, **458**
 significance level, 348, 369
American Nurses Association (ANA), 8
 Center for Research for Nursing, 8
 code of research ethics, 74
 Standards of Clinical Nursing Practice, 432
American Psychological Association, ethical guidelines and, 74
American Sociological Association, ethical guidelines and, 74
Analysis, **457**, *see also* Data analysis; Qualitative analysis; Quantitative analysis
 computers and, 351, 387
 content, 382, 394, **459**
 cost-benefit, 187, **460**
 data, 42, **460**, *see also* Data analysis
 discourse, 211, 212
 discriminant function, 363-364, **461**
 factor, 311, 364, 366, **462**
 impact, 187, **463**
 implementation, 186, **463**
 linear structural relations (LISREL), 365, **464**
 logit, 364
 meta-analysis, 134, **465**

multiple regression, 360, **465**, *see also* Multiple regression
 negative case, 314, **466**
 outcome, 186, **467**
 path, 365, **467**
 power, 244, 245, 348, **468**
 process, 186, **468**
 qualitative, 44, 380-395, **469**, *see also* Qualitative analysis
 quantitative, 42, 329-377, **469**, *see also* Quantitative analysis
 secondary, 262
 statistical, 42, 329-377, **471**, *see also* Quantitative analysis; Statistics
 styles of, qualitative, 382-383
 unit of, 134
Analysis of covariance (ANCOVA), 192, 361-363, 366, 372, **457**
Analysis of variance (ANOVA), 354-356, 359, **457**
 multivariate (MANOVA), 365, 366, **465**
 repeated measures, 355, 359
Analysis styles, qualitative, 382-383
Analytic phase of quantitative research, 42
ANCOVA. *See* Analysis of covariance
Anecdotes, literature reviews and, 129
Animal subjects, 75, 288
Anonymity, 82, 269, **457**
ANOVA. *See* Analysis of variance
Annual Review of Nursing Research, 8
Applied Nursing Research, 8
Applied research, 21-22, **457**
Assessment, psychometric, 309
Assessment phase of nursing process, 432
Associative relationship, 38
Assumptions, 12, **457**
 inferential statistics and, 350
 paradigms and, 13
 of scientific approach, 12
Assymetric distribution, 332
Attitudes, measurement of, 271
Attrition, 185, 194, **457**
Audit, inquiry, 315, **463**
Audit trail, 316, **457**
Author search, literature search and, 124